The Book of Life: Natural Healing

Natural Ways to Healthy Life

By Niddia Alexander

This book is a work of non-fiction. The information contained herein is intended for educational purposes only and is not a substitute for professional medical advice, diagnosis, or treatment. Always consult a qualified healthcare provider before making any changes to your diet, health routines, or lifestyle.

Published by:

Book of Life – Natural Healing

ISBN (Paperback): 979-8-9997306-6-4
ISBN (Hardcover): 978-1-970769-00-5
Library of Congress Control Number: 2025919915

Cover Design: Niddia Alexander
Interior Layout and Design: Niddia Alexander

Printed in the United States of America

First Edition – Volume 1

For more information or to contact the author, please visit:
https://authorniddiaalexander.com

THE BOOK OF LIFE – NATURAL HEALING A – C
VOL 1

Trust in the LORD with all your heart and lean not on your own understanding; in all your ways acknowledge him, and he will direct your path.
Proverbs 3 VS 5-6

Dedication

This book is dedicated to two extraordinary forces in my life whose unwavering support and guidance have been instrumental in bringing this work to fruition.

To God, the source of all wisdom and inspiration, I offer my deepest gratitude for choosing me for this sacred assignment. Your divine guidance has illuminated my path and filled my heart with purpose and conviction. May this book serve as a testament to Your grace and infinite wisdom, and may it be a source of hope, healing, and transformation for all who encounter its pages.

To my dear mother, whose love, encouragement, and unwavering support have been my constant source of strength throughout this journey. Your belief in me has been a beacon of light, guiding me through the challenges and triumphs of writing this book. Your dedication and sacrifice inspire me every day, and I am eternally grateful for your presence in my life.

With love and gratitude,

Niddia Alexander

For I know the plans I have for you," declares the LORD, "plans to prosper you and not to harm you, plans to give you hope and a future.

Jeremiah 29: 11

Acknowledgments

I would like to take this opportunity to express my heartfelt gratitude to the Almighty God for His divine guidance and inspiration throughout the journey of writing this book, “The Book of Life – Natural Healing” or "Natural Ways to a Healthy Life." It is with humility and reverence that I acknowledge His profound wisdom and grace, which have illuminated my path and empowered me to undertake this endeavor.

God's assignment and vision for this book have been a beacon of light, guiding my thoughts, words, and actions as I sought to impart knowledge and insights into the pursuit of a healthy and fulfilling life. His unwavering presence has provided me with strength, courage, and clarity, enabling me to navigate the complexities of health and wellness with diligence and compassion.

I am deeply grateful for the opportunity to serve as a vessel for His message of hope, healing and transformation. May His divine blessings continue to flow abundantly, touching the hearts and minds of all who engage with this work, and may it inspire positive change and empower individuals to embrace a lifestyle that nurtures both body and soul.

In closing, I offer my sincerest thanks to God for entrusting me with this sacred task and for blessing me with the resources, opportunities, and support needed to bring this vision to fruition. May His infinite love and grace guide us all on the path to wholeness and vitality.

With profound gratitude and humility,

Niddia Alexander.

Foreword

My name is Niddia Alexander, and I am honored to welcome you to the pages of this book. Before delving into the heart of its content, I feel compelled to introduce myself and shed light on the inspiration behind this transformative work on plant-based foods for natural healing.

As a mother of four beautiful children, I cherish every moment spent nurturing and motivating them to embrace the best versions of themselves. Alongside my role as a parent, I find solace in the simple joys of life – whether it's immersing myself in the wisdom of motivational speakers, indulging in the beauty of nature, or seeking refuge in the tranquil embrace of the beach.

While my passions may span from trading in the forex market to envisioning investment properties, one consistent thread defines my journey – a steadfast belief in the natural way of life. Whenever faced with ailments or discomforts, I instinctively turn to wholesome foods to restore balance and vitality to my body. For me, nourishing foods brimming with nutritional benefits have always been a cornerstone of well-being.

It was amidst this backdrop of reverence for nature and holistic living that I experienced a profound series of dreams and visions. Guided by the whispers of the Holy Spirit, I was entrusted with a divine assignment – to pen a book that would illuminate the path to health and wellness through plant-based nutrition. With unwavering faith and obedience, I embarked on this daunting task, surrendering myself to the guidance of a higher power.

Though initially daunted by the magnitude of the task before me, I found solace in the assurance that if God had called me to this mission, He would undoubtedly see me through it. Each morning, I approached my assignment with reverence, seeking divine guidance through prayer and worship. Along the way, I gleaned invaluable lessons and experienced the profound joy of being a conduit for a greater purpose.

As the words flowed onto the page, I realized that I was merely a vessel, channeling the wisdom and grace bestowed upon me by my Heavenly Father. All praise and gratitude belong to Him, for without His guidance, this book would not have come to fruition. It is my sincere prayer that the insights shared within these pages will empower you on your journey toward optimal health and wellness.

Luke 12 VS 48

"From everyone who has been given much, much will be demanded; and from the one who has been entrusted with much, much more will be asked."

This verse emphasizes the principle of accountability and stewardship. It suggests that those who have been given greater knowledge, resources or responsibility will be held to a higher standard. With privilege and blessing comes a greater expectation to use those blessings wisely and for the greater good.

CONTENTS

Introduction

In an era marked by the hustle and bustle of modern life, the pursuit of a healthy lifestyle has become an increasingly paramount endeavor for individuals seeking vitality, longevity and overall well-being. Amidst the myriad of trends, diets, and fads, one timeless truth stands unwavering: the profound impact of nature's bounty on our health and vitality.

In this book, titled "The Book of Life: Natural Healing," we embark on a journey to explore the transformative power of plant-based foods in nurturing a life of vitality and wellness. Rooted in ancient wisdom and modern science, this comprehensive guide offers a holistic approach to achieving optimal health through the consumption of nutrient-rich, plant-derived foods.

Drawing upon the latest research and centuries-old practices, "The Book of Life – Natural Healing" delves into the myriad benefits of embracing a plant-based lifestyle, from enhanced physical health to heightened mental clarity and spiritual well-being. Through a wealth of information, delicious recipes, and evidence-based insights, readers will discover the abundant riches that nature provides for nourishing the body, mind, and soul.

This book is not just a guide to healthy eating; it is a celebration of the inherent connection between humanity and our God-given natural world. It invites readers to rekindle their relationship with the earth, embracing the abundance of fruits, vegetables, grains, nuts, seeds, and legumes that sustain and nourish us at the deepest levels.

As we journey together through the pages of "The Book of Life – Natural Healing," let us awaken to the profound wisdom that lies within the embrace of plant-based wellness. May this book serve as a beacon of inspiration and empowerment, guiding us toward a life of radiant health, vitality, and harmony with the natural world.

Welcome to the transformative journey of "The Book of Life – Natural Healing: Embracing Plant-Based Wellness."

Warm regards,
Niddia Alexander

Ackee

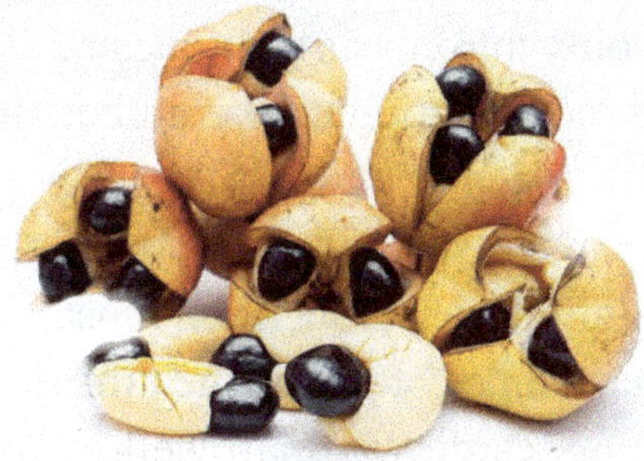

Ackee: A Tropical Treasure of Health Benefits and Culinary Delight

Ackee, with its vibrant appearance and unique flavor, is not just a delicious tropical fruit but also a nutritional powerhouse. Native to West Africa and prominently featured in Caribbean cuisine, ackee has gained popularity worldwide for its rich nutrient profile and versatile culinary uses. In this article, we'll explore the impressive health benefits of ackee and the various ways it can be enjoyed in the kitchen.

Nutrient-Rich Profile:

Ackee is a nutrient-dense fruit that provides an array of essential vitamins and minerals. Rich in vitamin C and vitamin A and a good source of potassium. Ackee contributes to immune support, vision health and proper electrolyte balance. Additionally, ackee contains healthy monounsaturated fats, making it a heart-friendly food.

Vitamin C:

Benefits: Ackee is a rich source of vitamin C, a powerful antioxidant that supports the immune system. Vitamin C is essential for collagen synthesis, promoting skin health, wound healing, and protecting cells from oxidative stress.

Vitamin A:

Benefits: Ackee contains significant amounts of vitamin A, crucial for maintaining healthy vision, skin, and mucous membranes. Vitamin A also plays a role in immune function and cell differentiation.

Potassium:

Benefits: Ackee is a good source of potassium, an essential mineral that helps regulate blood pressure, balance fluids in the body, and support proper muscle and nerve function. Adequate potassium intake is associated with a lower risk of cardiovascular diseases.

Ackee contains essential **electrolytes** that play a crucial role in maintaining proper bodily functions. **Electrolytes**, such as potassium, are vital for balancing fluids within cells, regulating blood pressure, and supporting nerve and muscle function. Ackee's significant potassium content contributes to its role as an electrolyte-rich food. Adequate intake of electrolytes is essential for hydration, especially in warm climates or during physical exertion. Including ackee in the diet not only introduces a unique and flavorful element but also provides a natural source of electrolytes, contributing to overall health and well-being.

Monounsaturated Fats:

Benefits: Ackee provides healthy monounsaturated fats, including oleic acid. These fats have been linked to heart health by helping reduce LDL cholesterol levels and promoting cardiovascular well-being. Monounsaturated fats are an important component of a heart-friendly diet.

Heart Health and Cholesterol Regulation:

One of the notable benefits of ackee is its potential impact on heart health. The monounsaturated fats in ackee, including oleic acid, have been associated with reducing levels of LDL cholesterol (often referred to as "bad" cholesterol). Maintaining healthy cholesterol levels is crucial for cardiovascular well-being and may reduce the risk of heart disease.

Rich Source of Protein:

Ackee is unique among fruits because it contains a moderate amount of protein. This makes ackee a valuable addition to plant-based diets, providing an alternative protein source for those who may not consume meat or other animal products. Protein is essential for muscle repair, immune function and overall body maintenance.

Historical Uses

Traditional Medicine in West Africa:

Historical Use: In West Africa, where ackee is native, the fruit has historical roots in traditional medicine. Various parts of the ackee tree were used to create herbal remedies believed to have medicinal properties. The bark, roots and leaves were employed to address ailments such as fever, digestive issues and skin conditions. These traditional uses reflected the acknowledgment of ackee's potential therapeutic benefits within local communities.

Culinary Staples in Jamaican Cuisine:

Historical Use: Ackee has been a culinary staple in Jamaican cuisine for centuries. Ackee and saltfish, a traditional Jamaican dish. Combine ackee with salted codfish, onions and various seasonings and this flavorful dish serves as a nutritious and filling meal, showcasing ackee's role as a dietary staple that provides sustenance and nourishment. The historical use of ackee in Jamaican cuisine reflects its cultural significance and importance as a food source.

Symbol of National Identity:

Historical Use: Ackee holds cultural and national significance in Jamaica, where it is the national fruit. Its distinctive appearance and historical use in Jamaican dishes have made ackee a symbol of national identity. Ackee and saltfish, in particular, are celebrated as a quintessential Jamaican national dish, representing the fusion of African, Caribbean, and European culinary influences. The historical use of ackee in this context goes beyond its nutritional benefits, highlighting its cultural importance and contribution to the identity of the Jamaican people.

Versatile Culinary Uses:

Beyond its health benefits, ackee is a star ingredient in a variety of culinary dishes, especially in Caribbean cuisine. Here are some creative ways ackee is used in the kitchen:

Ackee and Saltfish: A classic Jamaican dish, ackee and saltfish combined, the creamy texture of ackee with salted codfish, onions and various seasonings. It's a flavorful and hearty meal often enjoyed for breakfast or brunch.

Estimated Nutrition Facts (Per Serving – 1 cup)

- Calories: 320
- Protein: 18g
- Carbohydrates: 10g
- Fat: 24g
- Fiber: 2g
- Sodium: 650mg
- Vitamin C: 15% DV
- Iron: 20% DV

Note: Nutrition may vary depending on amount of oil and saltfish used.

Recipe 1: Traditional Jamaican Ackee and Saltfish

Servings: 4
Prep Time: 15 minutes
Cook Time: 25 minutes
Total Time: 40 minutes

Ingredients:

- 1 can of ackee (540 ml) drained and rinsed or 2 cups of fresh boiled ackee (must be ripe and properly cleaned)
- 1/2 lb (225g) salted codfish (saltfish)
- 2 tbsp cooking oil (olive, coconut or vegetable)
- 1 medium onion, thinly sliced
- 1 bell pepper (red or green), sliced
- 2 cloves garlic, minced
- 2 stalks scallion, chopped
- 1 medium tomato, diced
- 1 scotch bonnet pepper, finely chopped (optional)
- 1/4 tsp black pepper
- 2-3 sprigs thyme
- 1/4 tsp Jamaican all purpose seasoning (optional)

Instructions:

- **Prepare Saltfish:** Rinse codfish and boil in water for 10-15 minutes. Drain, cool, remove bones/skin, and flake.
- **Sauté Veggies:** In a skillet, heat oil. Add onion, garlic, bell pepper, tomato; sauté for 3-5 minutes.
- **Add Saltfish:** Mix in flaked fish and cook for 5 minutes.
- **Add Ackee:** Gently fold in ackee. Season with pepper and Jamaican all purpose seasoning. Simmer on low for 3-5 minutes.
- **Serve:** Enjoy with fried dumplings, yam, boiled banana, or rice.

Serving Suggestions

- Serve with boiled green bananas, dumplings, and yam for a traditional Jamaican breakfast.
- It also pairs well with fried plantains or festival (Jamaican cornmeal fritters).
- A side of avocado complements the creamy texture of ackee.

Estimated Nutrition Facts (Per Serving – 1 cup)

- **Calories: 270**
- **Protein: 7g**
- **Carbohydrates: 15g**
- **Fat: 22g**
- **Fiber: 5g**
- **Sodium: 320mg**
- **Vitamin A: 30% DV**
- **Vitamin C: 45% DV**

Servings: 3
Prep Time: 10 minutes
Cook Time: 20 minutes
Total Time: 30 minutes

Ingredients:

- 1 can of ackee (540 ml) drained and rinsed or 2 cups of fresh boiled ackee (must be ripe and properly cleaned)
- 2 tbsp olive or coconut oil
- 1 small onion, sliced
- 1 red bell pepper, sliced
- 1 zucchini, diced
- 1/2 cup mushrooms, sliced
- 1 tomato, chopped
- 2 cloves garlic, minced
- 1/2 tsp turmeric
- 1/2 tsp smoked paprika
- 1/4 tsp black pepper
- Sea salt to taste
- Fresh thyme or parsley for garnish

Instructions:

1. Prep Veggies: Slice all vegetables and drain the ackee.
2. Cook Aromatics: In a skillet, heat oil. Add onions and garlic; cook 3 minutes.
3. Add Veggies: Stir in zucchini, peppers, mushrooms. Cook 5-7 minutes.
4. Season: Add tomato, turmeric, paprika, pepper, and salt.
5. Add Ackee: Gently fold in ackee. Cook on low for 4-5 minutes.
6. Serve: Garnish with thyme or parsley. Great with rice, quinoa, or plantains.

Serving Suggestions

- Serve over brown rice, quinoa, or with roti or bammy.
- A drizzle of lime juice before serving brightens the flavors.
- Garnish with fresh parsley or thyme leaves.

Ackee Stir-Fry: Ackee's mild flavor makes it a versatile ingredient in stir-fries. Combine ackee with colorful vegetables, herbs and spices for a quick and nutritious meal.

Ackee Salad: Use ackee in salads to add a tropical twist. Combine it with fresh vegetables, greens and a zesty dressing for a refreshing and nutritious dish.

Ackee Patties and Wraps: Incorporate ackee into savory pastries like patties or wraps for a portable and flavorful snack.

Side Effects

Consuming ackee comes with potential side effects, primarily due to the presence of a toxin called hypoglycin. The unripe or underripe ackee fruit contains higher levels of hypoglycin, which can lead to a condition known as Vomiting Sickness. Symptoms may include vomiting, hypoglycemia (low blood sugar), and, in severe cases, seizures or coma. **Therefore, it is crucial to ensure that ackee is fully ripe and properly prepared before consumption. The seeds and outer arils should be discarded, and only the fully opened yellow ackee arils should be used for cooking.** Additionally, individuals with glucose metabolism disorders or those on certain medications should exercise caution and consult with healthcare professionals before including ackee in their diet to mitigate potential adverse effects.

Conclusion:

Ackee's unique combination of health benefits and culinary versatility makes it a standout fruit in the world of tropical produce. From its heart-friendly fats to its protein content and immune-boosting vitamins, ackee is a nutritious addition to any diet. Explore the diverse ways to enjoy ackee in your meals and embrace the goodness this tropical treasure brings to both your health and your taste buds.

Back to Table of Contents

Adzuki Beans

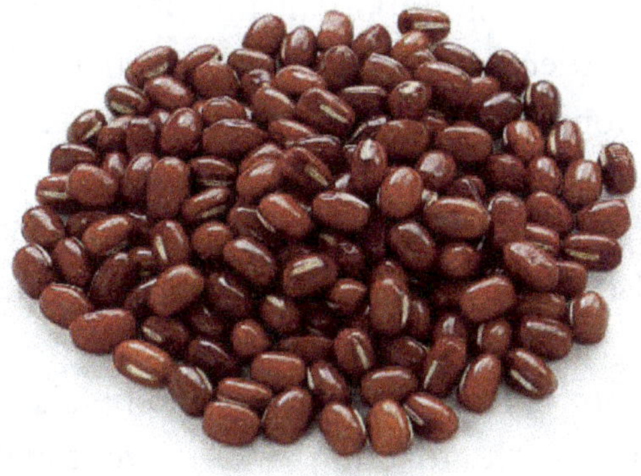

Exploring the Nutritional and Culinary Marvel: Adzuki Beans

Adzuki beans, also known as azuki or aduki beans, are small, red beans that have been a staple in Asian cuisine for centuries. These nutrient-dense legumes offer a host of health benefits and can be incorporated into a wide range of delicious dishes. Let's delve into the world of adzuki beans, uncovering their nutritional profile, remarkable benefits and diverse culinary uses.

Nutritional Profile of Adzuki Beans:

Adzuki beans are packed with essential nutrients, including:

Protein: Adzuki beans are a rich source of plant-based protein, making them an excellent option for vegetarians and vegans looking to meet their protein needs. A one-cup serving of cooked adzuki beans provides approximately 17 grams of protein, which is essential for muscle repair, growth and overall health.

Fiber: Adzuki beans are high in dietary fiber, both soluble and insoluble. Fiber aids digestion, promotes satiety and helps regulate blood sugar levels. Consuming adzuki beans can support digestive health, prevent constipation and reduce the risk of chronic diseases such as heart disease and diabetes.

Complex Carbohydrates: Adzuki beans are a good source of complex carbohydrates, which provide sustained energy and help stabilize blood sugar levels. They have a low glycemic index, making them suitable for individuals with diabetes or those looking to manage their weight.

Vitamins and Minerals:

Adzuki beans contain various vitamins and minerals, including folate, potassium, magnesium, iron, zinc, and manganese. These nutrients are essential for immune function, energy metabolism, bone health and overall well-being.

Folate (Vitamin B9): Folate is important for DNA synthesis, cell division, and the production of red blood cells. Adequate folate intake is crucial during pregnancy to prevent neural tube defects in the developing fetus. Folate also supports cardiovascular health and may reduce the risk of certain cancers.

Potassium: Potassium is an electrolyte that helps regulate fluid balance, nerve function and muscle contractions. It also supports heart health by helping to lower blood pressure and reduce the risk of stroke.

Magnesium: Magnesium is involved in over 300 biochemical reactions in the body, including energy production, muscle function and nerve transmission. Magnesium also supports bone health, heart health, and blood sugar regulation.

Iron: Iron is essential for oxygen transport, energy metabolism and the synthesis of hemoglobin and myoglobin. Adequate iron intake helps prevent iron deficiency anemia and supports immune function and cognitive health.

Zinc: Zinc is important for immune function, wound healing and DNA synthesis. It also supports growth and development, reproductive health and the maintenance of healthy skin, hair, and nails.

Copper: Copper is necessary for the formation of red blood cells, collagen synthesis and the absorption of iron. Copper also acts as an antioxidant and supports immune function, bone health and connective tissue health.

Manganese: Manganese is involved in bone formation, cartilage formation and the metabolism of carbohydrates, proteins, and cholesterol. Manganese also acts as an antioxidant and supports immune function and blood sugar regulation.

Phosphorus: Phosphorus is important for bone and teeth health, energy metabolism and cell membrane structure. Phosphorus also supports kidney function, nerve function and muscle contractions.

Vitamin B1 (Thiamine): Thiamine is important for energy metabolism, nerve function and carbohydrate metabolism. It also supports heart health, brain function and mood regulation.

Vitamin B2 (Riboflavin): Riboflavin is involved in energy production, antioxidant activity and the metabolism of fats, carbohydrates and proteins. Riboflavin also supports eye health, skin health and red blood cell production.

Vitamin B3 (Niacin): Niacin is important for energy metabolism, DNA repair and hormone synthesis. Niacin also supports heart health, brain function and skin health.

Vitamin B5 (Pantothenic Acid): Pantothenic acid is involved in energy metabolism, hormone synthesis and the production of neurotransmitters. Pantothenic acid also supports skin health, hair health and immune function.

Vitamin B6 (Pyridoxine): Pyridoxine is important for amino acid metabolism, neurotransmitter synthesis and immune function. Pyridoxine also supports heart health, brain function and hormone regulation.

Incorporating adzuki beans into your diet can help you meet your daily requirements for these essential vitamins and minerals, promoting overall health and well-being. Whether enjoyed in soups, salads, stews, or desserts, adzuki beans offer a delicious and nutritious addition to any meal.

Antioxidants:

Adzuki beans are rich in antioxidants, such as flavonoids and phenolic compounds, which help protect cells from oxidative damage and reduce inflammation in the body. Antioxidants play a crucial role in preventing chronic diseases and promoting longevity.

Anthocyanins: Anthocyanins are flavonoid pigments responsible for the red color of adzuki beans. They have strong antioxidant properties and may help reduce inflammation, improve cardiovascular health and support brain function. Anthocyanins also have potential anticancer effects and may protect against age-related cognitive decline.

Phenolic Acids: Adzuki beans contain various phenolic acids, including ferulic acid, caffeic acid and p-coumaric acid, among others. Phenolic acids have antioxidant and anti-inflammatory properties and may help reduce the risk of chronic diseases such as heart disease, diabetes, and certain cancers. They also support digestive health and immune function.

Flavonoids: Adzuki beans contain flavonoids, such as quercetin, kaempferol and myricetin, which have potent antioxidant and anti-inflammatory effects. Flavonoids may help improve cardiovascular health by reducing blood pressure, cholesterol levels and inflammation. They also support brain health, immune function and skin health.

Isoflavones: Adzuki beans contain isoflavones, such as genistein and daidzein, which have antioxidant and estrogen-like effects on the body. Isoflavones may help reduce the risk of hormone-related cancers, such as breast and prostate cancer. They also support bone health, cardiovascular health and menopausal symptoms.

Vitamin E: Adzuki beans are a good source of vitamin E, including tocopherols and tocotrienols, which have antioxidant properties and help protect cell membranes from oxidative damage. Vitamin E may help reduce the risk of heart disease, cancer and age-related eye disorders. It also supports immune function, skin health and hair health.

Saponins: Adzuki beans contain saponins, which are plant compounds with antioxidant and anti-inflammatory properties. Saponins may help lower cholesterol levels, regulate blood sugar levels and support immune function. They also have potential anticancer effects and may protect against certain infections.

Phytic Acid (Phytate): While often considered an anti-nutrient due to its ability to bind minerals, phytic acid also has antioxidant properties. Phytic acid may help reduce the risk of oxidative damage and inflammation in the body. It also supports digestive health and may have anticancer effects.

Incorporating adzuki beans into your diet can help increase your intake of these powerful antioxidants, promoting overall health and well-being. Whether enjoyed in soups, stews, salads, or desserts, adzuki beans offer a delicious and nutritious way to support your body's natural defense mechanisms against oxidative stress and chronic diseases.

Health Benefits of Adzuki Beans:

Heart Health: The high fiber and potassium content of adzuki beans support heart health by lowering cholesterol levels, regulating blood pressure and reducing the risk of cardiovascular disease. Consuming adzuki beans as part of a balanced diet may help prevent heart attacks, strokes, and other cardiovascular events.

Weight Management: Adzuki beans are low in fat and calories but high in fiber and protein, making them an excellent food choice for weight management. The fiber and protein in adzuki beans promote feelings of fullness and satiety, reducing overall calorie intake and aiding in weight loss or maintenance efforts.

Blood Sugar Control: The complex carbohydrates and soluble fiber in adzuki beans help stabilize blood sugar levels and improve insulin sensitivity. Including adzuki beans in meals can help prevent spikes and crashes in blood glucose levels, making them a valuable food for individuals with diabetes or those at risk of developing the condition.

Digestive Health: Adzuki beans are a natural source of dietary fiber, which supports digestive health by promoting regular bowel movements, preventing constipation and nourishing beneficial gut bacteria. Consuming adzuki beans can alleviate symptoms of digestive disorders like irritable bowel syndrome (IBS) and diverticulitis.

Nutritional Content

The approximate nutritional content in 1 cup (about 230 grams) of cooked adzuki beans is as follows:

- Carbohydrates: Approximately 44 grams
- Protein: Approximately 17 grams
- Fiber: Approximately 16 grams
- Fat: Approximately 0.5 grams

These values can vary slightly depending on factors such as cooking methods and specific varieties of adzuki beans.

Culinary Uses of Adzuki Beans:

Adzuki beans are incredibly versatile and can be used in various culinary applications, including:

Soups and Stews: Adzuki beans add texture, flavor and nutritional value to soups, stews and chili recipes. They can be combined with vegetables, herbs and spices to create hearty and satisfying dishes.

Salads: Adzuki beans can be tossed into salads for added protein and fiber. They pair well with leafy greens, tomatoes, cucumbers, and avocados, as well as with citrus-based dressings or vinaigrettes.

Desserts: Adzuki beans are commonly used in Asian desserts, such as sweet red bean paste or filling for pastries, buns and cakes. They can also be incorporated into puddings, custards and ice creams for a nutritious and delicious twist.

Rice and Grain Dishes: Adzuki beans can be mixed with rice, quinoa, or other grains to create flavorful and nutritious side dishes. They complement the earthy flavors of grains and add a protein boost to vegetarian or vegan meals.

Burgers and Patties: Adzuki beans can be mashed and formed into burgers or patties for a meatless alternative. Combined with breadcrumbs, herbs and spices, they make delicious and wholesome plant-based burgers that are perfect for grilling or pan-frying.

Here are two delicious recipes featuring adzuki beans:

Adzuki Bean and Vegetable Stir-Fry:

Ingredients:

- 1 cup cooked adzuki beans
- 2 cups mixed vegetables (such as bell peppers, broccoli, carrots, snap peas)
- 2 cloves garlic, minced
- 1 tablespoon ginger, minced
- 2 tablespoons soy sauce (or tamari for a gluten-free option)
- 1 tablespoon sesame oil
- 1 tablespoon rice vinegar
- 1 tablespoon maple syrup or honey
- Cooked rice or noodles for serving
- Optional toppings: sesame seeds, sliced green onions

Instructions:

1. Heat sesame oil in a large skillet or wok over medium-high heat. Add minced garlic and ginger, and sauté for 1-2 minutes until fragrant.
2. Add mixed vegetables to the skillet and stir-fry for 3-4 minutes until they start to soften.
3. Add cooked adzuki beans to the skillet, along with soy sauce, rice vinegar and maple syrup or honey. Stir to combine and cook for an additional 2-3 minutes until heated through.
4. Serve the stir-fry over cooked rice or noodles and garnish with sesame seeds and sliced green onions if desired. Enjoy this flavorful and nutritious dish!

Adzuki Bean Brownies:

Ingredients:

- 1 can (15 ounces) of cooked adzuki beans, drained and rinsed
- 1/4 cup cocoa powder
- 1/4 cup maple syrup or honey
- 1/4 cup almond butter or peanut butter
- 2 tablespoons coconut oil, melted
- 1 teaspoon vanilla extract
- 1/2 teaspoon baking powder
- Pinch of salt
- 1/4 cup dark chocolate chips (optional)

Instructions:

1. Preheat your oven to 350°F (175°C) and grease or line a baking dish with parchment paper.
2. In a food processor, combine the cooked adzuki beans, cocoa powder, maple syrup or honey, almond butter or peanut butter, melted coconut oil, vanilla extract, baking powder, and salt. Blend until smooth and creamy, scraping down the sides as needed.
3. If using, fold the dark chocolate chips into the brownie batter.
4. Pour the brownie batter into the prepared baking dish and spread it out evenly.
5. Bake in the preheated oven for 20-25 minutes, or until the edges are set and a toothpick inserted into the center comes out clean.
6. Remove from the oven and let the brownies cool completely before slicing into squares.
7. Enjoy these decadent and fudgy adzuki bean brownies as a healthier alternative to traditional brownies!

These recipes showcase the versatility of adzuki beans and how they can be incorporated into both savory and sweet dishes for a nutritious and delicious meal or snack. Experiment with these recipes and feel free to customize them with your favorite ingredients and flavors!

How to Grow Adzuki Beans from Seed to Harvest

Adzuki beans are easy to grow in warm climates and well-suited for backyard gardens.

Quick Facts

- **Botanical Name:** Vigna angularis
- **Plant Type:** Warm-season annual legume
- **Time to Harvest:** 90–120 days
- **Soil pH:** 6.0–7.5
- **Sunlight:** Full sun (6–8 hours/day)

1. Preparing to Plant

Climate & Location

- Grows best in temperatures between 65–85°F (18–29°C).

- Prefers dry, warm climates during flowering and pod formation.
- Avoid areas with heavy rainfall, especially during flowering.

Soil Requirements

- Light, well-drained loamy soil is ideal.
- Avoid waterlogged or clay-heavy soils.
- Enrich with compost or aged manure before planting.

Soil Prep

- Till the soil to a depth of 6–8 inches.
- Mix in organic compost to improve drainage and nutrient content.

2. Planting the Seeds

When to Plant

Plant after the last frost, once soil temperature is at least 60°F (16°C).

How to Plant

- Soak seeds overnight in water to speed germination (optional).
- Sow seeds 1 inch deep and 2–3 inches apart.
- Space rows 18–24 inches apart.

Tip: Do not fertilize with high nitrogen—too much will encourage leaves instead of pods.

3. Watering & Care

Watering

- Keep soil consistently moist but not soggy during germination.
- Once established, water moderately—about 1 inch per week.
- Reduce watering as pods begin to mature to avoid mold.

Thinning & Weeding

- Thin to 6 inches apart once seedlings have 2–3 sets of leaves.
- Weed regularly but carefully—adzuki roots are shallow and delicate.

4. Flowering & Pollination

- Adzuki beans produce small yellow flowers, usually after 45–60 days.
- They are self-pollinating, but insect activity can improve yields.

5. Pest & Disease Management
Common Pests

- Aphids
- Spider mites
- Bean beetles

Solutions:

- Use neem oil or insecticidal soap.
- Encourage ladybugs and beneficial insects.

Diseases:

- Root rot (from overwatering)
- Powdery mildew (in humid conditions)

Prevention:

- Space plants well for airflow.
- Avoid watering leaves late in the day.

6. Harvesting
When to Harvest:

- 90–120 days after planting.
- Pods turn brown and dry when ready.
- Shake the pod—you'll hear the beans rattle inside.

How to Harvest

Cut pods from plant or pull up the whole plant and hang upside down to dry. Shell beans by hand once pods are crispy dry.

7. Storing Adzuki Beans

- Store shelled, dry beans in an airtight container in a cool, dry place.
- They can last up to 1 year when properly stored.

Bonus Tips

- **Companion Plants:** Corn, cucumber, or spinach.
- **Avoid:** Onions or garlic (can inhibit bean growth).

- **Successive Sowing:** Stagger planting every 2–3 weeks for an extended harvest.

In **conclusion**, adzuki beans are a versatile and nutrient-dense ingredient that offers a myriad of health benefits and culinary possibilities. Whether enjoyed in savory dishes or sweet treats, adzuki beans are a valuable addition to any diet, providing protein, fiber, vitamins, minerals, and antioxidants to support overall health and well-being. Embrace the goodness of adzuki beans and explore the endless ways to incorporate them into your favorite recipes for a nutritious and flavorful dining experience.

If you have specific health concerns, allergies, or conditions, it's advisable to consult with a healthcare professional or a registered dietitian before making significant changes to your diet.

Back to Table of Contents

Alfalfa

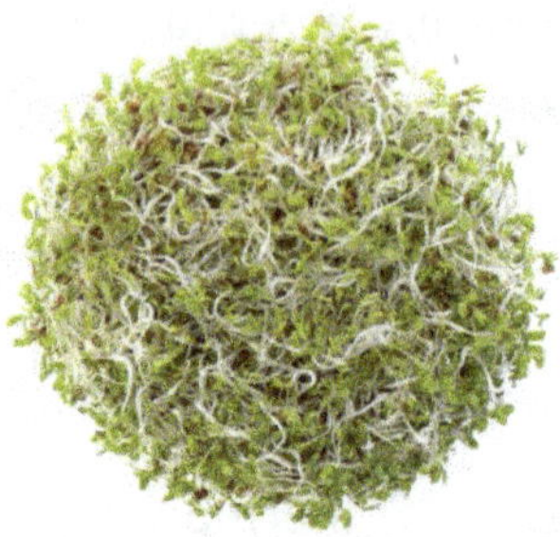

A Nutrient-Rich Superfood with Countless Benefits and Uses

Alfalfa (Medicago sativa) is a perennial flowering plant that belongs to the legume family Fabaceae. It is widely cultivated as a forage crop and is valued for its high nutritional content and ability to improve soil fertility. Alfalfa is characterized by its trifoliate leaves and clusters of small purple flowers. It is commonly used as feed for livestock, including cattle, horses, and poultry, due to its high protein and fiber content. Additionally, alfalfa is popular in human diets as sprouts or as a component of salads and sandwiches, owing to its crisp texture and mild flavor. Beyond its agricultural significance, alfalfa is also utilized in traditional medicine for its purported health benefits, which include aiding digestion, promoting detoxification, and supporting overall wellness.

Nutritional Powerhouse:

Alfalfa is celebrated for its rich nutritional content, offering a wide array of vitamins, minerals, and phytonutrients. Here's a glimpse of the nutrients found in alfalfa:

Vitamins:

Alfalfa is a rich source of vitamins, including vitamin A, vitamin C, vitamin E, and various B vitamins. These vitamins contribute to skin health, immune function, and overall well-being.

Vitamin A:

- Important for vision, immune function, and skin health.

Vitamin C:

- An antioxidant that supports immune function, aids in collagen formation, and helps the body absorb iron.

Vitamin E:

- A fat-soluble antioxidant that protects cells from oxidative damage.

Vitamin K:

- Essential for blood clotting and bone health.

Vitamin B1 (Thiamine):

- Crucial for energy metabolism and the proper functioning of the nervous system.

Vitamin B2 (Riboflavin):

- Plays a key role in energy production, cell growth, and the maintenance of healthy skin.

Vitamin B3 (Niacin):

- Essential for DNA repair, energy metabolism, and the proper functioning of the nervous system.

Vitamin B5 (Pantothenic Acid):

- Involved in the synthesis of fatty acids, amino acids, and other important molecules.

Vitamin B6 (Pyridoxine):

- Important for brain development, the production of neurotransmitters, and the metabolism of amino acids.

Folate (Vitamin B9):

- Important for DNA synthesis and cell division. Adequate folate intake is particularly important during pregnancy for fetal development.

Vitamin B12 (Cobalamin):

- While vitamin B12 is primarily found in animal products, alfalfa may contain small amounts. However, it's important to note that alfalfa is not a reliable source of vitamin B12.

Alfalfa's vitamin content contributes to its overall nutritional value and makes it a valuable addition to a well-balanced diet. Including alfalfa in various forms, such as sprouts or supplements, can provide a range of essential vitamins for overall health and well-being.

Minerals:

Essential minerals such as calcium, iron, magnesium, potassium, and phosphorus are abundant in alfalfa. These minerals play a crucial role in bone health, blood circulation, and maintaining electrolyte balance.

Calcium:

- Essential for bone and teeth health, muscle function, and nerve transmission.

Iron:

- Important for the formation of hemoglobin, which carries oxygen in the blood.

Magnesium:

- Crucial for muscle and nerve function, energy metabolism, and bone health.

Phosphorus:

- Vital for bone and teeth health, energy production, and the synthesis of DNA and RNA.

Potassium:

- Important for maintaining proper heart and muscle function, regulating fluid balance, and supporting overall cardiovascular health.

Sodium:

- While sodium is generally present in smaller amounts, it plays a role in maintaining fluid balance and nerve function.

Zinc:

- Important for immune function, wound healing, and DNA synthesis.

Copper:

- Involved in the formation of red blood cells, maintenance of bones and nerves, and the immune system.

Manganese:

- Plays a role in bone formation, blood clotting, and reducing inflammation.

Selenium:

- An antioxidant that supports thyroid function and immune system health.

Chromium:

- Involved in glucose metabolism and may play a role in maintaining stable blood sugar levels.

Molybdenum:

- A trace element that participates in various enzymatic reactions in the body.

Boron:

- May play a role in bone health and the metabolism of certain minerals.

The specific mineral content of alfalfa can vary based on factors such as growing conditions, plant maturity, and soil composition. Incorporating alfalfa into the diet, whether through alfalfa sprouts, supplements, or herbal teas, can provide a range of essential minerals that contribute to overall health and well-being.

Proteins and Amino Acids:

Alfalfa contains a notable amount of protein, providing a valuable plant-based protein source. It also contains essential amino acids, supporting muscle development and various bodily functions.

Antioxidants:

Phytochemicals in alfalfa, including flavonoids and carotenoids, act as antioxidants, helping to neutralize free radicals and reduce oxidative stress in the body.

Flavonoids:

- These compounds, including quercetin, kaempferol, and myricetin, exhibit antioxidant properties and are associated with various health benefits.

Carotenoids:

- Alfalfa contains carotenoids like beta-carotene, lutein, and zeaxanthin. These compounds have antioxidant and anti-inflammatory effects, supporting eye health and overall well-being.

Chlorophyll:

- The vibrant green color of alfalfa is due to chlorophyll, which not only gives plants their color but also possesses antioxidant and anti-inflammatory properties. Chlorophyll is believed to aid in detoxification.

Saponins:

- Saponins are plant compounds with antioxidant properties. They may have immune-boosting effects and potentially contribute to the prevention of certain diseases.

Coumarins:

- Alfalfa contains coumarins, which are antioxidants with potential anti-inflammatory and cardiovascular benefits.

Phytosterols:

- These plant compounds have antioxidant and cholesterol-lowering properties. They may contribute to heart health and overall well-being.

Vitamin C:

- While already mentioned in the vitamins list, it's worth noting that vitamin C is a potent antioxidant found in alfalfa. It plays a crucial role in scavenging free radicals and supporting immune function.

Vitamin E:

- Another antioxidant present in alfalfa, vitamin E protects cells from oxidative damage and supports overall skin health.

Polyphenols:

- Polyphenolic compounds, including phenolic acids, are found in alfalfa and contribute to its antioxidant activity. They have potential health-promoting effects.

Superoxide Dismutase (SOD):

- Alfalfa is known to contain enzymes like superoxide dismutase, which helps neutralize harmful free radicals in the body.

The combination of these antioxidants in alfalfa contributes to its potential to combat oxidative stress, reduce inflammation, and support overall health. It's essential to include a variety of antioxidant-rich foods in your diet to benefit from their synergistic effects and promote well-being.

Chlorophyll:

Alfalfa's vibrant green color is indicative of its chlorophyll content. Chlorophyll has been associated with detoxification and may have anti-inflammatory and immune-boosting properties.

Health Benefits:

Nutrient Density:

- The diverse range of vitamins and minerals in alfalfa contributes to its overall nutrient density, supporting various aspects of health, from bone strength to immune function.

Digestive Health:

- Alfalfa has been traditionally used to promote digestive health. Its fiber content supports regular bowel movements and a healthy digestive system.

Anti-Inflammatory Properties:

- Some studies suggest that the bioactive compounds in alfalfa may possess anti-inflammatory properties, which can be beneficial in managing inflammation-related conditions.

Cholesterol Management:

- Preliminary research indicates that alfalfa may have a role in managing cholesterol levels, potentially contributing to cardiovascular health.

Blood Sugar Control:

- There is evidence to suggest that certain compounds in alfalfa may help regulate blood sugar levels, making it a potential ally for those with diabetes or those at risk.

Nutritional Content

Alfalfa is typically not consumed in cooked form like other legumes, such as beans or lentils. Instead, it is commonly consumed as sprouts or dried leaves. However, if you were to consider the nutritional content of 1 cup of raw alfalfa sprouts, here's an approximate breakdown:

- Carbohydrates: About 0.7 grams
- Protein: About 1 gram
- Fiber: About 0.6 grams
- Fat: About 0.1 grams

These values may vary slightly depending on factors such as growing conditions and the specific stage of growth at which the sprouts are harvested. Alfalfa sprouts are often prized for their nutritional density, containing a range of vitamins, minerals, and phytochemicals. However, they are very low in calories and macronutrients compared to other foods.

Culinary and Herbal Uses:

Alfalfa Sprouts:

- Alfalfa sprouts are a popular addition to salads, sandwiches, and wraps. They add a crunchy texture and a mild, nutty flavor.

Tea Infusions:

- Dried alfalfa leaves and flowers can be used to make herbal tea infusions. This tea is believed to have mild diuretic properties and is often consumed for its potential detoxifying effects.

Supplements:

- Alfalfa supplements, available in various forms such as capsules or powders, are commonly used to ensure a consistent intake of its nutritional benefits.

Livestock Feed:

- Alfalfa is a significant crop in agriculture, commonly used as feed for livestock due to its high nutritional value.

Alfalfa's mild and nutty flavor makes it a versatile ingredient that can be incorporated into various dishes. ***Here are two recipes featuring alfalfa:***

Alfalfa and Avocado Salad:

Ingredients:

- 2 cups fresh alfalfa sprouts
- 1 ripe avocado, sliced
- 1 cup cherry tomatoes, halved
- 1 cucumber, sliced
- 1/4 cup red onion, thinly sliced
- 2 tablespoons extra-virgin olive oil
- 1 tablespoon balsamic vinegar
- Salt and pepper to taste
- Optional: Feta cheese crumbles for garnish

Instructions:

1. **Prepare Vegetables:**
    - In a large bowl, combine alfalfa sprouts, avocado slices, cherry tomatoes, cucumber, and red onion.
2. **Make the Dressing:**
    - In a small bowl, whisk together olive oil, balsamic vinegar, salt, and pepper.
3. **Combine and Toss:**
    - Pour the dressing over the salad ingredients. Gently toss the salad to ensure even coating.
4. **Garnish:**
    - If desired, sprinkle feta cheese crumbles over the top.
5. **Serve:**
    - Serve the refreshing Alfalfa and Avocado Salad as a side dish or a light and nutritious lunch.

Alfalfa Pesto Pasta:

Ingredients:

- 2 cups fresh alfalfa sprouts
- 2 cups fresh basil leaves

- 1/2 cup grated Parmesan cheese
- 1/2 cup pine nuts, toasted
- 2 cloves garlic
- 1/2 cup extra-virgin olive oil
- Salt and pepper to taste
- 12 ounces pasta of your choice (spaghetti or linguine work well)
- Optional: Cherry tomatoes for garnish

Instructions:

1. **Prepare Pesto:**
    - In a food processor, combine alfalfa sprouts, basil, Parmesan cheese, pine nuts, and garlic. Pulse until finely chopped.
2. **Add Olive Oil:**
    - With the food processor running, gradually add the olive oil until the mixture forms a smooth pesto.
3. **Cook Pasta:**
    - Cook the pasta according to package instructions. Drain and set aside.
4. **Combine Pasta and Pesto:**
    - In a large mixing bowl, toss the cooked pasta with the alfalfa pesto until well coated.
5. **Adjust Seasoning:**
    - Season with salt and pepper to taste. Add more olive oil if needed.
6. **Garnish and Serve:**
    - Garnish with cherry tomatoes and additional Parmesan cheese if desired. Serve the Alfalfa Pesto Pasta as a delightful and flavorful main dish.

These recipes showcase the versatility of alfalfa, allowing you to enjoy its unique texture and nutritional benefits in a variety of dishes.

How to Grow Alfalfa from Seed to Reaping

Alfalfa, often called the "Queen of Forages," is a nutrient-dense legume used for sprouts, animal feed, and natural soil enrichment. It's a hardy perennial known for deep roots and nitrogen-fixing ability.

Quick Facts

- **Botanical Name:** Medicago sativa
- **Plant Type:** Perennial legume (often grown as an annual in home gardens)
- **Time to Harvest:**
    - Sprouts: 5–7 days
    - Forage/Leaf Harvest: 60–70 days

Soil pH: 6.5–7.5
Sunlight: Full sun (minimum 6 hours/day)

1. Preparing to Plant

Choosing a Location

- Needs full sun.
- Choose an area with well-drained, fertile soil.

Soil Preparation

- Till soil 6–8 inches deep to remove weeds and loosen roots.
- Incorporate organic compost to enhance structure.
- Ensure pH is neutral to slightly alkaline. Use lime to raise pH if needed.
- Avoid acidic or compacted soils.

Inoculating Seeds (Optional but beneficial)

- Coat seeds with rhizobium inoculant for alfalfa to promote nitrogen fixation.
- Especially important if alfalfa hasn't been grown in that soil before.

2. Planting Alfalfa Seeds

When to Plant

- Spring (after last frost) or late summer (6–8 weeks before first frost).
- Soil temperature should be at least 65°F (18°C).

How to Plant

- Sow seeds ¼ inch deep.
- Broadcast seeds evenly or plant in rows.
- Use ¼ pound of seed per 100 square feet (for dense cover).

Watering After Planting

- Lightly water immediately after sowing.
- Keep soil moist (not soggy) during germination (5–10 days).

3. Caring for Alfalfa

Watering

- Water 1–2 times/week depending on rainfall.
- Deep watering is better than frequent light watering.
- Once established, alfalfa is drought-tolerant thanks to its deep root system.

Weed Control

- Weed early—alfalfa seedlings are slow to establish.
- After 3–4 weeks, plants form a canopy that suppresses weeds.

Fertilizing

- Use a phosphorus- and potassium-rich fertilizer (not nitrogen).
- Test soil if unsure—too much nitrogen discourages root nodulation.

4. Flowering & Growth

- Alfalfa produces purple flowers and grows 2–3 feet tall.
- Begins flowering around 6–8 weeks after planting.

5. Harvesting Alfalfa

Sprouts (Microgreens Use)

- Place seeds in a sprouting jar or tray.
- Rinse seeds 2–3 times daily.
- Ready in 5–7 days when sprouts are 1–3 inches tall.

Field or Garden Harvest (For Leaves or Hay)

- **First cutting:** When 10%–20% of plants are in bloom (around 60–70 days).
- Use garden shears or a scythe to cut 2–3 inches above the ground.
- Allow regrowth for up to 3–4 cuttings per growing season.

6. Drying and Storage

For Drying (Hay or Tea)

- Dry cuttings in a well-ventilated, shaded area.
- Turn frequently to prevent mold.
- Once fully dry, store in airtight containers or breathable bags.

For Sprouts

- Once harvested, refrigerate in a sealed container for up to 1 week.

7. Soil Benefits and Regrowth

- Alfalfa fixes nitrogen in the soil, making it ideal for crop rotation.
- Deep taproots break up compacted soil and draw up nutrients.

Pest & Disease Prevention
Pests

- Aphids
- Alfalfa weevils
- Cutworms

Remedy: Use neem oil or beneficial insects like ladybugs.
Diseases

- Root rot (from waterlogging)
- Leaf spot

Prevention:

- Good drainage
- Crop rotation every 3–4 years
- Proper spacing

Companion Planting Tips

- Good companions: Clover, corn, cucumbers
- Avoid planting with: Onions, garlic, or potatoes (can inhibit alfalfa growth)

Conclusion:

Alfalfa, with its nutrient-rich composition and diverse applications, stands as a powerhouse in the world of superfoods. Whether incorporated into culinary creations, consumed as herbal tea, or utilized as a nutritional supplement, alfalfa offers a broad spectrum of health benefits. If you have specific health concerns, allergies, or conditions, it's advisable to consult with a healthcare professional or a registered dietitian before making significant changes to your diet.

As we continue to explore the potential of this versatile plant, alfalfa remains a testament to the valuable intersection of agriculture, nutrition, and traditional medicine, offering a host of advantages for those seeking to enhance their well-being naturally.

Back to Table of Contents

Almond

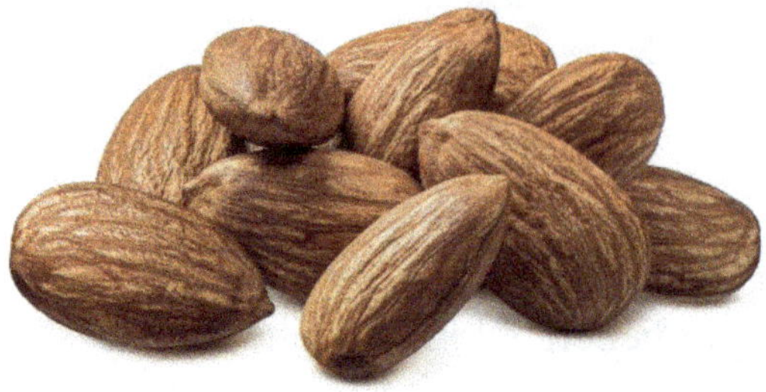

The Nutty Marvel: Health Benefits and Versatility of Almonds

Almonds, the delectable nuts that have been cherished for centuries, are not only a culinary delight but also a powerhouse of nutrition. Prized for their delicate flavor and crunchy texture, almonds have transcended their role as a mere snack to become a versatile and nutrient-rich addition to a well-balanced diet. In this article, we'll explore the myriad benefits and diverse uses that make almonds a staple in both kitchens and holistic health practices.

Nutrient-Rich Powerhouse:

Almonds are a nutrient-dense food, packed with essential vitamins, minerals, and antioxidants. They are an excellent source of vitamin E, a potent antioxidant that helps protect cells from oxidative damage. Almonds also provide a healthy dose of magnesium, copper, and phosphorus, contributing to overall well-being.

Vitamins:

Vitamin E: Almonds are particularly rich in vitamin E, specifically in the form of alpha-tocopherol, which is a potent antioxidant that helps protect cells from oxidative damage.

Vitamin B2 (Riboflavin): Almonds contain riboflavin, a B-vitamin that plays a role in energy metabolism and supports the body's antioxidant mechanisms.

Vitamin B3 (Niacin): Niacin is involved in energy metabolism and may have cardiovascular benefits. Almonds provide a small amount of niacin.

Vitamin B9 (Folate): Almonds contain folate, which is essential for cell division and the formation of DNA.

Minerals:

Magnesium: Almonds are a good source of magnesium, a mineral that plays a crucial role in various physiological functions, including muscle and nerve function, blood glucose control, and bone health.

Phosphorus: Phosphorus is important for bone health, and almonds contribute to the overall phosphorus intake in the diet.

Copper: Almonds contain copper, a trace mineral involved in the formation of red blood cells and the maintenance of healthy bones and nerves.

Manganese: Manganese is a trace mineral that plays a role in bone formation and helps the body process carbohydrates, amino acids, and cholesterol.

Zinc: Almonds provide a small amount of zinc, which is important for immune function, wound healing, and DNA synthesis.

Iron: While almonds contain iron, it is a non-heme iron, which is less easily absorbed by the body compared to heme iron found in animal products.

Antioxidants:

Phytochemicals: Almonds contain various phytochemicals, including flavonoids and polyphenols, which have antioxidant properties. These compounds help neutralize free radicals in the body, reducing oxidative stress.

L-arginine: Almonds contain L-arginine, an amino acid that can contribute to improved vascular function and heart health.

It's important to note that the nutrient content can vary depending on factors such as almond variety and preparation methods. While almonds are a nutritious addition to a balanced diet, it's advisable to consume them as part of a diverse and varied eating plan to ensure a broad spectrum of essential nutrients.

Heart Health:

Incorporating almonds into your diet may contribute to heart health. Almonds are rich in monounsaturated fats, which are heart-healthy fats that may help reduce bad cholesterol levels. Additionally, their magnesium content supports cardiovascular health by promoting proper blood flow and regulating blood pressure.

Weight Management:

Despite being calorie-dense, almonds can be a valuable asset for weight management. Their combination of healthy fats, protein, and fiber provides a satisfying and satiating snack that may help control appetite, preventing overeating and supporting weight loss efforts.

Blood Sugar Control:

Almonds have a low glycemic index, meaning they have a minimal impact on blood sugar levels. Including almonds in meals or snacks can contribute to better blood sugar control, making them a smart choice for individuals managing diabetes or those looking to stabilize energy levels throughout the day.

Bone Health:

The magnesium and phosphorus content in almonds plays a crucial role in maintaining strong and healthy bones. These minerals contribute to bone density and help prevent conditions like osteoporosis.

Nutritional Content

In 1 cup (approximately 143 grams) of almonds, you can expect to find roughly the following nutritional content:

- Carbohydrates: About 20 grams

- Protein: About 30 grams
- Fiber: About 12 grams
- Fat: About 55 grams

Almonds are a nutrient-dense food, rich in healthy fats, protein, fiber, vitamins, and minerals. They are particularly known for their high content of monounsaturated fats, which are beneficial for heart health, as well as their significant protein and fiber content, which can contribute to feelings of fullness and satiety.

Versatile Culinary Uses:

Almonds are remarkably versatile in the kitchen. They can be enjoyed in various forms, including raw, roasted, sliced, or ground into almond flour. Almond butter and almond milk have become popular alternatives for those seeking dairy-free options, adding a rich and creamy texture to recipes.

Here are two delicious and nutritious recipes that incorporate almonds:

Almond-Crusted Baked Salmon

Ingredients:

- 4 salmon fillets
- 1 cup almonds, finely chopped
- 1/2 cup whole wheat breadcrumbs
- 2 tablespoons Dijon mustard
- 1 tablespoon honey
- 1 tablespoon olive oil
- Salt and pepper to taste
- Lemon wedges for serving

Instructions:

1. Preheat the oven to 400°F (200°C) and line a baking sheet with parchment paper.
2. In a bowl, mix chopped almonds and breadcrumbs. Season with salt and pepper.
3. In a separate small bowl, whisk together Dijon mustard, honey, and olive oil.
4. Dip each salmon fillet into the mustard mixture, ensuring it's well coated.
5. Press the coated side of each salmon fillet into the almond and breadcrumb mixture, coating it evenly.
6. Place the almond-crusted salmon fillets on the prepared baking sheet.
7. Bake in the preheated oven for 12-15 minutes or until the salmon is cooked through and the crust is golden brown.
8. Serve the almond-crusted salmon with lemon wedges for a burst of citrusy flavor.

Almond and Spinach Pesto Pasta

Ingredients:

- 8 oz (225g) whole wheat or gluten-free pasta
- 2 cups fresh spinach leaves

- 1 cup fresh basil leaves
- 1/2 cup almonds, toasted
- 2 cloves garlic, minced
- 1/2 cup nutritional yeast (or grated Parmesan for non-vegan option)
- 1/2 cup olive oil
- Salt and pepper to taste
- Cherry tomatoes (optional, for garnish)
- Red pepper flakes (optional, for extra heat)

Instructions:

1. Cook the pasta according to package instructions. Drain and set aside.
2. In a food processor, combine spinach, basil, toasted almonds, minced garlic, and nutritional yeast.
3. Pulse the ingredients while gradually adding olive oil until you reach a smooth consistency. Season with salt and pepper to taste.
4. Toss the pesto sauce with the cooked pasta until evenly coated.
5. Garnish with cherry tomatoes and red pepper flakes if desired.
6. Serve the almond and spinach pesto pasta warm, and enjoy a flavorful, nutrient-packed meal.

These almond-infused recipes not only provide a delightful crunch but also deliver a dose of healthy fats, protein, and other essential nutrients. Enjoy the goodness of almonds in both savory and pasta dishes!

Skincare Benefits:

Almond oil, derived from pressed almonds, is a common ingredient in skincare products. Rich in vitamin E and monounsaturated fats, almond oil moisturizes and nourishes the skin, promoting a healthy complexion. It is often used in massage oils and as a natural remedy for dry skin.

Brain Health:

The presence of nutrients like riboflavin (vitamin B2) and L-carnitine in almonds contributes to brain health. These elements may support neurological function and cognitive performance.

How to Grow Almond from Seed to Reaping

Quick Facts

- Botanical name: Prunus dulcis
- Tree type: Deciduous, fruit and nut tree
- Grows in: USDA Zones 7–9
- Time to bear nuts: 3–5 years from planting
- Full harvest: Around year 5–7

- Life span: 25–30 years

1. Preparing the Seed

Choose the Right Almond

- Use raw, unsalted, unpasteurized almond seeds (ideally from a trusted organic source or directly from a tree).

- Most store-bought almonds are pasteurized and won't germinate.

Stratify the Seeds

Almond seeds need a cold period (stratification) to break dormancy.

Method:

Crack open the shell slightly without damaging the nut.

- Soak seeds in lukewarm water for 24–48 hours.
- Place seeds in a damp paper towel inside a plastic bag.
- Store in refrigerator at 34–41°F (1–5°C) for 6–8 weeks.
- Check weekly to ensure they remain moist and mold-free.
- After 6–8 weeks, look for a tiny root emerging — it's ready to plant.

2. Planting Almond Seedlings

Best Time to Plant

- After the last frost in early spring.

How to Plant (Indoors or Outdoors)

1. Potting soil or outdoor soil should be:

- Well-drained
- Loamy with pH 6.0–7.5

2. Plant seed 1–2 inches deep, root side down.
3. Water thoroughly, keeping the soil moist but not soggy.
4. Place in a sunny location (full sun is crucial).

Almond trees need 6–8 hours of direct sunlight daily.

3. Transplanting to the Ground

Once your seedling reaches 12–18 inches tall (after 3–4 months), transplant to a permanent outdoor location.

Spacing

- Minimum 15–20 feet apart for standard trees.
- Plant near another almond tree (or compatible pollinator like peach) if your variety is not self-pollinating.

Soil Preparation

- Dig a hole twice the size of the root ball.
- Mix compost with native soil.
- Place tree in hole, backfill and water deeply.

4. Caring for the Almond Tree

Watering

- Young trees: Water every 7–10 days deeply.
- Mature trees: Every 2–4 weeks, depending on rainfall.
- Avoid overwatering—roots don't like soggy soil.

Pruning

- First year: Train a central leader and 3–5 main branches.
- After: Prune annually to remove dead or crowded branches and encourage airflow.

Fertilization

- Apply balanced organic fertilizer in early spring.
- Don't over-fertilize, especially with nitrogen.

5. Pest & Disease Management

Common Pests:

- Aphids
- Spider mites
- Peach twig borers

Solution: Neem oil, beneficial insects, regular inspections.

Common Diseases:

- Leaf curl
- Rust
- Root rot

Solution:

- Use copper fungicide during dormant season.
- Ensure well-drained soil and good air circulation.

6. Flowering and Pollination

- Flowers bloom in early spring, even before leaves emerge.
- Some varieties are self-pollinating (like 'All-in-One'), but most need a second compatible almond tree.
- Bees are essential for pollination—avoid using pesticides during bloom time.

7. Harvesting Almonds

Timeframe

- You can expect your first light harvest in year 3–4, full harvest by year 5–6.
- Almonds are usually ready to harvest in late summer (August–September).

Signs of Readiness

- The hull (outer casing) splits open to reveal the shell.
- Shake or gently knock branches—mature almonds will fall.
- Pick them up and remove the hull immediately.

Drying

Lay nuts in a single layer in the sun for 7–10 days.
Store dried almonds in a cool, dry, dark place.

Additional Notes
Benefits of Growing Almonds

- High in healthy fats, vitamin E, and fiber
- Supports pollinators
- Enhances soil when mulched with leaves and pruned material

Sustainability Tips

- Mulch to conserve water
- Use companion planting (e.g., lavender, comfrey) to deter pests

Conclusion:

In conclusion, almonds stand as a testament to the harmonious blend of taste and nutrition. From supporting heart health to enhancing culinary creations, almonds have earned their reputation as a wholesome and delightful addition to our daily lives. Whether enjoyed as a convenient snack, incorporated into meals, or harnessed for their skin-nourishing properties, the almond continues to play a significant role in promoting overall health and well-being. If you have specific health concerns, allergies, or conditions, it's advisable to consult with a healthcare professional or a registered dietitian before making significant changes to your diet.

Embrace the nutty marvel and let the myriad benefits of almonds enrich your life in more ways than one.

Back to Table of Contents

Aloe Vera

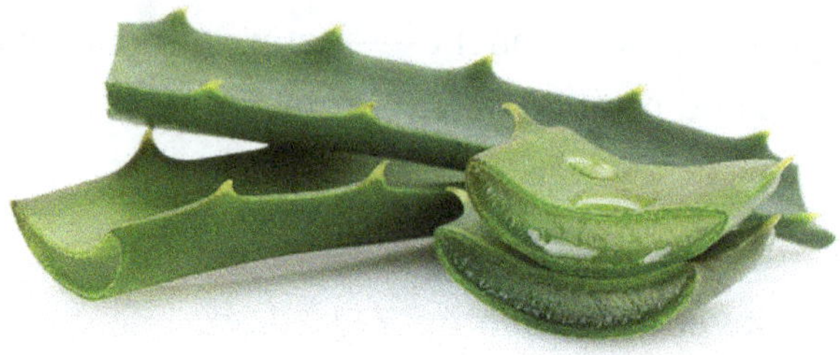

The Healing Power of Aloe Vera

In the realm of natural remedies, few plants hold the esteemed reputation of Aloe vera. Revered for its myriad health benefits and versatile applications, Aloe vera has cemented its place as a household staple, adorning windowsills, skincare routines, and medicinal cabinets alike. Originating from the arid regions of North Africa, Aloe vera's robust succulent leaves house a treasure trove of healing compounds, making it a botanical powerhouse with a legacy spanning millennia.

Aloe vera is a succulent plant species that has been widely recognized for its historical benefits and diverse uses. This resilient plant has a rich history dating back thousands of years, with its origins traced to the Arabian Peninsula. Over time, aloe vera has become a staple in various cultures, appreciated for its medicinal, cosmetic, and therapeutic properties. In this document, we will explore the historical significance and benefits of aloe vera, shedding light on its cultural, traditional, and contemporary uses.

Aloe vera is a botanical powerhouse teeming with an array of vitamins, minerals, enzymes, and antioxidants, each contributing to its remarkable health-promoting properties. Rich in vitamins A, C, and E, this succulent plant nourishes the body with essential nutrients, bolstering immune function and supporting skin health. Its mineral content, including calcium, magnesium, and potassium, fortifies bones, muscles, and nerve function, while enzymes like lipase and cellulase aid digestion and promote gastrointestinal wellness. Furthermore, aloe vera boasts a diverse array of antioxidants such as polyphenols and flavonoids, which combat oxidative stress, reduce inflammation, and shield cells from damage, offering comprehensive protection against chronic diseases and promoting overall vitality and well-being.

Vitamins:

- **Vitamin A:** Supports healthy vision, skin, and immune function.
- **Vitamin C:** Boosts immunity, promotes collagen production, and acts as an antioxidant to protect cells from damage.
- **Vitamin E:** Acts as an antioxidant, protecting cells from damage caused by free radicals.
- **Vitamin B12:** Essential for nerve function and the production of DNA and red blood cells.

- **Folic Acid (Vitamin B9):** Important for cell division and the prevention of birth defects during pregnancy.
- **Choline:** Supports brain health and aids in nerve signaling.
- **Niacin (Vitamin B3):** Helps convert food into energy and supports skin health.

Minerals:

- **Calcium:** Essential for bone health, muscle function, and nerve signaling.
- **Magnesium:** Supports muscle and nerve function, regulates blood sugar levels, and aids in energy production.
- **Zinc:** Important for immune function, wound healing, and DNA synthesis.
- **Copper:** Needed for the formation of red blood cells and collagen, and supports immune function.
- **Iron:** Essential for the production of hemoglobin, which carries oxygen in the blood.
- **Sodium:** Regulates fluid balance and helps transmit nerve impulses.
- **Potassium:** Important for heart health, muscle function, and fluid balance.
- **Chromium:** Helps regulate blood sugar levels by enhancing the action of insulin.
- **Manganese:** Necessary for bone formation, metabolism, and antioxidant defense.

Enzymes:

- **Amylase:** Aids in the digestion of carbohydrates.
- **Lipase:** Helps digest fats and support lipid metabolism.
- **Catalase:** Protects cells from oxidative stress by breaking down hydrogen peroxide.
- **Alkaline Phosphatase:** Supports bone health and plays a role in DNA synthesis.
- **Cellulase:** Aids in the digestion of cellulose, a type of fiber found in plants.
- **Bradykinase:** Known for its anti-inflammatory properties and ability to promote wound healing.

Antioxidants:

- **Polyphenols:** Protect cells from damage caused by free radicals and reduce inflammation.
- **Flavonoids:** Have antioxidant and anti-inflammatory properties, supporting heart health and reducing the risk of chronic diseases.
- **Tannins:** Possess antimicrobial properties and can help with diarrhea and other gastrointestinal issues.
- **Anthraquinones:** Have laxative effects and may promote wound healing.
- **Saponins:** Exhibit anti-inflammatory and immune-modulating effects.
- **Lignins:** Help enhance the absorption of nutrients and may have antioxidant properties.

Benefits and Common Uses:

- **Skin Health:** Aloe vera is widely used for its soothing and moisturizing properties, making it effective for treating sunburns, rashes, and dry skin conditions.
- **Digestive Health:** Enzymes like cellulase and bradykinase support digestion and can help alleviate symptoms of digestive disorders like acid reflux and irritable bowel syndrome (IBS).
- **Immune Support:** Vitamins, minerals, and antioxidants in aloe vera bolster immune function, helping the body defend against infections and illness.
- **Wound Healing:** Aloe vera's antibacterial and anti-inflammatory properties promote wound healing and reduce the risk of infection.
- **Oral Health:** Aloe vera is used in natural toothpaste and mouthwashes for its antimicrobial properties, which can help prevent gum disease and promote oral hygiene.

Overall, the vitamins, minerals, enzymes, and antioxidants found in aloe vera contribute to its multifaceted health benefits, making it a valuable addition to both internal and external health and wellness routines.

Historical Roots of Aloe Vera

The history of aloe vera can be traced to ancient civilizations, where it was revered for its healing properties. Ancient Egyptians referred to aloe vera as the "plant of immortality" and used it in various aspects of daily life. Historical records indicate that Cleopatra herself attributed her legendary beauty to the use of aloe vera. The plant was depicted in hieroglyphs on the walls of temples, signifying its importance in religious and medicinal practices.

The Greeks and Romans also embraced aloe vera for its therapeutic attributes. The famous Greek physician Dioscorides documented its medicinal uses in his influential work "De Materia Medica." Aloe vera found its way into the annals of traditional Chinese medicine, where it was valued for its ability to balance the body's energy and promote overall well-being.

Medicinal Uses Through the Ages

Aloe vera's historical benefits are deeply intertwined with its medicinal uses. The gel extracted from the plant's leaves has been employed to treat a myriad of ailments. In traditional medicine, aloe vera was used to heal wounds, soothe burns, reduce dental plaque, prevent wrinkles, manage blood sugar levels and alleviate skin conditions. The gel contains compounds with anti-inflammatory, antibacterial, and antioxidant properties, making it a valuable remedy for skin-related issues.

As civilizations advanced, aloe vera continued to play a role in medical practices. Arab traders introduced aloe vera to Europe during the medieval period, where it gained popularity for its healing properties. In the 18th and 19th centuries, aloe vera became a key ingredient in various pharmaceutical preparations. Its use expanded beyond topical applications to include internal remedies for digestive issues and overall health.

Cultivating Wellness, Naturally

Cultivating Aloe vera at home is a straightforward endeavor, as it thrives in arid conditions and requires minimal maintenance. Whether grown in pots indoors or in sunny garden beds, Aloe vera's fleshy leaves provide a readily available source of healing gel. Simply slice open a leaf to access the gel's soothing properties or blend it into a nourishing juice for internal consumption.

Aloe Vera in the Modern World

In the contemporary era, aloe vera has transcended cultural and geographical boundaries to become a global phenomenon. Its historical benefits are now supported by scientific research, reaffirming its efficacy in various applications. Aloe vera is a common ingredient in cosmetic and skincare products due to its moisturizing and anti-aging properties. Additionally, the plant's juice is consumed for its potential digestive benefits.

Aloe Vera Juice: A Gooey Elixir

Aloe vera juice, derived from the plant's leaf flesh, is thick liquid rich in polyphenols and antioxidants, offering various health benefits.

Aloe vera can be prepared in various ways to harness its medicinal and cosmetic benefits. **Here are a few common methods:**

Aloe Vera Gel:

Harvest a mature aloe vera leaf.
Cut the leaf lengthwise to expose the inner gel.
Scoop out the gel using a spoon or knife.
Blend the gel to achieve a smooth consistency.
The resulting gel can be applied topically on the skin for soothing and healing effects.

Aloe Vera Juice:

Extract the gel from a mature aloe vera leaf.
Mix the gel with water or fruit juice using a blender.
Strain the mixture to remove any pulp or latex.
The resulting liquid is aloe vera juice, which can be consumed for its potential digestive benefits. Ensure moderation due to its laxative properties.

Aloe Vera Extract/Oil:

Blend aloe vera gel with a carrier oil like coconut or olive oil.

Allow the mixture to sit for a period, letting the oil absorb the beneficial compounds from the aloe vera.

Strain the mixture to separate the oil from any remaining solid particles.

The resulting aloe vera extract or oil can be used for moisturizing the skin or as an ingredient in cosmetic formulations.

Aloe Vera Capsules or Supplements:

Extract the gel from aloe vera leaves.

Process the gel into a concentrated form suitable for encapsulation.

Encapsulate the concentrated aloe vera extract into capsules or prepare it as a supplement.

Aloe vera capsules or supplements are often taken orally for various health benefits. It's important to follow recommended dosages and consult with a healthcare professional.

People predominantly use aloe vera topically, leveraging its historical effectiveness in treating sores, burns, and skin conditions. Oral use is also promoted for various health concerns, including weight loss, diabetes, and inflammatory bowel diseases.

Aloe vera is a versatile plant with various medicinal benefits. **Here are a few different medicinal benefits of aloe vera:**

Skin Healing and Burns:

Aloe vera is renowned for its ability to soothe and heal the skin. The gel extracted from its leaves contains compounds that accelerate wound healing, making it effective for treating burns, sunburns, and minor skin irritations. The cooling sensation and anti-inflammatory properties of aloe vera help reduce pain and promote skin regeneration.

Moisturization and Hydration:

Aloe vera is an excellent natural moisturizer. Its gel is rich in water content, which helps hydrate and nourish the skin without leaving a greasy residue. Regular application of aloe vera gel can contribute to smoother, softer skin, making it a popular ingredient in various skincare products.

Anti-Inflammatory and Arthritis Relief:

Aloe vera possesses anti-inflammatory properties that can be beneficial for conditions involving inflammation, such as arthritis. Consuming aloe vera or using its gel topically may help alleviate joint pain and stiffness associated with inflammatory conditions, providing relief for those with arthritis.

Digestive Health:

Aloe vera has been traditionally used to promote digestive health. Its latex, derived from the inner leaf skin, contains compounds with laxative effects that may aid in relieving constipation. However, it's crucial to use aloe vera for this purpose under proper guidance, as excessive consumption can lead to side effects.

Antibacterial and Antifungal Properties:

Aloe vera exhibits antibacterial and antifungal properties, making it effective in treating minor skin infections. The gel can be applied topically to wounds or cuts to prevent infection and promote healing. Additionally, aloe vera's antimicrobial properties contribute to its role in maintaining oral hygiene, and it is sometimes used in natural toothpaste formulations.

As we navigate the 21st century, aloe vera continues to evolve, finding new applications in the fields of biotechnology and agriculture. Researchers are exploring the plant's potential in wound healing, tissue engineering, and as a sustainable source of bioactive compounds. Aloe vera stands as a testament to the enduring significance of traditional remedies in the modern world, bridging the gap between ancient wisdom and contemporary science.

It's crucial to note that when preparing aloe vera at home, attention should be given to cleanliness and proper processing to avoid contamination. Additionally, while aloe vera offers numerous health benefits, individuals should be cautious when using aloe vera internally, as excessive consumption may lead to adverse effects. Always consult with healthcare professionals before incorporating aloe vera into your diet or skincare routine.

In conclusion, aloe vera's historical journey is one of resilience and adaptability. From its revered status in ancient civilizations to its widespread use in modern times, the plant has proven its versatility and efficacy. The historical benefits of aloe vera, rooted in cultural practices and traditional medicine, continue to shape its role in today's global landscape.

Back to Table of Contents

Amaranth

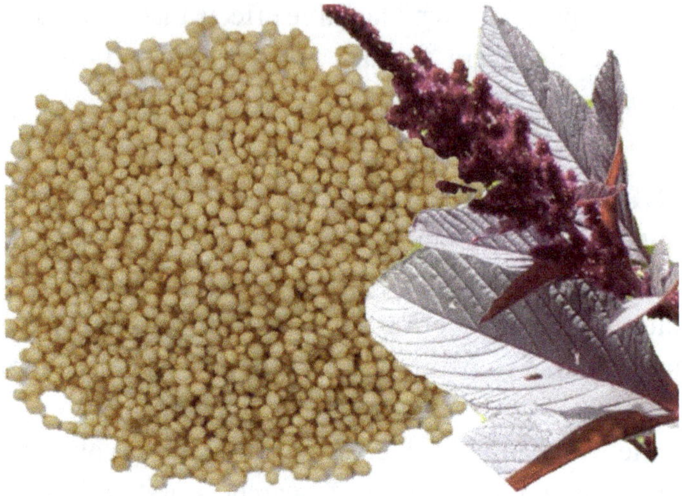

The Marvelous Amaranth: Unveiling Its Benefits and Diverse Uses

Amaranth, a tiny yet powerful grain, has been cultivated for thousands of years and is renowned for its exceptional nutritional profile and versatility. This ancient pseudo-grain, revered by various cultures, has recently experienced a resurgence in popularity due to its numerous health benefits and culinary adaptability. In this article, we'll explore the impressive advantages and diverse uses of amaranth.

Nutritional Powerhouse:

Amaranth stands out as a nutritional powerhouse, offering a host of essential nutrients that contribute to overall well-being. Some key nutritional components include:

Protein: Amaranth is exceptionally high in protein, making it an excellent plant-based source for individuals looking to boost their protein intake. It contains all essential amino acids, making it a complete protein source.

Dietary Fiber: Rich in dietary fiber, amaranth promotes digestive health, aids in weight management, and helps regulate blood sugar levels.

Vitamins:

Amaranth contains various vitamins, including vitamin A, vitamin C, vitamin K, folate, and riboflavin, contributing to a well-rounded nutrient profile.

Vitamin A: Essential for vision, immune function, and skin health, vitamin A is present in amaranth in the form of beta-carotene.

Vitamin C: A powerful antioxidant, vitamin C supports immune function, helps the body absorb iron, and promotes healthy skin.

Vitamin K: Vitamin K is crucial for blood clotting and bone health. Amaranth provides a significant amount of vitamin K, contributing to these essential functions.

Vitamin E: An antioxidant that helps protect cells from damage caused by free radicals, vitamin E is present in amaranth in varying amounts.

Folate (Vitamin B9): Folate is essential for DNA synthesis and cell division. Adequate folate intake is particularly important during pregnancy for fetal development.

Thiamine (Vitamin B1): Thiamine plays a key role in energy metabolism and the proper functioning of the nervous system.

Riboflavin (Vitamin B2): Riboflavin is involved in energy production, cell growth, and the maintenance of healthy skin.

Niacin (Vitamin B3): Niacin is essential for DNA repair, energy metabolism, and the proper functioning of the nervous system.

Vitamin B6: Pyridoxine, or vitamin B6, is crucial for brain development, the production of neurotransmitters, and the metabolism of amino acids.

Pantothenic Acid (Vitamin B5): Pantothenic acid is involved in the synthesis of fatty acids, amino acids, and other important molecules.

Amaranth's diverse vitamin profile contributes to its overall nutritional benefits, making it a valuable addition to a balanced and nutrient-rich diet.

Minerals:

It is a good source of essential minerals such as calcium, iron, magnesium, phosphorus, and potassium, vital for bone health, energy metabolism, and overall vitality.

Calcium: Essential for bone and teeth health, blood clotting, and muscle function.

Iron: Important for the formation of hemoglobin, which carries oxygen in the blood.

Magnesium: Crucial for muscle and nerve function, blood glucose control, and bone health.

Phosphorus: Vital for bone and teeth health, energy metabolism, and acid-base balance.

Potassium: Important for maintaining proper heart and muscle function and balancing fluid levels in the body.

Zinc: Essential for immune function, wound healing, and DNA synthesis.

Copper: Involved in the formation of red blood cells, maintenance of bones and nerves, and the immune system.

Manganese: Plays a role in bone formation, blood clotting, and reducing inflammation.

Selenium: An antioxidant that supports thyroid function and immune system health.

Sodium: While sodium is typically present in small amounts, it is important for maintaining fluid balance and nerve function.

Phytosterols: While not a mineral, phytosterols are plant compounds found in amaranth that may contribute to heart health by lowering cholesterol levels.

Amaranth's diverse mineral profile makes it a valuable addition to a balanced and nutrient-rich diet. Incorporating amaranth into meals provides not only essential minerals but also a host of other nutrients, including vitamins, fiber, and protein. It is particularly beneficial for those seeking plant-based sources of key minerals.

Health Benefits:

Heart Health: The high fiber content in amaranth supports heart health by helping to lower cholesterol levels and reduce the risk of cardiovascular diseases.

Bone Health: Amaranth's rich calcium and magnesium content contribute to maintaining strong and healthy bones, reducing the risk of osteoporosis.

Weight Management: The combination of protein and fiber in amaranth promotes satiety, making it a valuable addition to weight management and control programs.

Antioxidant Properties: Amaranth contains antioxidants, including vitamin C and polyphenols, which help neutralize free radicals and protect the body from oxidative stress.

Nutritional Content

In 1 cup (about 246 grams) of cooked amaranth, you can expect to find approximately:

- Carbohydrates: Around 46-47 grams
- Protein: Approximately 9-10 grams
- Fiber: Roughly 5-6 grams
- Fat: About 3-4 grams

Please note that these values are approximate and can vary slightly based on factors such as cooking method and specific variety of amaranth.

Culinary Uses:

Amaranth's versatility extends to the culinary realm, where it can be incorporated into a wide range of dishes. Here are some popular culinary uses:

Whole Grain Dish: Cooked amaranth can be enjoyed as a whole grain dish, similar to rice or quinoa. Its nutty flavor and slightly crunchy texture make it a delightful addition to salads, stir-fries, or as a side dish.

Flour and Baking: Amaranth flour is a gluten-free alternative that can be used in baking. It adds a unique taste and nutritional boost to bread, pancakes, muffins, and other baked goods.

Porridge or Breakfast Bowl: Amaranth porridge is a nutritious and satisfying breakfast option. Cooked amaranth can be mixed with milk or plant-based alternatives, topped with fruits, nuts, and honey.

Popped Amaranth: Similar to popcorn, amaranth can be popped and used as a crunchy topping for salads, yogurt, or desserts.

Vegetarian Burgers and Patties: Amaranth can be combined with vegetables and spices to create delicious vegetarian burgers or patties, providing a protein-packed meat alternative.

Amaranth's versatility allows it to be used in a variety of dishes, from savory to sweet. ***Here are two delicious recipes featuring amaranth:***

Amaranth and Vegetable Stir-Fry:

Ingredients:

- 1 cup amaranth, rinsed and drained
- 2 cups mixed vegetables (bell peppers, broccoli, carrots, snap peas, etc.), chopped
- 2 tablespoons olive oil
- 3 cloves garlic, minced
- 1 tablespoon ginger, grated
- 2 tablespoons soy sauce
- 1 tablespoon sesame oil
- 1 tablespoon rice vinegar
- 1 tablespoon maple syrup or honey
- Salt and pepper to taste
- Sesame seeds for garnish (optional)

Instructions:

1. Cook amaranth according to package instructions. Typically, you'll need to bring 2.5 cups of water to a boil, add amaranth, reduce heat, cover, and simmer for 20-25 minutes until water is absorbed.
2. In a large skillet or wok, heat olive oil over medium-high heat. Add minced garlic and grated ginger, sautéing for about 1-2 minutes until fragrant.
3. Add chopped vegetables to the skillet and stir-fry until they are tender-crisp.
4. In a small bowl, whisk together soy sauce, sesame oil, rice vinegar, and maple syrup. Pour the sauce over the vegetables and stir to coat evenly.
5. Add the cooked amaranth to the skillet and toss everything together until well combined.
6. Season with salt and pepper to taste. Garnish with sesame seeds if desired.
7. Serve the amaranth and vegetable stir-fry hot, and enjoy a nutrient-packed, flavorful meal.

Amaranth Breakfast Porridge:

Ingredients:

- 1/2 cup amaranth
- 1 1/2 cups milk (dairy or plant-based)
- 1 tablespoon maple syrup or honey
- 1/2 teaspoon vanilla extract
- Fresh fruit (berries, sliced banana) for topping
- Nuts or seeds (almonds, chia seeds) for topping

Instructions:

1. In a saucepan, combine amaranth, milk, maple syrup (or honey), and vanilla extract.

2. Bring the mixture to a boil, then reduce the heat to low, cover, and simmer for about 20-25 minutes or until the amaranth is cooked and the mixture has thickened.
3. Stir occasionally to prevent sticking.
4. Once cooked, remove from heat and let it sit, covered, for a few minutes.
5. Serve the amaranth porridge in bowls, topped with fresh fruit and nuts or seeds of your choice.
6. Drizzle with additional maple syrup if desired.
7. Enjoy a warm and nutritious amaranth breakfast porridge to kick-start your day.

These recipes showcase the versatility of amaranth, whether used in a savory stir-fry or a comforting breakfast porridge. Feel free to customize these recipes with your favorite vegetables, fruits, or toppings.

Tips Incorporating Amaranth

Transitioning to a plant-based diet using amaranth can be a rewarding journey, as amaranth is a highly nutritious grain rich in protein, fiber, and essential nutrients. Here are two ways you can transition to a plant-based diet using amaranth and overcome challenges:

1. **Incorporate Amaranth into Everyday Meals:**
    - Start by incorporating amaranth into your favorite meals to make the transition to a plant-based diet more seamless. For example, you can cook amaranth and use it as a substitute for rice, quinoa, or oats in recipes.
    - Add cooked amaranth to soups, stews, and chili to increase their nutritional content and add texture. Amaranth has a slightly nutty flavor and a creamy texture when cooked, making it a versatile addition to savory dishes.
    - Use amaranth flour in baking recipes to make plant-based bread, muffins, pancakes, and other baked goods. Amaranth flour adds a nutritious boost to baked goods and can help improve their texture and flavor.
2. **Experiment with New Amaranth-Based Recipes:**
    - Explore new recipes and meal ideas that feature amaranth as the main ingredient. Look for plant-based cookbooks, websites, or cooking blogs for inspiration.
    - Use amaranth as a base for salads, grain bowls, and porridge, and top it with a variety of vegetables, fruits, nuts, seeds, and herbs for added flavor and nutrition.
    - Incorporate amaranth into sweet dishes, such as puddings, smoothies, and desserts, to satisfy your sweet tooth while still adhering to a plant-based diet.

By incorporating amaranth into everyday meals and experimenting with new recipes and meal ideas, you can transition to a plant-based diet while enjoying the delicious flavors and health benefits of this nutritious grain. Overcoming challenges may involve adjusting your cooking techniques, taste preferences, and meal planning strategies to accommodate a plant-based lifestyle. With creativity and exploration, you can embrace the versatility and nutritional value of amaranth and thrive on a plant-based diet.

1. How to Grow Amaranth from Seed to Reaping

- **Type:** Warm-season annual
- **Uses:** Edible leaves (like spinach), grain-like seeds, ornamental flowers
- **Climate:** Thrives in warm temperatures, frost-sensitive
- **Soil pH:** 6.0–7.5

2. Choosing Your Variety

Amaranth has many types:

- Leaf amaranth (Amaranthus tricolor) — grown mainly for greens
- Grain amaranth (Amaranthus caudatus, A. cruentus, A. hypochondriacus) — grown for seeds
- Ornamental amaranth — mainly decorative but still edible

3. Sowing Seeds

When to Plant

- Plant outdoors after all danger of frost has passed and soil is warm (≥ 65°F / 18°C).
- Indoors: Start seeds 3–4 weeks before transplanting if you want an early start.

How to Plant

1. Prepare the soil — loosen, remove weeds, add compost for nutrition.
2. Direct sow or start indoors:

- **Direct sow:** Sprinkle seeds thinly in rows or broadcast over an area.
- **Indoors:** Plant seeds ¼ inch deep in trays or small pots.

3. Spacing:

- For leaf harvest: Space plants 6–8 inches apart.
- For grain harvest: Space 10–12 inches apart, rows 18–24 inches apart.

4. **Cover lightly** — seeds need light to germinate, so barely cover with fine soil.

5. **Water gently** — keep soil consistently moist until germination (5–10 days).

4. Growing Conditions

- **Sunlight:** Full sun (at least 6 hours/day).
- **Water:** Moderate; water deeply but let topsoil dry slightly between waterings.
- **Fertilizer:** Balanced organic fertilizer or compost at planting; amaranth doesn't need heavy feeding.
- **Weeding:** Weed early — once established, amaranth outcompetes most weeds.
- **Thinning:** Once seedlings are 2–3 inches tall, thin to desired spacing.

5. Harvesting Leaves

- Begin harvesting young leaves when plants are 4–6 inches tall (20–30 days after germination).
- Pinch or cut leaves from the top to encourage bushy growth.
- For continuous harvest, take only a few leaves from each plant at a time.

6. Harvesting Seeds (Reaping)
When Seeds Are Ready

- 90–120 days after planting.
- Flower heads will turn brown/dry, and seeds will become firm and easily fall when rubbed.
- Wait for a few dry days in a row before harvesting.

How to Harvest

1. Cut the entire seed head with pruning shears.
2. Place seed heads in a paper bag or large container.
3. Let them dry indoors for 1–2 weeks in a well-ventilated area.
4. Rub or shake the heads to release seeds.
5. Winnow (blow away) chaff using a gentle breeze or fan.

7. Storage

- **Leaves:** Store fresh in a fridge for up to 5 days or blanch and freeze.
- **Seeds:** Store in airtight jars in a cool, dry place for up to 1 year.

8. Pests & Problems

- Aphids and flea beetles can attack young plants — use neem oil or insecticidal soap.
- Excess water can cause root rot; keep soil well-drained.

Pro Tips for Success

- Sow every 2–3 weeks for continuous leaf harvest.
- Mulch around plants to retain moisture and reduce weeds.
- For better grain yield, avoid heavy nitrogen feeding — it encourages leaf over seed production.

In conclusion, amaranth emerges as a nutritional gem with an array of health benefits and culinary possibilities. Whether you're seeking a nutrient-dense addition to your diet or looking to diversify your culinary repertoire, amaranth offers a satisfying solution. If you have specific health concerns, allergies, or conditions, it's advisable to consult with a healthcare professional or a registered dietitian before making significant changes to your diet.

Embrace the versatility of amaranth and explore the myriad ways this ancient grain can contribute to both your health and your palate. Incorporating amaranth into your meals is a delightful journey into the world of wholesome nutrition and delicious flavors.

Back to Table of Contents

Angelica Root:

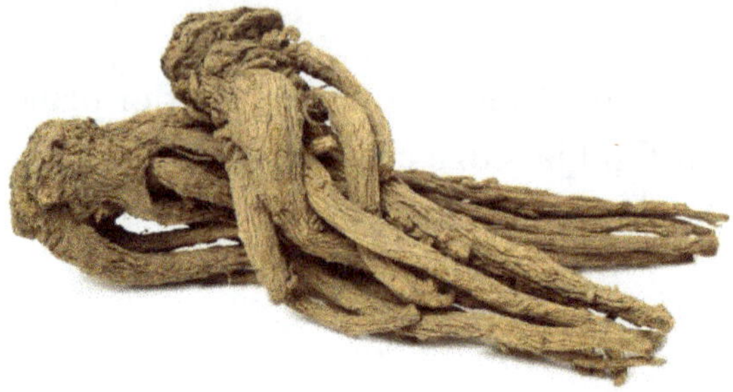

The Benefits and Versatile Uses of a Botanical Marvel

Angelica root, derived from the Angelica archangelica plant, has a long history of traditional use in herbal medicine and culinary practices. With a unique aroma and a host of potential health benefits, angelica root is a botanical marvel that deserves attention. In this article, we will explore the various benefits and versatile uses of angelica root, shedding light on its rich history and contemporary applications.

Botanical Background:

Angelica archangelica, commonly known as garden angelica or wild celery, is a large, aromatic plant belonging to the Apiaceae family. The plant is native to regions of Northern Europe, Siberia, and Greenland. Angelica root, extracted from the plant's thick taproot, has been revered for centuries for its potential medicinal and culinary properties.

Benefits of Angelica Root:

Digestive Aid:

- Angelica root has been traditionally used to support digestive health. It may help alleviate symptoms such as indigestion, bloating, and flatulence. The root is believed to stimulate the production of digestive juices and enzymes, promoting a healthy digestive process.

Anti-Inflammatory Properties:

- Compounds found in angelica root, including coumarins and flavonoids, exhibit anti-inflammatory properties. This makes angelica root a potential remedy for conditions involving inflammation, such as arthritis or muscle pain.

Respiratory Support:

- Angelica root has been employed as a respiratory tonic in traditional herbal medicine. It is believed to have expectorant properties, helping to clear the respiratory passages and alleviate symptoms of coughs and colds.

Menstrual and Menopausal Support:

- Some herbal practitioners suggest that angelica root may be beneficial for women's health. It is believed to have properties that may help regulate menstrual cycles and ease symptoms associated with menopause.

Stress and Anxiety Relief:

- The calming properties of angelica root have been explored for their potential in stress and anxiety relief. It is thought to have a soothing effect on the nervous system, promoting relaxation.

Vitamins and Minerals

Angelica root is not particularly known for being a rich source of vitamins compared to fruits and vegetables. However, it does contain trace amounts of certain vitamins. Here are a few vitamins and minerals found in angelica root and their associated benefits:

Vitamin B6 (Pyridoxine):

Benefits:

- **Metabolism Support:** Vitamin B6 is involved in the metabolism of proteins, carbohydrates, and fats, contributing to the conversion of food into energy.
- **Neurotransmitter Synthesis:** Vitamin B6 is important for the synthesis of neurotransmitters, supporting proper nerve function and mood regulation.

Vitamin C:

Benefits:

- **Immune Support:** Vitamin C is essential for the proper functioning of the immune system. It stimulates the production of white blood cells and helps the body defend against infections.
- **Antioxidant Defense:** As a powerful antioxidant, vitamin C helps neutralize free radicals in the body, protecting cells from oxidative **damage.**

Vitamin E:

Benefits:

- **Antioxidant Protection:** Vitamin E is an antioxidant that helps protect cells from oxidative stress. It plays a role in maintaining skin health and supporting the immune system.

Vitamin K:

Benefits:

- **Blood Clotting:** Vitamin K is essential for blood clotting, which is crucial for wound healing and overall blood vessel health.
- **Bone Health:** Vitamin K plays a role in bone metabolism and may contribute to maintaining bone density.

Minerals

Potassium:

Benefits:

- **Heart Health:** Potassium is essential for maintaining heart health by helping to regulate blood pressure. Adequate potassium intake is associated with a lower risk of hypertension and cardiovascular diseases.

Calcium:

Benefits:

- **Bone and Teeth Health:** Calcium is crucial for the development and maintenance of strong bones and teeth. It also plays a role in muscle function, blood clotting, and nerve transmission.

Phosphorus:

Benefits:

- **Bone Health:** Phosphorus is a key component of bones and teeth, contributing to their strength and structure. It also plays a role in energy metabolism and the formation of DNA.

Magnesium:

Benefits:

- **Muscle and Nerve Function:** Magnesium is involved in muscle and nerve function, helping to regulate muscle contractions and support the transmission of nerve signals. It also plays a role in bone health and energy metabolism.

While angelica root contains these vitamins and minerals in small amounts, it is not a primary source for meeting daily vitamin requirements. Including a variety of nutrient-rich foods in your diet is essential for obtaining adequate vitamin and mineral intake.

Versatile Uses of Angelica Root

Culinary Applications:

In culinary practices, angelica root is used as a flavoring agent, particularly in the preparation of liqueurs, bitters, and certain desserts. The root's unique, slightly sweet and musky aroma adds depth to culinary creations.

Preparation:

- Use fresh or dried angelica root as a flavoring agent in culinary dishes.
- Crush or finely chop the root and add it to soups, stews, or sauces.
- Use it in the preparation of desserts or as an aromatic addition to beverages.

Tinctures and Extracts:

Angelica root can be prepared as tinctures or extracts, preserving its beneficial compounds. These extracts are often used in herbal formulations for various health purposes.

Preparation:

- Combine dried angelica root with a high-proof alcohol (such as vodka or brandy) in a glass jar.
- Let the mixture sit for several weeks, shaking the jar occasionally.
- Strain the liquid to separate the infused alcohol from the solid plant material.

Here are two recipes featuring angelica root:

Angelica Root Infused Syrup:

- ***Ingredients:***
  - 1 cup water
  - 1 cup granulated sugar
  - 1/4 cup dried angelica root
- ***Instructions:***
  1. In a saucepan, combine water and sugar over medium heat, stirring until the sugar dissolves completely.
  2. Add dried angelica root to the saucepan and bring the mixture to a gentle simmer.
  3. Let the mixture simmer for 10-15 minutes, allowing the flavors of the angelica root to infuse into the syrup.
  4. Remove the saucepan from heat and let the syrup cool to room temperature.
  5. Strain the syrup through a fine mesh sieve or cheesecloth to remove the angelica root pieces.
  6. Transfer the infused syrup to a clean glass jar or bottle for storage.
  7. Use the angelica root syrup to sweeten cocktails, beverages, or drizzle over desserts for a unique flavor twist.

Herbal Tea

Angelica root can be used to prepare herbal tea. The tea is believed to have a calming effect and may be consumed for its potential digestive benefits.

Angelica Root Tea:

- ***Ingredients:***
  - 1 tablespoon dried angelica root
  - 1 cup hot water
  - Optional: honey or lemon for flavor
- ***Instructions:***
  1. Place dried angelica root in a teapot or heatproof mug.
  2. Pour hot water over the angelica root, covering it completely.
  3. Let the angelica root steep in hot water for 5-10 minutes, allowing the flavors to infuse into the tea.
  4. Strain the tea through a fine mesh sieve or tea strainer into another cup.
  5. Add honey or lemon to taste, if desired.

6. Enjoy the soothing and aromatic angelica root tea as a warm beverage, either on its own or as part of your herbal tea rotation.

These recipes highlight the versatility of angelica root and offer delightful ways to incorporate its unique flavor and potential health benefits into your culinary and wellness routines.

Aromatherapy:

The essential oil derived from angelica root is used in aromatherapy for its grounding and balancing properties. It is often included in blends designed to promote relaxation and stress relief.

Preparation:

- Dry angelica root by cutting it into small pieces and allowing it to air dry.
- Combine the dried root with other aromatic herbs or flowers.
- Place the mixture in sachets or use it as potpourri in different areas of your home.

Conclusion:

Angelica root stands as a testament to the rich interplay between nature and human well-being. With its potential digestive, anti-inflammatory, and calming properties, angelica root has found its way into traditional medicine and culinary traditions. Whether sipped as a herbal tea, incorporated into recipes, or enjoyed in aromatherapy blends, angelica root invites us to explore the diverse ways in which botanical wonders can enhance our lives. As with any herbal remedy, it's advisable to consult with a healthcare professional before incorporating angelica root into your wellness routine, especially if you have specific health concerns or are pregnant.

Back to Table of Contents

Apples

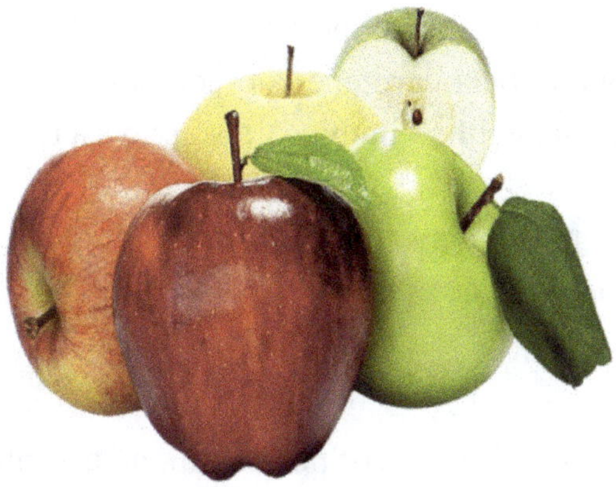

Exploring the Versatility and Health Benefits of Apples

Apples, with their crisp texture, sweet flavor, and vibrant colors, have long been celebrated as one of nature's most beloved fruits. Beyond their delicious taste, apples are packed with essential nutrients and offer a multitude of health benefits. From snacking to baking, apples are a versatile fruit that can be enjoyed in various forms, making them a staple in kitchens around the world. Let's delve into the many benefits and uses of apples:

Nutritional Powerhouse:

Apples are not only delicious but also incredibly nutritious, earning them a spot as a superfood in many dietary guidelines. Here are some key nutrients found in apples:

Fiber: Apples are an excellent source of dietary fiber, both soluble and insoluble. Fiber aids digestion, promotes satiety, and helps regulate blood sugar levels.

Vitamins: Apples contain various vitamins, including vitamin C, vitamin A, vitamin K, and some B vitamins like B6. These vitamins support immune function, vision, blood clotting, and overall wellbeing.

Antioxidants: Apples are rich in antioxidants, such as flavonoids and polyphenols, which help combat oxidative stress and reduce the risk of chronic diseases, including heart disease and cancer.

Minerals: While apples are not particularly high in minerals, they contain small amounts of potassium, calcium, and magnesium, which contribute to bone health and muscle function.

Vitamins:

Vitamin C: Ascorbic acid, or vitamin C, is abundant in apples. It acts as a powerful antioxidant, helping to protect cells from damage caused by free radicals. Vitamin C also supports immune function, collagen synthesis, and wound healing.

Vitamin A: Apples contain beta-carotene, a precursor to vitamin A, which is essential for vision, immune function, and skin health. Vitamin A also plays a role in maintaining healthy bones and teeth.

Vitamin K: Although present in small amounts, apples contain vitamin K, which is important for blood clotting and bone health.

Minerals:

Potassium: Apples are a good source of potassium, an essential mineral that helps regulate fluid balance, nerve transmission, and muscle function. Potassium also supports heart health by helping to maintain healthy blood pressure levels.

Calcium: While not as abundant as in dairy products, apples contain small amounts of calcium, which is crucial for bone and teeth health, muscle function, and nerve transmission.

Magnesium: Apples provide trace amounts of magnesium, which plays a role in over 300 biochemical reactions in the body, including energy production, muscle and nerve function, and protein synthesis.

Antioxidants:

Flavonoids: Apples are rich in various flavonoids, including quercetin, catechin, and epicatechin, which have potent antioxidant properties. Flavonoids help neutralize free radicals, reduce inflammation, and may lower the risk of chronic diseases such as heart disease and cancer.

Polyphenols: Polyphenols are another group of antioxidants found in apples, with compounds like chlorogenic acid and phloridzin being particularly abundant. Polyphenols help protect cells from oxidative damage, support heart health, and may have anti-inflammatory effects.

Phytochemicals: Apples contain other phytochemicals, such as procyanidins and triterpenoids, which contribute to their antioxidant and anti-inflammatory properties. These compounds may also play a role in promoting digestive health and reducing the risk of certain cancers.

Health Benefits:

Incorporating apples into your diet can offer numerous health benefits:

Heart Health: The soluble fiber in apples, particularly pectin, helps lower cholesterol levels and reduce the risk of heart disease. Additionally, the antioxidants in apples may protect against cardiovascular damage.

Weight Management: Apples are low in calories and high in fiber, making them a satisfying snack that can help control appetite and support weight loss or maintenance goals.

Digestive Health: The fiber content in apples promotes healthy digestion and regular bowel movements, preventing constipation and supporting gut health.

Blood Sugar Control: The fiber and polyphenols in apples help regulate blood sugar levels, making them a suitable fruit choice for individuals with diabetes or those aiming to manage blood sugar levels.

Cancer Prevention: Some studies suggest that the antioxidants in apples may have protective effects against certain types of cancer, including colorectal cancer.

Nutritional Content

The nutritional content of 1 cup (about 125 grams) of raw, sliced apples typically includes:

- Carbohydrates: Approximately 25 grams
- Protein: Approximately 0.5 grams
- Fiber: Approximately 4 grams
- Fat: Negligible (less than 0.5 grams)
- Sugar: Approximately 19 grams

Keep in mind that these values can vary slightly depending on the specific variety of apples and how it's prepared.

Versatile Culinary Uses:

Apples can be enjoyed in numerous culinary applications, adding flavor, texture, and nutritional value to dishes. Here are some popular uses of apples:

Snacking: Apples make for a convenient and portable snack that can be enjoyed on its own or paired with nut butter, cheese, or yogurt for added flavor and protein.

Baking: Apples are a versatile ingredient in baking, adding natural sweetness and moisture to cakes, muffins, pies, and crisps. They can also be dried or turned into applesauce for baking recipes.

Salads: Sliced or diced apples add a refreshing crunch and sweetness to salads, balancing out savory flavors and complementing ingredients like greens, nuts, and cheese.

Cooking: Apples can be cooked into savory dishes such as soups, stews, and sauces, where their natural sweetness can enhance the flavor profile of the dish.

Beverages: Apples are commonly juiced or blended into smoothies, providing a naturally sweet base and nutritional boost to drinks.

Here are two delicious recipes that incorporate apples:

Classic Homemade Apple Pie:

Ingredients:

- 6-8 medium-sized apples, peeled, cored, and thinly sliced (use your favorite variety, such as Granny Smith or Honeycrisp)
- 1/2 cup granulated sugar

- 1/4 cup packed brown sugar
- 2 tablespoons all-purpose flour
- 1 teaspoon ground cinnamon
- 1/4 teaspoon ground nutmeg
- 1/4 teaspoon salt
- 1 tablespoon lemon juice
- 1 package store-bought or homemade pie crust (for a double crust pie)
- 2 tablespoons unsalted butter, cut into small cubes
- 1 egg, beaten (for egg wash)
- Optional: Vanilla ice cream or whipped cream, for serving

Instructions:

1. Preheat your oven to 375°F (190°C).
2. In a large mixing bowl, combine the sliced apples, granulated sugar, brown sugar, flour, cinnamon, nutmeg, salt, and lemon juice. Toss until the apples are evenly coated with the mixture.
3. Roll out one pie crust and place it into a 9-inch pie dish. Trim any excess dough from the edges.
4. Spoon the apple mixture into the prepared pie crust, spreading it out evenly. Dot the top of the apples with cubed butter.
5. Roll out the second pie crust and place it over the filling. Trim any excess dough and crimp the edges to seal the pie.
6. Cut slits in the top crust to allow steam to escape during baking. Brush the crust with beaten egg wash for a golden finish.
7. Place the pie on a baking sheet to catch any drips and bake in the preheated oven for 45 to 55 minutes, or until the crust is golden brown and the filling is bubbling.
8. Remove the pie from the oven and let it cool on a wire rack for at least 30 minutes before slicing.
9. Serve warm or at room temperature with a scoop of vanilla ice cream or a dollop of whipped cream, if desired.

Apple Cinnamon Oatmeal Breakfast Bake:

Ingredients:

- 2 cups old-fashioned rolled oats
- 1/4 cup packed brown sugar
- 1 teaspoon ground cinnamon
- 1/2 teaspoon baking powder
- 1/4 teaspoon salt
- 2 cups milk (dairy or non-dairy)
- 1 large egg

- 2 tablespoons unsalted butter, melted
- 2 teaspoons vanilla extract
- 2 medium-sized apples, peeled, cored, and diced
- 1/2 cup chopped nuts (such as walnuts or pecans), optional

Instructions:

1. Preheat your oven to 375°F (190°C). Grease an 8x8-inch baking dish with butter or cooking spray.
2. In a large mixing bowl, combine the rolled oats, brown sugar, ground cinnamon, baking powder, and salt.
3. In another bowl, whisk together the milk, egg, melted butter, and vanilla extract until well combined.
4. Pour the wet ingredients into the dry ingredients and mix until evenly combined.
5. Gently fold in the diced apples and chopped nuts, if using.
6. Pour the oatmeal mixture into the prepared baking dish and spread it out evenly.
7. Bake in the preheated oven for 35 to 40 minutes, or until the top is golden brown and the oatmeal is set.
8. Remove from the oven and let it cool for a few minutes before serving.
9. Serve slices of the apple cinnamon oatmeal bake warm, optionally drizzled with maple syrup or topped with a dollop of yogurt.

These recipes highlight the delicious versatility of apples, whether enjoyed in a classic dessert like apple pie or incorporated into a wholesome breakfast bake. Enjoy these comforting and flavorful dishes any time of the year!

Historical Uses:

Apples have a rich history and have been utilized in various ways throughout the ages. Here are two historical uses of apples:

Symbolism and Mythology:

- Apples have played significant roles in mythology and symbolism across different cultures throughout history. In Greek mythology, apples were associated with the goddess of discord, Eris, who famously threw a golden apple marked "for the fairest" into a gathering of gods and goddesses, sparking the events that led to the Trojan War.
- In Norse mythology, apples were believed to grant immortality and were associated with the goddess Idunn, who guarded the golden apples of youth, which the gods ate to maintain their eternal youthfulness.
- In Christian tradition, the apple became associated with the biblical story of Adam and Eve in the Garden of Eden. While the Bible does not specifically mention apples, they have been traditionally depicted as the forbidden fruit from the Tree of Knowledge, leading to the expulsion of Adam and Eve from paradise.

Medicinal Uses:

- Apples have a long history of being used for medicinal purposes in various cultures around the world. In ancient Greece and Rome, apples were believed to have medicinal properties and were prescribed by physicians to treat a range of ailments, including digestive issues, fevers, and skin conditions.
- Traditional Chinese medicine also recognizes the therapeutic properties of apples. They are believed to have cooling and moistening effects on the body, making them useful for treating conditions such as dry coughs, thirst, and constipation. Apple peel is particularly valued in Chinese medicine for its fiber content and potential health benefits.
- In medieval Europe, apples were used in various remedies and tonics to promote health and well-being. They were believed to aid digestion, improve appetite, and cleanse the body of toxins. Additionally, apple cider vinegar was used topically as a disinfectant and internally as a tonic.

These historical uses of apples highlight their cultural significance and versatility beyond their culinary appeal. From mythological symbolism to medicinal applications, apples have left an indelible mark on human history and continue to be valued for their diverse range of uses.

Tips on Growing Apple

Growing an apple tree from seed to fruit-bearing maturity is a long process that typically takes several years. Here's a detailed breakdown of the stages and timeframes involved in growing an apple tree:

1. **Germination**: Apple seeds need to be stratified before germination, which involves exposing them to cold temperatures to simulate winter conditions. This process can take anywhere from 2 to 4 months.
2. **Seedling Stage**: After stratification, apple seeds will germinate and grow into seedlings. During this stage, the seedlings will develop their primary leaves and root systems. This stage usually lasts for about 1 to 2 years.
3. **Transplanting**: Once the apple seedlings have grown large enough and developed sturdy root systems, they can be transplanted into their permanent growing location, such as a garden or orchard. This typically occurs when the seedlings are around 1 to 2 years old.
4. **Juvenile Stage**: After transplanting, the apple trees enter a juvenile stage where they focus on vegetative growth rather than fruit production. This stage can last for several years, depending on factors such as the apple tree variety, growing conditions, and pruning practices. In general, apple trees reach maturity and start bearing fruit between 3 to 8 years after planting, with dwarf and semi-dwarf varieties typically bearing fruit earlier than standard-sized trees.
5. **Fruit Production**: Once apple trees reach maturity, they begin to produce flowers and fruit. The time it takes for an apple tree to produce its first significant crop can vary depending

on factors such as tree health, growing conditions, and weather conditions. In general, apple trees may start producing small yields of fruit as early as 3 to 4 years after planting, with full production typically achieved by 5 to 8 years.

6. **Mature Tree**: A mature apple tree can continue to produce fruit for many years, with some varieties remaining productive for several decades under optimal growing conditions. With proper care, pruning, and maintenance, apple trees can provide a reliable harvest of delicious fruit year after year.

Overall, growing an apple tree from seed to fruit-bearing maturity is a long-term commitment that requires patience, attention to detail, and proper care. While it may take several years for apple trees to reach full production, the reward of homegrown apples is well worth the wait.

Conclusion:

In summary, apples are not only delicious but also incredibly nutritious, offering a wide array of health benefits. From promoting heart health to supporting digestion and weight management, apples are a valuable addition to a healthy diet. Whether enjoyed fresh, baked, or incorporated into various recipes, the versatility of apples makes them a beloved fruit enjoyed by people of all ages. So next time you reach for a snack or plan a meal, consider adding apples to your menu for a tasty and nutritious boost to your day.

If you have specific health concerns, allergies, or conditions, it's advisable to consult with a healthcare professional or a registered dietitian before making significant changes to your diet.

Back to Table of Contents

Apple Cider Vinegar

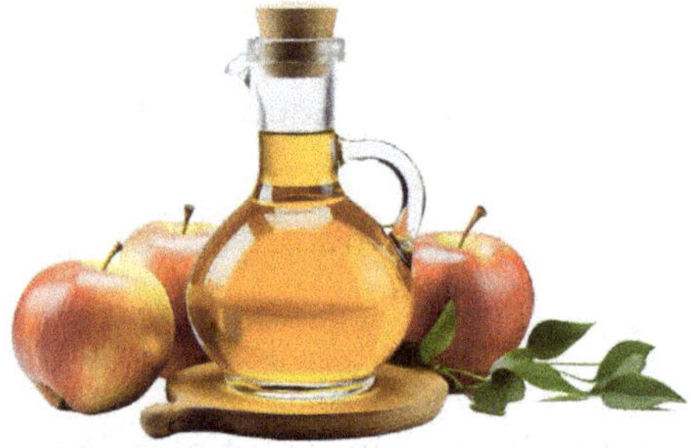

The Power of Apple Cider Vinegar

Apple cider vinegar (ACV) has long been celebrated as a versatile elixir, valued for its myriad health benefits and culinary applications. Derived from fermented apple juice, this amber-colored liquid has earned a reputation as a natural remedy for various ailments and a staple in countless households worldwide. Let's delve into the remarkable benefits and diverse uses of apple cider vinegar.

Nutritional Profile and Composition

At the heart of apple cider vinegar's potency lies its rich nutritional profile. While its exact composition can vary slightly depending on factors like fermentation time and apple variety, ACV typically contains acetic acid, vitamins, minerals, and beneficial plant compounds such as polyphenols.

Vitamins:

Vitamin C: Boosts immune function, promotes collagen production, and acts as an antioxidant to protect cells from damage caused by free radicals.

Vitamin A: Supports vision health, immune function, and skin integrity.

Vitamin E: Acts as an antioxidant, protecting cells from oxidative stress, and may support heart health and skin health.

Vitamin K: Essential for blood clotting and bone health.

Vitamin B1 (Thiamine): Supports energy metabolism, nervous system function, and may enhance mood and cognitive function.

Vitamin B2 (Riboflavin): Supports energy production, cellular function, and may help maintain healthy skin and eyes.

Vitamin B3 (Niacin): Supports energy metabolism, nervous system function, and may help lower cholesterol levels.

Vitamin B6: Supports brain health, immune function, and the production of neurotransmitters.

Vitamin B12 (in trace amounts): Important for red blood cell formation, nerve function, and DNA synthesis.

Minerals:

Potassium: Helps regulate blood pressure, fluid balance, and muscle function.

Calcium: Essential for bone and teeth health, muscle function, and nerve transmission.

Magnesium: Supports muscle and nerve function, energy production, and bone health.

Phosphorus: Important for bone and teeth health, energy metabolism, and cell structure.

Iron: Essential for oxygen transport, energy production, and immune function.

Sodium: Regulates fluid balance, nerve function, and muscle contractions.

Zinc: Supports immune function, wound healing, and DNA synthesis.

Manganese: Acts as an antioxidant, supports bone health, and plays a role in metabolism.

Antioxidants and Polyphenols:

Polyphenols (Flavonoids and Phenolic Acids): Possess antioxidant properties, protecting cells from oxidative damage and reducing inflammation.

Quercetin: Anti-inflammatory and antioxidant properties, may support heart health and immune function.

Catechins: Antioxidant compounds found in tea, may help protect against heart disease and cancer.

Epicatechin: Found in cocoa and tea, may support heart health and improve blood flow.

Chlorogenic Acid: Found in coffee and certain fruits, may help regulate blood sugar levels and support weight loss.

Gallic Acid: Antioxidant and anti-inflammatory properties, may have potential anticancer effects.

Caffeic Acid: Antioxidant and anti-inflammatory properties, may help protect against oxidative stress-related diseases.

These vitamins, minerals, and antioxidants found in apple cider vinegar contribute to its potential health benefits, including supporting digestion, regulating blood sugar levels, promoting heart health, strengthening the immune system, and providing antioxidant protection against oxidative stress and inflammation. However, it's important to consume ACV in moderation and as part of a balanced diet to maximize its potential benefits.

Health Benefits of Apple Cider Vinegar

Digestive Health: ACV is celebrated for its ability to support digestive function. The acetic acid in vinegar may aid in the breakdown of food, facilitating better nutrient absorption and reducing bloating and indigestion.

Blood Sugar Regulation: Research suggests that consuming apple cider vinegar may help regulate blood sugar levels, making it particularly beneficial for individuals with diabetes or those aiming to manage their insulin sensitivity.

Weight Management: Incorporating ACV into your diet may assist in weight management efforts. Some studies indicate that vinegar consumption can promote feelings of fullness and reduce calorie intake, potentially aiding in weight loss over time.

Heart Health: The polyphenols found in apple cider vinegar possess antioxidant properties that may help lower blood pressure and cholesterol levels, thereby supporting heart health and reducing the risk of cardiovascular disease.

Skin and Hair Care: Diluted ACV can serve as a natural toner for the skin, helping to balance pH levels, minimize acne, and clarify complexion. Additionally, rinsing hair with diluted vinegar can enhance shine, remove product buildup, and soothe scalp irritation.

Practical Uses of Apple Cider Vinegar

Culinary Delight:

From salad dressings and marinades to sauces and soups, apple cider vinegar adds a tangy flavor dimension to a wide array of dishes. It can also be used to pickle vegetables or create refreshing beverages like switchel or shrubs.

Here are two recipes that feature apple cider vinegar as a key ingredient:

Apple Cider Vinegar Salad Dressing:

Ingredients:

- 1/4 cup apple cider vinegar
- 1/2 cup extra virgin olive oil
- 1 tablespoon Dijon mustard
- 1 clove garlic, minced
- 1 teaspoon honey or maple syrup (optional)
- Salt and black pepper to taste

Instructions:

1. In a small bowl or jar, combine apple cider vinegar, olive oil, Dijon mustard, minced garlic, and honey or maple syrup (if using).
2. Whisk or shake vigorously until the ingredients are well combined and the dressing is emulsified.
3. Season with salt and black pepper to taste.
4. Serve immediately over your favorite salad greens or store in a sealed container in the refrigerator for up to one week.

Honey Garlic Apple Cider Vinegar Chicken:

Ingredients:

- 4 boneless, skinless chicken breasts
- 1/4 cup apple cider vinegar
- 2 tablespoons honey
- 2 tablespoons soy sauce (or tamari for gluten-free option)
- 3 cloves garlic, minced
- 1 teaspoon grated ginger
- 1 tablespoon olive oil
- Salt and black pepper to taste
- Fresh parsley or green onions for garnish (optional)

Instructions:

1. In a small bowl, whisk together apple cider vinegar, honey, soy sauce, minced garlic, and grated ginger to make the marinade.
2. Place the chicken breasts in a shallow dish or resealable plastic bag and pour the marinade over them. Ensure the chicken is evenly coated. Marinate in the refrigerator for at least 30 minutes, or up to 4 hours for maximum flavor.
3. Heat olive oil in a large skillet over medium-high heat. Remove the chicken from the marinade, shaking off any excess, and season with salt and black pepper.
4. Add the chicken to the skillet and cook for 6-8 minutes per side, or until golden brown and cooked through. The internal temperature should reach 165°F (75°C).
5. Once cooked, transfer the chicken to a serving platter and tent with foil to keep warm.
6. Pour the remaining marinade into the skillet and bring to a simmer. Cook for 3-4 minutes, or until slightly thickened.
7. Pour the sauce over the chicken and garnish with fresh parsley or green onions, if desired. Serve hot with your favorite side dishes, such as steamed vegetables or rice.

These recipes showcase the versatility of apple cider vinegar, whether used in a tangy salad dressing or as a flavorful marinade for chicken. Enjoy experimenting with these delicious and nutritious dishes in your kitchen!

Household Cleaner: Harness the cleaning power of apple cider vinegar to tackle household chores. Diluted vinegar makes an effective, eco-friendly cleaner for countertops, glass surfaces, and floors, cutting through grease and grime with ease.

Natural Deodorizer: Banish unpleasant odors from your home by placing bowls of diluted ACV in areas prone to lingering smells, such as the kitchen or bathroom. Its acidic properties help neutralize odors without relying on synthetic fragrances.

Preservative: Extend the shelf life of fruits and vegetables by soaking them in a solution of water and apple cider vinegar. This simple preservation method can help inhibit microbial growth and maintain freshness.

Natural Remedies: Beyond its culinary and cleaning applications, apple cider vinegar can be used topically to soothe insect bites, alleviate sunburn, or as a foot soak to combat foot odor and fungal infections.

Precautions and Considerations

While apple cider vinegar offers numerous benefits, it's essential to use it responsibly and in moderation. Consuming undiluted vinegar can be harsh on tooth enamel and the delicate tissues of the digestive tract. Always dilute vinegar before ingestion and consult with a healthcare professional, especially if you have underlying health conditions, allergies or are taking medications.

In conclusion, apple cider vinegar stands as a testament to the age-old adage that "food is medicine." Its versatility, coupled with a plethora of health-enhancing properties, renders it a valuable addition to any wellness arsenal. Whether utilized in the kitchen, bathroom, or beyond, ACV continues to captivate enthusiasts worldwide, offering a potent blend of tradition, science, and natural goodness.

Back to Table of Contents

Apricots

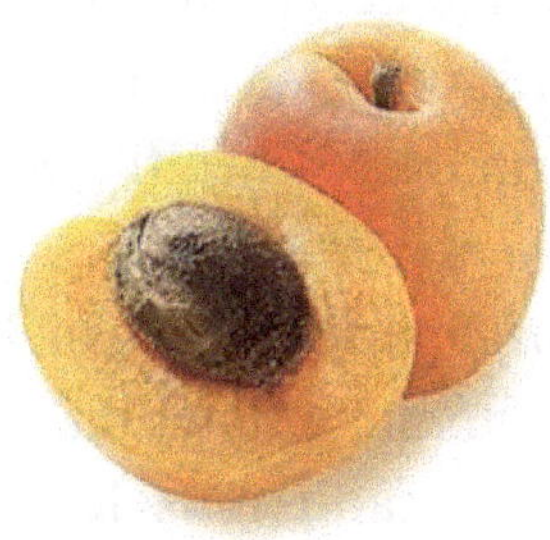

The Golden Goodness of Apricots: Benefits and Uses

Apricots, scientifically known as Prunus armeniaca, are the small, golden fruits that come from the apricot tree, a member of the Rosaceae family. Originating from Central Asia, apricots have traveled across the globe and are now enjoyed for their sweet, juicy flesh and numerous health benefits. Beyond their delightful taste, apricots are packed with essential nutrients, making them a valuable addition to a wholesome diet. In this article, we explore the benefits and versatile uses of this golden-hued fruit.

Nutritional Profile:

Apricots are nutrient-dense fruits, providing an array of vitamins, minerals, and antioxidants in a small package. Here's a glimpse of the nutritional profile of apricots:

Vitamins:

Vitamin A (as beta-carotene): Essential for vision health, immune function, and skin health. Beta-carotene, a precursor to vitamin A, acts as an antioxidant, helping to protect cells from damage.

Vitamin C: Important for immune function, collagen production (for healthy skin), and as an antioxidant, helping to protect cells from oxidative stress. It also aids in the absorption of iron.

Vitamin E (alpha-tocopherol): Acts as an antioxidant, protecting cells from oxidative damage. It also plays a role in immune function and skin health.

Vitamin K: Necessary for blood clotting and bone health. It helps regulate calcium levels in the body and may also have anti-inflammatory properties.

Minerals:

Potassium: Important for maintaining fluid balance, nerve transmission, muscle contraction, and blood pressure regulation. It supports heart health and helps prevent muscle cramps.

Copper: Essential for the formation of red blood cells, connective tissue, and the functioning of the nervous system. It also acts as an antioxidant and may help with iron absorption.

Manganese: Involved in bone formation, blood sugar regulation, and the metabolism of carbohydrates, amino acids, and cholesterol.

Magnesium: Necessary for muscle and nerve function, blood sugar regulation, blood pressure control, and the synthesis of proteins, bone, and DNA.

Phosphorus: Important for bone and teeth health, energy metabolism, and cell membrane structure.

Iron: Essential for the formation of hemoglobin, which carries oxygen in the blood. It's also involved in energy metabolism and immune function.

Calcium: Crucial for bone and teeth health, muscle function, nerve transmission, and blood clotting.

Zinc: Involved in immune function, wound healing, DNA synthesis, and cell division. It also acts as an antioxidant and may support reproductive health.

Antioxidants:

Beta-carotene: Converted to vitamin A in the body, beta-carotene acts as an antioxidant, protecting cells from damage caused by free radicals. It may help reduce the risk of certain chronic diseases, including heart disease and cancer.

Lutein and Zeaxanthin: Carotenoids that accumulate in the retina and may help protect against age-related macular degeneration (AMD) and cataracts.

Cryptoxanthin: Another carotenoid with antioxidant properties that may help reduce the risk of inflammatory conditions and certain cancers.

Lycopene: A carotenoid with antioxidant properties that may help reduce the risk of certain cancers, particularly prostate cancer.

Anthocyanins: Plant pigments responsible for the red, purple, and blue colors of certain fruits and vegetables. They have antioxidant properties and may help reduce inflammation, improve heart health, and protect against age-related decline in brain function.

Flavonoids (such as quercetin and kaempferol): Plant compounds with antioxidant and anti-inflammatory properties that may help reduce the risk of chronic diseases, including heart disease and certain cancers.

These nutrients work together to support overall health, including immune function, heart health, eye health, skin health, and bone health, while also providing protection against oxidative stress and inflammation. Incorporating apricots into your diet can be a delicious way to reap these benefits.

Health Benefits:

Eye Health:

Apricots are rich in beta-carotene and lutein, antioxidants known for promoting eye health and reducing the risk of age-related macular degeneration.

Heart Health:

The potassium content in apricots supports heart health by helping regulate blood pressure and reducing the risk of cardiovascular diseases.

Digestive Health:

Apricots are a good source of dietary fiber, which aids digestion, prevents constipation, and promotes a healthy gut.

Skin Health:

The combination of vitamin A and vitamin C in apricots contributes to healthy skin by promoting collagen production and protecting against oxidative damage.

Immune Support:

The high vitamin C content in apricots boosts the immune system, helping the body fend off infections and illnesses.

Nutritional Content

In 1 cup (about 155 grams) of sliced apricots, you can expect to find approximately:

- Carbohydrates: Around 17 grams
- Protein: Approximately 1.5 grams
- Fiber: Roughly 3 grams
- Fat: About 0.5 grams

Please note that these values are approximate and can vary slightly based on factors such as the variety of apricots and their ripeness.

Culinary Uses:

Fresh Snacking: Enjoy apricots fresh as a convenient and delicious snack. Their sweet and juicy flesh makes them a satisfying and healthy treat on their own.

Dried Apricots: Dried apricots are a convenient and portable snack. They can also be added to trail mixes, cereals, or used in baking for a natural sweetness.

Apricot Jams and Preserves: Apricots can be transformed into flavorful jams and preserves, which can be spread on toast, used as a topping for desserts, or incorporated into savory dishes.

Baking and Desserts: Apricots add a sweet and tangy flavor to various baked goods, including pies, tarts, muffins, and cakes.

Savory Dishes: Apricots can be used in savory dishes, especially in Middle Eastern and Mediterranean cuisines. They pair well with meats, salads, and couscous, providing a unique sweetness to the savory profile.

Here are two delicious recipes that showcase the sweet and versatile nature of apricots:

Apricot and Almond Granola Bars

Ingredients:

- 1 cup dried apricots, chopped
- 1 cup rolled oats
- 1/2 cup almonds, chopped
- 1/4 cup honey or maple syrup
- 1/4 cup almond butter
- 1/4 cup coconut oil, melted
- 1/2 teaspoon vanilla extract
- 1/4 teaspoon salt

Instructions:

1. Preheat the oven to 350°F (175°C) and line a baking dish with parchment paper.
2. In a food processor, combine dried apricots, rolled oats, and chopped almonds. Pulse until well combined but still slightly chunky.
3. In a small saucepan over low heat, combine honey or maple syrup, almond butter, melted coconut oil, vanilla extract, and salt. Stir until well combined and smooth.
4. Pour the wet mixture over the apricot-oat-almond mixture in the food processor. Pulse until everything is evenly mixed.
5. Press the mixture firmly into the prepared baking dish.
6. Bake in the preheated oven for 15-20 minutes or until the edges are golden brown.
7. Allow the bars to cool completely before cutting into squares or bars.

Grilled Apricot and Chicken Skewers

Ingredients:

- 1 pound boneless, skinless chicken breasts, cut into chunks
- 1 cup fresh apricots, halved and pitted
- 1/4 cup olive oil
- 2 tablespoons balsamic vinegar
- 2 tablespoons honey
- 1 teaspoon Dijon mustard
- Salt and pepper to taste
- Wooden skewers, soaked in water for 30 minutes

Instructions:

1. In a bowl, whisk together olive oil, balsamic vinegar, honey, Dijon mustard, salt, and pepper to create the marinade.
2. Place the chicken chunks in a resealable plastic bag and pour half of the marinade over them. Seal the bag and refrigerate for at least 30 minutes.
3. Preheat the grill to medium-high heat.
4. Thread marinated chicken chunks and apricot halves alternately onto the soaked wooden skewers.

5. Grill the skewers for about 8-10 minutes, turning occasionally, until the chicken is cooked through and the apricots are lightly caramelized.
6. Brush the skewers with the remaining marinade during the last few minutes of grilling.
7. Serve the grilled apricot and chicken skewers hot, garnished with fresh herbs if desired.

These recipes highlight the sweetness and versatility of apricots, whether used in a wholesome granola bar or paired with savory grilled chicken. Enjoy these apricot-infused dishes as a delightful addition to your meals!

Tips on Growing Apricots

🌱 1. Selecting & Preparing the Seed

1. Choose fresh apricot pits: Take pits from fully ripe, healthy, organic apricots (store-bought ones may be treated not to sprout).
2. Clean the pit: Remove any fruit flesh and let it dry for a day.
3. Crack or stratify:

   - Some growers carefully crack the shell to remove the seed inside (riskier but faster).
   - Or, stratify (mimic winter dormancy): place the whole pit in moist sand or peat moss inside a plastic bag, and refrigerate for 6–8 weeks.

2. Germinating the Seed

- After stratification, check for sprouting.
- Plant the sprouted seed in a small pot:
  - Depth: About 2 inches deep.
  - Soil: Well-drained, loamy soil with compost.
  - Location: Bright spot with indirect sun.
- Water gently—keep soil moist but not soggy.

3. Transplanting Outdoors

- **Best time:** After the last frost in spring, when seedlings are 6–8 inches tall.
- **Site selection:**

    - Full sun (at least 6–8 hours daily).
    - Well-drained soil (apricots dislike waterlogged roots).
    - Space trees about 15–20 feet apart.

- **Planting hole:** Dig a hole twice as wide and the same depth as the root ball. Mix compost into the backfill soil.
- Water deeply after planting.

4. Growing & Care

Watering

- Young trees: Water weekly during dry spells.
- Mature trees: Deep water every 10–14 days in dry weather.

Fertilizing

- In early spring, apply balanced fertilizer (10-10-10) or compost.
- Avoid excessive nitrogen (leads to leafy growth but fewer fruits).

Pruning

- Prune in late winter/early spring to shape the tree and remove crossing or diseased branches.
- Apricots bear fruit on short spurs on 2–3 year old wood, so avoid heavy pruning of those areas.

Pest/Disease Management

- Common pests: Aphids, borers, mites.
- Diseases: Brown rot, bacterial canker.
- Use neem oil or insecticidal soap for pests. Good air circulation prevents fungal issues.

5. Flowering & Pollination

- Apricots bloom early in spring.

- Many varieties are self-pollinating, but having a second tree nearby increases yield.
- Protect blossoms from late frost with row covers if needed.

6. Harvesting (Reaping)

- Apricots usually begin fruiting in 3–5 years from seed (sometimes longer).
- Fruits ripen in early to mid-summer depending on the variety and location.
- Signs of ripeness:
    - Fruits turn golden-orange with a reddish blush.
    - Slightly soft to touch and come off easily when twisted.
    - Sweet, fruity aroma.
- Harvest gently to avoid bruising.

7. Storage & Use

- Fresh apricots last 3–5 days at room temperature or up to a week in the fridge.
- Can be dried, canned, or made into jams for long-term use.

Quick Timeline Recap

- Year 0: Stratify and sprout seed.
- Year 1: Seedling growth, transplant outdoors.
- Year 2–3: Tree develops structure, prune and maintain.
- Year 3–5: First fruits appear.
- Year 5+: Regular harvests each summer.

Conclusion:

Incorporating apricots into your diet not only satisfies your taste buds with their natural sweetness but also provides a plethora of health benefits. Additionally, individuals with known allergies or sensitivities should exercise caution and seek guidance from a medical professional.

Whether enjoyed fresh, dried, or incorporated into a variety of culinary creations, apricots stand out as a versatile and nutrient-rich fruit. Make room for the golden goodness of apricots in your daily meals and savor the delightful combination of flavor and nutrition that this fruit brings to the table.

Back to Table of Contents

Arugula

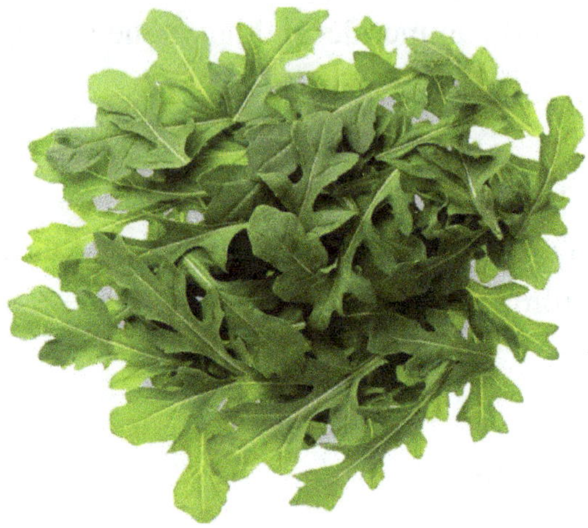

Nutrient-Rich Elegance: The Benefits and Uses of Arugula

Arugula, scientifically known as Eruca sativa, is a leafy green vegetable that has gained popularity for its distinctive peppery flavor and nutritional richness. Often featured in salads, sandwiches, and various culinary creations, arugula offers a delightful combination of taste and health benefits. Let's delve into the diverse advantages and creative uses of this vibrant green.

Nutritional Profile

Arugula is a nutritional powerhouse, packed with essential vitamins, minerals, and phytochemicals. Here's a glimpse of its impressive nutritional profile:

Vitamins:

Vitamin A: Supports healthy vision, immune function, and skin health.
Vitamin C: Acts as an antioxidant, boosts immune function, supports collagen production, and aids in wound healing.
Vitamin K: Essential for blood clotting, bone health, and may help prevent osteoporosis.
Folate (Vitamin B9): Important for DNA synthesis, cell division, and may help prevent neural tube defects during pregnancy.
Vitamin E: Acts as an antioxidant, protects cells from damage, and supports immune function.

Minerals:

Calcium: Essential for bone and teeth health, muscle function, and nerve signaling.
Potassium: Helps maintain fluid balance, supports heart health, and regulates blood pressure.
Magnesium: Important for muscle function, nerve function, bone health, and energy production.
Iron: Essential for the production of red blood cells and oxygen transport in the body.
Phosphorus: Important for bone and teeth health, energy metabolism, and cell signaling.

Antioxidants:

Beta-carotene: Converted to vitamin A in the body, acts as an antioxidant, and may help protect against certain chronic diseases.
Lutein and zeaxanthin: Carotenoids that support eye health and may help reduce the risk of age-related macular degeneration.
Quercetin: A flavonoid with antioxidant and anti-inflammatory properties, may help reduce inflammation and lower the risk of chronic diseases.
Kaempferol: Another flavonoid with antioxidant and anti-inflammatory properties, may help protect against heart disease and certain cancers.

Benefits of consuming arugula include:

- Supporting overall immune function and reducing inflammation due to its high antioxidant content.
- Promoting bone health and reducing the risk of osteoporosis due to its vitamin K and calcium content.
- Supporting heart health and regulating blood pressure due to its potassium content.
- Providing essential nutrients for energy production and overall vitality.

Health Benefits:

Incorporating arugula into your diet can offer a range of health benefits:

Heart Health: The combination of potassium and antioxidants in arugula contributes to heart health by supporting blood pressure regulation and reducing oxidative stress.

Bone Health: The high vitamin K and calcium content in arugula are essential for bone health, promoting bone density and reducing the risk of fractures.

Cancer Prevention: The presence of phytochemicals like glucosinolates in arugula has been associated with potential cancer-preventive effects, particularly against certain types of cancers.

Weight Management: Arugula is low in calories and high in fiber, making it a great addition to a weight-conscious diet. The fiber promotes satiety, aiding in weight management.

Ancient Medicinal Herb:

- **Historical Use:** Arugula has a history as a medicinal herb dating back to ancient times. It was valued for its believed medicinal properties and was used to treat various ailments.
- **Benefits:** The peppery leaves of arugula were thought to have digestive benefits, aiding in the alleviation of indigestion and promoting overall digestive health. Additionally, the presence of certain compounds may have contributed to its use in traditional medicine for various health concerns.

Roman Culinary Delight:

- **Historical Use:** Arugula was a popular ingredient in Roman cuisine, where it was consumed both for its flavor and potential health benefits.
- **Benefits:** Romans appreciated arugula not only for its distinct peppery taste but also for its potential digestive benefits. The inclusion of arugula in meals might have contributed to improved digestion and overall well-being.

Middle Ages Culinary Herb:

- **Historical Use:** During the Middle Ages, arugula was cultivated in monastic gardens and featured prominently in culinary preparations across Europe.
- **Benefits:** Arugula's consumption during this period likely provided essential vitamins and minerals, contributing to improved nutrition. Its aromatic and flavorful nature made it a valuable addition to the limited culinary options of the time.

Traditional Mediterranean Remedy:

- **Historical Use:** In various Mediterranean cultures, arugula was historically considered more than just a culinary herb. It found its place in traditional remedies and tonics.
- **Benefits:** Arugula's potential detoxifying properties and the presence of antioxidants might have contributed to its use in traditional remedies aimed at promoting overall health. It was believed to have cleansing effects on the body, supporting liver function and general well-being.

These historical uses of arugula highlight its multifaceted role in ancient cultures, ranging from a medicinal herb to a culinary delight. The perceived benefits of arugula, whether related to digestion, nutrition, or overall health, have contributed to its enduring presence in diverse historical contexts.

Nutritional Content

In 1 cup (about 20 grams) of raw arugula, you can expect to find approximately:

- Carbohydrates: Around 0.7 grams
- Protein: Approximately 0.3 grams
- Fiber: Roughly 0.3 grams
- Fat: About 0.2 grams

Arugula is a low-calorie leafy green vegetable that is often used in salads and as a garnish due to its peppery flavor and crisp texture. It is rich in vitamins A, C, and K, as well as folate, calcium, and potassium.

Culinary Uses:

Arugula's distinctive peppery taste adds a flavorful kick to various dishes. Here are some creative ways to enjoy the versatility of arugula in the kitchen:

Salads: Arugula is a classic addition to salads, complementing other greens and ingredients with its unique flavor. Pair it with fruits, nuts, and cheese for a delightful salad experience.

Pesto: Create a flavorful arugula pesto by blending arugula with nuts, Parmesan cheese, garlic, and olive oil. Use it as a sauce for pasta, sandwiches, or as a dip.

Pizza Topping: Add a handful of fresh arugula to your pizza after baking for a burst of freshness and a peppery contrast to the savory flavors.

Sandwiches and Wraps: Include arugula in sandwiches and wraps for a crunchy texture and a zesty flavor that elevates the overall taste.

Here are two delicious recipes that incorporate arugula:

Arugula and Pear Salad with Goat Cheese and Walnuts:

Ingredients:

- 4 cups arugula
- 2 ripe pears, thinly sliced
- 1/2 cup crumbled goat cheese
- 1/4 cup chopped walnuts
- 2 tablespoons extra virgin olive oil
- 1 tablespoon balsamic vinegar
- Salt and pepper to taste

Instructions:

1. In a large salad bowl, combine the arugula, sliced pears, crumbled goat cheese, and chopped walnuts.
2. In a small bowl, whisk together the extra virgin olive oil and balsamic vinegar to make the dressing. Season with salt and pepper to taste.
3. Drizzle the dressing over the salad and toss gently to coat all the ingredients evenly.
4. Serve immediately as a refreshing and nutritious salad.

Arugula and Prosciutto Pizza:

Ingredients:

- 1 pre-made pizza dough (or homemade if preferred)
- 1/2 cup pizza sauce

- 2 cups shredded mozzarella cheese
- 2 cups arugula
- 4 slices prosciutto
- 1 tablespoon olive oil
- Salt and pepper to taste
- Optional: grated Parmesan cheese for topping

Instructions:

1. Preheat your oven according to the instructions for the pizza dough.
2. Roll out the pizza dough on a floured surface to your desired thickness.
3. Spread the pizza sauce evenly over the dough, leaving a small border around the edges.
4. Sprinkle the shredded mozzarella cheese over the sauce.
5. Tear the prosciutto slices into smaller pieces and distribute them evenly over the cheese.
6. Bake the pizza in the preheated oven according to the dough instructions, until the crust is golden and the cheese is melted and bubbly.
7. While the pizza is baking, toss the arugula with olive oil, salt, and pepper in a bowl to lightly coat.
8. Once the pizza is done, remove it from the oven and top it with the dressed arugula.
9. Optionally, sprinkle some grated Parmesan cheese over the top for extra flavor.
10. Slice the pizza and serve hot, enjoying the combination of savory prosciutto, melted cheese, and fresh arugula.

These recipes showcase the versatility of arugula and how it can be used in both salads and cooked dishes to add a peppery flavor and nutritional boost to your meals. Enjoy!

Conclusion: Arugula's combination of bold flavor and nutritional benefits makes it a versatile and valuable addition to a well-balanced diet. Whether you're aiming to enhance your health or elevate your culinary creations, arugula stands out as a leafy green that brings both elegance and nourishment to the table. Embrace the peppery goodness of arugula and explore countless ways to enjoy its benefits in your meals.

If you have specific health concerns, allergies, or conditions, it's advisable to consult with a healthcare professional or a registered dietitian before making significant changes to your diet.

Back to Table of Contents

Asafoetida

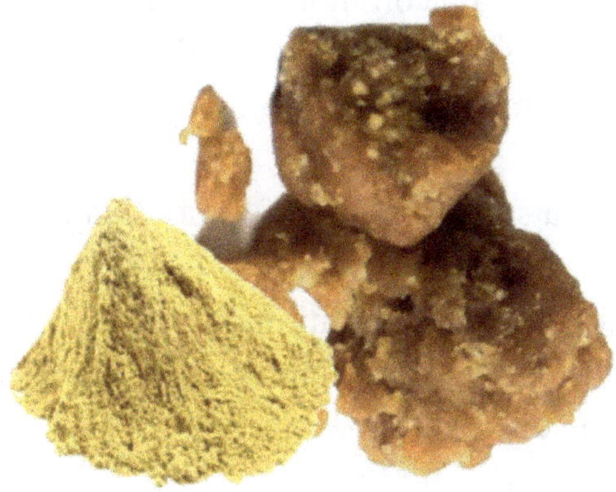

Benefits and Versatile Uses of the Resinous Wonder

Asafoetida, derived from the Ferula assa-foetida plant, is a unique and pungent resin that has been a staple in culinary and traditional medicine for centuries. Often referred to as the "Devil's Dung" due to its strong aroma, Asafoetida is prized for its distinct flavor profile and a myriad of health benefits. This article delves into the rich history and the diverse applications of the Asafoetida plant.

Culinary Delight:

One of the primary uses of Asafoetida is as a culinary spice, especially in Indian cuisine. Despite its initially strong and pungent smell, when added to dishes, Asafoetida imparts a savory and umami flavor. It is commonly used in vegetarian and lentil-based dishes to enhance the overall taste. Asafoetida is a key component of many spice blends, adding depth and complexity to the flavor profile.

Asafoetida is typically used as a spice in cooking, and it is not usually consumed directly. However, there are ways to incorporate asafoetida into dishes to enjoy its unique flavor. Here are four ways in which asafoetida can be prepared for consumption:

Tempering (Tadka):

- ***Process:*** In Indian cuisine, tempering is a common method for using asafoetida. Heat oil or ghee in a pan, add mustard seeds, cumin seeds, and a pinch of asafoetida. Allow the spices to sizzle in the hot oil before adding them to cooked dishes.
- ***Usage:*** Tempering enhances the flavor of dals, curries, and rice dishes. The aromatic asafoetida complements other spices, creating a well-balanced and flavorful meal.

Sprinkling on Cooked Dishes:

- ***Process**:* After a dish is cooked, sprinkle a small amount of powdered asafoetida directly over the food.
- ***Usage:*** This method is common in lentil-based dishes, rice, and vegetable preparations. It allows for a more controlled distribution of the asafoetida flavor and adds a finishing touch to the meal.

Asafoetida Water:

- ***Process:*** Dissolve a small amount of asafoetida powder in warm water to create a solution.
- ***Usage:*** Asafoetida water is traditionally used in Indian cuisine to sprinkle over cooked lentils, beans, and vegetables. It imparts the flavor evenly and adds a distinct taste to the dish.

Asafoetida Paste:

- ***Process:*** Mix asafoetida powder with a small amount of water to form a thick paste.
- ***Usage:*** Asafoetida paste is convenient for adding the spice to dishes where an even distribution is desired. It can be stirred into gravies, sauces, or marinades for a consistent flavor profile.

It's important to note that asafoetida is potent, and only a small amount is needed to add its characteristic flavor to dishes. Additionally, the spice is usually cooked with other ingredients rather than being consumed on its own. Experimenting with these preparation methods will allow you to enjoy the unique taste of asafoetida in a variety of culinary creations.

Digestive Aid:

Asafoetida has long been recognized for its digestive properties. It contains compounds that help alleviate digestive issues, including bloating and gas. Traditionally, it has been used to aid in the digestion of heavy or hard-to-digest foods, making it a popular choice in many traditional remedies for indigestion.

Volatile Oils:

- *Contribution:* Asafoetida contains volatile oils, including compounds such as umbelliferone and ferulic acid. These oils contribute to the spice's distinct aroma and are believed to have digestive properties.
- *Digestive Benefits:* Volatile oils in asafoetida are thought to stimulate the production of digestive enzymes, facilitating the breakdown of food in the digestive tract. This can help alleviate issues such as bloating and indigestion.

Coumarins:

- *Contribution:* Coumarins are a class of compounds found in asafoetida.
- *Digestive Benefits:* Coumarins have been studied for their potential to have anti-flatulent properties, reducing the formation of gas in the digestive system. As a result, asafoetida may help relieve gas-related discomfort and bloating.

Resin Compounds (Gum Resin):

- *Contribution:* Asafoetida contains resin compounds, which are extracted from the sap of the plant's roots.
- *Digestive Benefits:* The resin compounds in asafoetida are believed to possess anti-inflammatory properties. In the context of digestive health, these properties may contribute to soothing inflammation in the digestive tract, potentially providing relief from conditions like irritable bowel syndrome (IBS).

Respiratory Health:

In traditional medicine, Asafoetida has been used to address respiratory issues. It is believed to have expectorant properties, making it beneficial for individuals dealing with respiratory congestion, asthma, or bronchitis. Asafoetida is often used in combination with other herbs to create remedies for respiratory health.

Bronchodilator Effects:

- *Contribution:* Asafoetida is believed to have bronchodilator effects, which can help widen the airways in the respiratory system.
- *Expectorant Benefits:* Conditions like asthma involve constriction of the airways, making breathing challenging. The bronchodilator effects of asafoetida may aid in relaxing and widening the air passages, potentially easing respiratory symptoms and promoting the expulsion of mucus.

Anti-inflammatory and Antimicrobial:

Asafoetida contains compounds with anti-inflammatory and antimicrobial properties. This makes it a valuable ingredient in traditional medicine for addressing various health concerns. It is believed to have the potential to reduce inflammation and fight against certain types of infections.

Anti-Inflammatory Compounds:

- *Contribution:* Asafoetida contains compounds with anti-inflammatory properties, including volatile oils and resin compounds.
- *Expectorant Benefits:* In respiratory conditions such as asthma and bronchitis, inflammation of the airways can lead to difficulty in breathing and the production of excess mucus. The anti-inflammatory properties of asafoetida may help soothe inflammation in the respiratory tract, making it easier to expel mucus and facilitating clearer airways.

Blood Pressure Regulation:

Some studies suggest that Asafoetida may play a role in helping regulate blood pressure. The compounds present in Asafoetida are thought to have vasodilatory effects, which could contribute to maintaining healthy blood pressure levels. However, further research is needed to fully understand and validate these potential benefits.

Ferulic Acid:

- *Contribution:* Asafoetida contains ferulic acid, a phenolic compound with antioxidant properties.
- *Potential Benefits:* Ferulic acid has been studied for its potential to have a positive impact on cardiovascular health. Antioxidants may help protect blood vessels from damage and contribute to overall heart health.

Coumarins:

- *Contribution:* Asafoetida contains coumarins, which are aromatic compounds with diverse biological activities.
- *Potential Benefits:* Coumarins have been studied for their potential vasodilatory effects, which means they may help dilate blood vessels. Vasodilation can contribute to improved blood flow and, in turn, may have implications for blood pressure regulation.

Sulfur Compounds:

- *Contribution:* Asafoetida contains sulfur compounds, including allyl disulfide and others.
- *Potential Benefits:* Some sulfur compounds found in foods have been associated with cardiovascular benefits, including potential effects on blood pressure. However, more research is needed to understand the specific mechanisms and impact of these compounds.

External Applications:

Beyond internal uses, Asafoetida has been used externally in certain traditional practices. It is believed to have antispasmodic properties, and poultices or pastes containing Asafoetida have been applied to alleviate muscle spasms and joint pain.

In conclusion, the Asafoetida plant stands as a testament to the diverse benefits and applications found in nature. From its role in spicing up culinary creations to its contributions to traditional medicine, Asafoetida continues to be a versatile and valued resource. As we explore the depths of its flavor and harness its potential for health and well-being. Individuals with respiratory conditions or allergic should consult healthcare professionals for guidance on appropriate management and treatment options. The Asafoetida plant remains a fascinating and integral part of cultural and culinary traditions around the world.

Back to Table of Contents

Ashwagandha

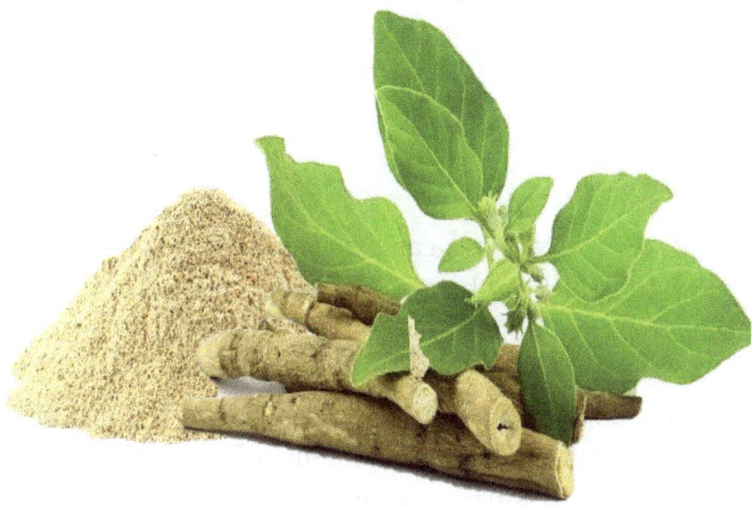

Unveiling the Wonders of the Ayurvedic Adaptogen

Ashwagandha, scientifically known as Withania somnifera, is a revered herb in Ayurvedic medicine that has gained widespread popularity for its myriad health benefits. Often referred to as an adaptogen, ashwagandha is known for its ability to help the body adapt to stress and promote overall well-being. In this article, we will delve into the benefits and diverse uses of ashwagandha, exploring its rich history and contemporary applications.

Ancient Roots and Traditional Uses:

Ashwagandha has deep roots in Ayurveda, the ancient system of medicine that originated in India. The Sanskrit name "Ashwagandha" translates to "smell of horse," suggesting that the herb imparts the strength and vigor of a horse. Traditionally, ashwagandha has been used to address a variety of health concerns, including stress, anxiety, fatigue, and immune support.

Benefits of Ashwagandha:

Adaptogenic Properties:

- Ashwagandha is classified as an adaptogen, a group of herbs that help the body adapt to stressors. It is believed to modulate the body's stress response by balancing cortisol levels, promoting a sense of calm, and improving resilience to stress.

Cognitive Function and Mental Health:

- Research suggests that ashwagandha may have neuroprotective effects and could support cognitive function. It has been explored for its potential to enhance memory, improve concentration, and alleviate symptoms of anxiety and depression.

Energy and Vitality:

- Ashwagandha is traditionally associated with promoting energy and vitality. It is believed to nourish and strengthen the nervous and immune systems, providing a holistic approach to overall well-being.

Immune Support:

- The immune-modulating properties of ashwagandha make it a valuable ally for immune support. It is thought to enhance the activity of immune cells, offering a natural defense against infections and illnesses.

Anti-Inflammatory Effects:

- Ashwagandha contains compounds with anti-inflammatory properties, making it a potential remedy for conditions involving inflammation. This includes inflammatory joint disorders and other inflammatory conditions.

Diverse Uses of Ashwagandha:

Supplements and Extracts:

- Ashwagandha supplements, available in various forms such as capsules, powders, and tinctures, are commonly used to ensure consistent and convenient intake of the herb's benefits.

Ayurvedic Formulations:

- In traditional Ayurvedic medicine, ashwagandha is often included in formulations known as "rasayanas" or rejuvenating tonics. These formulations aim to promote vitality, longevity, and overall health.

Stress Management:

- Ashwagandha is frequently used as a natural remedy for stress management. Whether in the form of teas, supplements, or tonics, it is sought after for its calming effects on the nervous system.

Topical Applications:

- Ashwagandha oil is used topically in Ayurveda for massages. It is believed to nourish the skin, relax muscles, and contribute to overall well-being.

Ashwagandha can be prepared in various ways to harness its benefits. Here are a few common methods of preparing Ashwagandha:

Ashwagandha Tea:

Preparation:

- Steep dried Ashwagandha root or powder in hot water.
- Allow it to steep for about 10-15 minutes.
- Strain the tea and sweeten with honey or your preferred sweetener if desired.

- **Uses:**
  - Consumed as a calming tea to promote relaxation and manage stress. Ashwagandha tea is often favored for its earthy flavor.

Ashwagandha Tincture or Extract:

Preparation:

- Combine dried Ashwagandha root with a high-proof alcohol (such as vodka or brandy) in a glass jar.
- Let the mixture sit for several weeks, shaking the jar occasionally.
- Strain the liquid to separate the infused alcohol from the solid plant material.

- **Uses:**
  - Ashwagandha tinctures or extracts can be taken in small doses and are convenient for those who prefer concentrated forms of the herb.

Ashwagandha Powder in Smoothies or Recipes:

Preparation:

- Mix Ashwagandha powder into smoothies, beverages, or recipes.
- Start with a small amount and adjust the dosage based on personal preference.

- **Uses:**
  - Blended into smoothies or added to recipes to incorporate Ashwagandha into daily nutrition. This method provides flexibility in how the herb is consumed.

Here are two recipes featuring ashwagandha:

Ashwagandha Golden Milk:

- ***Ingredients:***
  - 1 cup milk (plant-based preferred)
  - 1/2 teaspoon ground turmeric
  - 1/4 teaspoon ground cinnamon
  - 1/4 teaspoon ground ginger
  - 1/4 teaspoon ground cardamom
  - 1/8 teaspoon ground black pepper
  - 1 teaspoon ashwagandha powder
  - Honey or maple syrup (optional, for sweetness)
- ***Instructions:***
  1. In a small saucepan, heat the milk over medium heat until it begins to simmer.

2. Add the turmeric, cinnamon, ginger, cardamom, black pepper, and ashwagandha powder to the milk.
3. Whisk the mixture gently to combine the ingredients evenly.
4. Allow the golden milk to simmer for 5-7 minutes, stirring occasionally.
5. Remove the saucepan from heat and strain the golden milk into a mug to remove any spices that haven't dissolved completely.
6. Sweeten with honey or maple syrup, if desired.
7. Serve warm and enjoy as a soothing and nourishing beverage.

Ashwagandha Energy Balls:

- ***Ingredients:***
  - 1 cup rolled oats
  - 1/2 cup almond butter or peanut butter
  - 1/4 cup honey or maple syrup
  - 2 tablespoons chia seeds
  - 2 tablespoons ground flaxseed
  - 1 teaspoon ashwagandha powder
  - 1/2 teaspoon ground cinnamon
  - Pinch of sea salt
  - Optional: shredded coconut or cocoa powder for coating
- ***Instructions:***
  1. In a large mixing bowl, combine rolled oats, almond butter, honey or maple syrup, chia seeds, ground flaxseed, ashwagandha powder, cinnamon, and sea salt.
  2. Stir the mixture until well combined and a sticky dough forms.
  3. Using your hands, roll the dough into small balls, about 1 inch in diameter.
  4. Optional: Roll the energy balls in shredded coconut or cocoa powder for added flavor and texture.
  5. Place the energy balls on a baking sheet lined with parchment paper and refrigerate for at least 30 minutes to firm up.
  6. Once firm, store the energy balls in an airtight container in the refrigerator for up to one week.
  7. Enjoy these nutrient-packed ashwagandha energy balls as a healthy and convenient snack on the go.

These recipes offer delicious and convenient ways to incorporate ashwagandha into your diet, providing potential health benefits while satisfying your taste buds.

Conclusion:

Ashwagandha's rise to prominence in the world of herbal medicine is a testament to its remarkable adaptogenic properties and holistic health benefits. From stress management to immune support and cognitive well-being, ashwagandha continues to capture the interest of those seeking natural remedies for a balanced and vibrant life. As with any herbal supplement, it's advisable to consult with a healthcare professional before incorporating ashwagandha into your routine, especially if you have specific health concerns or are pregnant. Embrace the ancient wisdom of Ayurveda and discover the potential wonders of ashwagandha on your journey to optimal health and vitality.

Back to Table of Contents

Asparagus

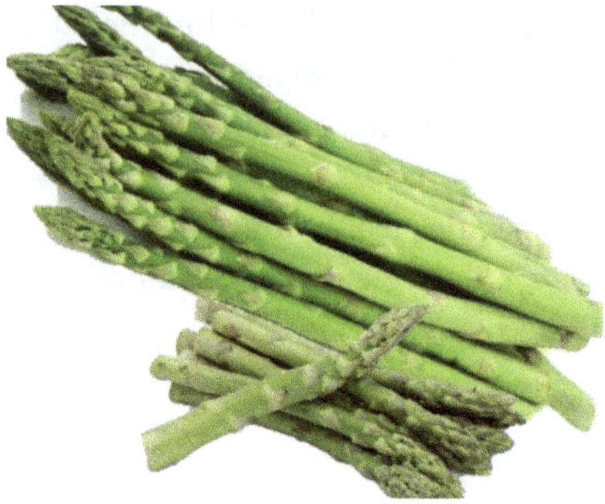

The Green Elegance: Unveiling the Health Benefits and Culinary Delights of Asparagus

Asparagus, with its slender stalks and distinctive flavor, is not just a culinary delight but also a nutritional powerhouse. This versatile vegetable has been cherished for centuries, not only for its delectable taste but also for the myriad health benefits it offers. In this article, we will explore the nutritional virtues, health advantages, and diverse culinary uses that make asparagus a green gem on our plates.

Nutritional Profile:

Asparagus is renowned for its rich array of nutrients, providing a low-calorie option packed with essential vitamins and minerals. A one-cup (134g) serving of cooked asparagus contains:

Fiber:

- Asparagus is a good source of dietary fiber, supporting digestive health and promoting a feeling of fullness.

Vitamins:

Asparagus is particularly rich in vitamins, including vitamin K, vitamin A, vitamin C, vitamin E, and various B vitamins such as folate (vitamin B9).

Vitamin K:

- **Benefits:** Essential for blood clotting, vitamin K also plays a role in bone metabolism by assisting in the regulation of calcium. Adequate vitamin K intake is crucial for maintaining bone density and preventing fractures.

Vitamin A:

- **Benefits:** Vitamin A is essential for vision, immune function, and skin health. Asparagus contains beta-carotene, a precursor to vitamin A, which contributes to maintaining healthy skin and mucous membranes.

Vitamin C:

- **Benefits:** As a powerful antioxidant, vitamin C in asparagus helps protect cells from oxidative stress. It supports the immune system, aids in the absorption of non-heme iron, and contributes to the synthesis of collagen for skin health.

Vitamin E:

- **Benefits:** Vitamin E is a potent antioxidant that protects cells from oxidative damage. It contributes to maintaining healthy skin, eyes, and the immune system.

Vitamin B1 (Thiamine):

- **Benefits:** Thiamine is crucial for energy metabolism, supporting the conversion of carbohydrates into usable energy. It also plays a role in maintaining proper nerve function.

Vitamin B2 (Riboflavin):

- **Benefits:** Riboflavin is essential for energy production and metabolism. It plays a role in converting food into usable energy and contributes to the health of the skin, eyes, and nerve functions.

Vitamin B3 (Niacin):

- **Benefits:** Niacin is important for energy production, DNA repair, and skin health. It also helps regulate cholesterol levels and supports overall cardiovascular health.

Vitamin B5 (Pantothenic Acid):

- **Benefits:** Pantothenic acid is involved in the synthesis of fatty acids and is essential for the metabolism of carbohydrates, proteins, and fats. It also plays a role in supporting adrenal function.

Vitamin B6 (Pyridoxine):

- **Benefits:** Vitamin B6 is involved in various metabolic processes, including amino acid metabolism and neurotransmitter synthesis. It contributes to the formation of red blood cells and supports the immune system.

Folate (Vitamin B9):

- **Benefits:** Folate is crucial for DNA synthesis and cell division. Adequate folate intake is particularly important during pregnancy as it helps prevent neural tube defects in the developing fetus. Folate also supports overall cellular function.

Minerals:

Asparagus provides essential minerals like potassium, phosphorus, magnesium, and iron, contributing to overall well-being.

Potassium:

- **Benefits:** Potassium is crucial for maintaining proper fluid balance, nerve transmission, and muscle contraction. It also helps regulate blood pressure and supports heart health.

Phosphorus:

- **Benefits:** Phosphorus is essential for bone and teeth formation, energy metabolism, and the synthesis of DNA and RNA. It also plays a role in maintaining the pH balance of body fluids.

Calcium:

- **Benefits:** While asparagus contains smaller amounts of calcium compared to dairy products, calcium is essential for bone and teeth formation, blood clotting, and muscle function.

Magnesium:

- **Benefits:** Magnesium is involved in over 300 enzymatic reactions in the body, including energy metabolism, muscle and nerve function, and bone health. It also contributes to the regulation of blood pressure.

Sodium:

- **Benefits:** Sodium is an essential electrolyte that helps maintain fluid balance, supports nerve function, and plays a role in muscle contraction.

Iron:

- **Benefits:** Iron is vital for the formation of hemoglobin, the oxygen-carrying protein in red blood cells. Adequate iron intake helps prevent anemia and supports overall energy metabolism.

Zinc:

- **Benefits:** Zinc is involved in immune function, wound healing, and the synthesis of DNA. It also plays a role in taste and smell perception.

Copper:

- **Benefits:** Copper acts as a cofactor for various enzymes involved in energy metabolism, connective tissue formation, and the protection against oxidative stress.

Manganese:

- **Benefits:** Manganese is a trace element that serves as a cofactor for enzymes involved in bone formation, blood clotting, and reducing oxidative stress.

Selenium:

- **Benefits:** Selenium is an essential trace element that functions as part of antioxidant enzymes, helping protect cells from oxidative damage. It also supports immune function.

Health Benefits:

Rich in Antioxidants:

- Asparagus contains antioxidants, including vitamin C and beta-carotene, which help neutralize free radicals in the body, potentially reducing the risk of chronic diseases.

Supports Digestive Health:

- The fiber content in asparagus aids in digestion, supports a healthy gut microbiome, and may help prevent constipation.

Loaded with Folate (Vitamin B9):

- Asparagus is an excellent source of folate, a crucial nutrient for cell division, DNA synthesis, and the prevention of neural tube defects during pregnancy.

Heart Health:

- Potassium in asparagus helps regulate blood pressure, while the presence of folate contributes to cardiovascular health by reducing homocysteine levels.

Anti-Inflammatory Properties:

- Asparagus contains anti-inflammatory compounds that may help reduce inflammation in the body, contributing to overall health.

Nutritional Content

In 1 cup (about 134 grams) of cooked asparagus, you can expect to find approximately:

- Carbohydrates: Around 5-6 grams
- Protein: Approximately 3-4 grams
- Fiber: Roughly 2-3 grams
- Fat: Less than 1 gram

Asparagus is a low-calorie vegetable that is rich in essential nutrients such as vitamins A, C, E, and K, as well as folate, potassium, and antioxidants. These values are approximate and can vary slightly based on factors such as cooking method and the specific variety of asparagus.

Culinary Uses:

Grilled Asparagus:

- Toss asparagus spears in olive oil, sprinkle with salt and pepper, and grill until tender. Grilled asparagus makes for a flavorful side dish or a topping for salads and pastas.

Asparagus Risotto:

- Incorporate finely chopped asparagus into a creamy risotto. The vibrant green color and distinct flavor add a refreshing twist to this classic dish.

Asparagus Soup:

- Blend cooked asparagus with broth and seasonings to create a velvety asparagus soup. Garnish with a dollop of yogurt or a sprinkle of fresh herbs.

Asparagus Salad:

- Shave raw asparagus into thin ribbons and toss them in a salad with cherry tomatoes, feta cheese, and a light vinaigrette for a crisp and refreshing dish.

Here are two delicious and nutritious recipes featuring Asparagus:

Lemon Garlic Roasted Asparagus:

Ingredients:

- 1 bunch of asparagus, tough ends trimmed

- 2 tablespoons olive oil
- 3 cloves garlic, minced
- 1 lemon, zest and juice
- Salt and pepper to taste
- Grated Parmesan cheese (optional, for serving)

Instructions:

1. Preheat the oven to 400°F (200°C).
2. Place the trimmed asparagus on a baking sheet.
3. In a small bowl, mix olive oil, minced garlic, lemon zest, and lemon juice.
4. Drizzle the lemon-garlic mixture over the asparagus, ensuring even coating.
5. Sprinkle with salt and pepper to taste.
6. Roast in the preheated oven for 12-15 minutes or until the asparagus is tender but still crisp.
7. Optional: Sprinkle with grated Parmesan cheese before serving.

Asparagus and Mushroom Quiche:

Ingredients:

- 1 refrigerated pie crust or homemade pie crust
- 1 bunch of asparagus, tough ends trimmed and cut into bite-sized pieces
- 1 cup mushrooms, sliced
- 1 cup shredded Gruyère or Swiss cheese
- 4 large eggs
- 1 cup milk or half-and-half
- Salt and pepper to taste
- 1 tablespoon olive oil

Instructions:

1. Preheat the oven to 375°F (190°C).
2. Roll out the pie crust and press it into a pie dish.
3. In a skillet, heat olive oil over medium heat. Sauté the mushrooms and asparagus until tender. Season with salt and pepper.
4. Spread the sautéed vegetables evenly over the pie crust.
5. In a bowl, whisk together eggs and milk. Season with salt and pepper.
6. Pour the egg mixture over the vegetables in the pie crust.
7. Sprinkle shredded cheese on top.
8. Bake in the preheated oven for 30-35 minutes or until the quiche is set and golden brown.
9. Allow the quiche to cool for a few minutes before slicing and serving.

These recipes showcase the delicious and versatile nature of asparagus, whether roasted with a burst of lemon and garlic or incorporated into a savory quiche with mushrooms and cheese. Enjoy the vibrant flavors and nutritional benefits of asparagus in these delightful dishes.

Conclusion:

Asparagus, celebrated for both its exquisite taste and nutritional bounty, stands as a testament to the wonders of fresh, wholesome produce. Whether grilled, sautéed, steamed, or enjoyed raw, asparagus brings a burst of flavor and a myriad of health benefits to your table. If you have specific health concerns, allergies, or conditions, it's advisable to consult with a healthcare professional or a registered dietitian before making significant changes to your diet.

So, embrace this green elegance and savor the goodness that asparagus adds to both your culinary adventures and your journey towards a healthier lifestyle.

Back to Table of Contents

Avocado

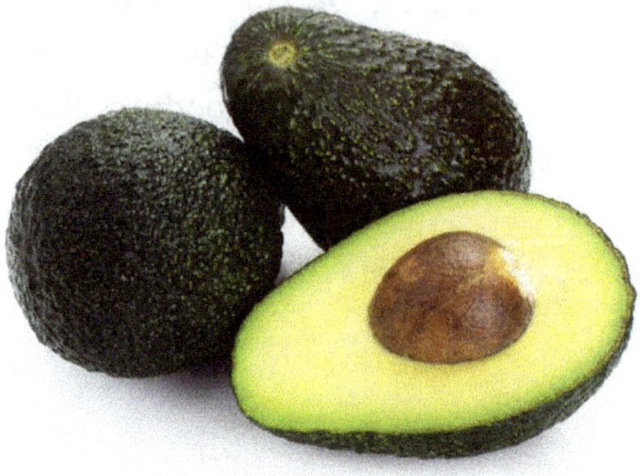

Embracing the Green Gold

Avocado, with its creamy texture and distinct flavor, has earned its reputation as a nutritional powerhouse and a culinary delight. This versatile fruit goes beyond being a favorite toast topper, offering an array of health benefits that make it a valuable addition to a well-balanced diet. In this article, we will explore the nutritional richness, health advantages, and diverse culinary uses of the beloved avocado.

Nutritional Value of Avocado:

Healthy Monounsaturated Fats:

- Avocados are rich in monounsaturated fats, specifically oleic acid.
- Monounsaturated fats are heart-healthy and may contribute to reducing bad cholesterol levels while increasing good cholesterol, promoting cardiovascular health.

Abundance of Nutrients:

Avocados are nutrient-dense fruits that offer a wide array of vitamins, minerals, and antioxidants, contributing to their reputation as a superfood. Here's a list of some of the key nutrients found in avocados and their benefits:

Vitamins:

Vitamin K: Vitamin K plays a crucial role in bone metabolism and may contribute to bone health by aiding in calcium absorption and bone mineralization. Vitamin K is also essential for blood clotting, promoting wound healing and reducing the risk of excessive bleeding.

Vitamin C: Acts as an antioxidant, supports immune function, and aids in collagen synthesis.

Vitamin E: Vitamin E is a powerful antioxidant that helps protect cells from oxidative damage caused by free radicals.

- **Skin Health:** The antioxidant properties of vitamin E contribute to skin health, helping to maintain its elasticity and protect against premature aging.

Vitamin B6: Important for metabolism, brain health, and immune function.
Folate (Vitamin B9): Essential for DNA synthesis and cell division, especially important during pregnancy for fetal development.
Vitamin A: Supports vision health, immune function, and skin health.

Minerals:

Potassium: Avocados are a rich source of potassium, which helps regulate blood pressure by balancing the effects of sodium. Adequate potassium intake is associated with a lower risk of hypertension and stroke.

- **Electrolyte Balance:** Potassium is essential for maintaining proper electrolyte balance in the body, supporting nerve and muscle function.

Magnesium: Important for muscle and nerve function, bone health, and energy metabolism.
Copper: Necessary for the production of red blood cells, collagen synthesis, and iron absorption.
Iron: Essential for oxygen transport in the blood and energy production.
Zinc: Important for immune function, wound healing, and DNA synthesis.

Antioxidants:

Carotenoids (including lutein and zeaxanthin): Support eye health and may help reduce the risk of age-related macular degeneration.
Glutathione: Acts as a powerful antioxidant, protecting cells from oxidative damage and supporting detoxification processes.
Polyphenols (including flavonoids): Have antioxidant and anti-inflammatory properties, potentially reducing the risk of chronic diseases such as heart disease and cancer.
Vitamin E: As mentioned earlier, acts as an antioxidant, protecting cells from oxidative damage.

Benefits of consuming avocados include:

- Supporting heart health due to their high potassium content and healthy fat profile, which may help lower cholesterol levels and reduce the risk of heart disease.
- Promoting eye health and reducing the risk of age-related macular degeneration due to the presence of carotenoids like lutein and zeaxanthin.
- Providing essential nutrients for overall health and well-being, including vitamins, minerals, and antioxidants that support various bodily functions.

Incorporating avocados into your diet can be as simple as adding slices to salads, spreading avocado on toast, or blending it into smoothies. Enjoying avocados regularly can contribute to a balanced and nutritious eating pattern, providing a wide range of health benefits.

Dietary Fiber Content:

- Avocados are an excellent source of dietary fiber.
- Dietary fiber aids digestion, promotes a feeling of fullness, and helps regulate blood sugar levels. This makes avocados a valuable component for those seeking weight management and blood sugar control.

Health Benefits of Avocado:

Heart Health Support:

- The monounsaturated fats in avocados contribute to heart health by reducing the risk of cardiovascular diseases.
- Avocado's potassium content helps regulate blood pressure, and its anti-inflammatory properties may contribute to overall heart health.

Weight Management and Satiety:

- The combination of healthy fats and fiber in avocados promotes a feeling of satiety.
- Including avocados in meals may help control appetite, potentially aiding in weight management by reducing overall calorie intake.

Antioxidant Properties:

- Avocados contain antioxidants, including lutein and zeaxanthin, which are beneficial for eye health.
- Antioxidants help protect cells from oxidative stress, supporting the body's defense against chronic diseases and promoting overall well-being.

Nutritional Content

In 1 cup (about 150 grams) of sliced avocado, you can expect to find approximately:

- Carbohydrates: Around 12-13 grams
- Protein: Approximately 2-3 grams
- Fiber: Roughly 10-11 grams
- Fat: About 21-22 grams

Avocado is a nutrient-dense fruit that is particularly rich in heart-healthy monounsaturated fats, making it a valuable source of energy and essential fatty acids. Additionally, avocados provide dietary fiber, vitamins, and minerals, including potassium, vitamin K, vitamin E, and folate. These values are approximate and can vary based on factors such as the size and variety of the avocado.

Culinary Uses of Avocado:

Classic Guacamole:

- Avocado is the star ingredient in the beloved guacamole, a flavorful dip made with mashed avocados, tomatoes, onions, lime, and cilantro.
- Guacamole is a versatile accompaniment for chips, tacos, or as a topping for various dishes.

Avocado Toast and Sandwiches:

- Avocado's creamy texture makes it an ideal spread for toast or a flavorful addition to sandwiches.
- Pairing avocado with whole-grain bread creates a satisfying and nutritious meal.

Salads and Bowls:

- Sliced or diced avocados enhance the nutritional content and taste of salads and grain bowls.
- Avocados add a creamy texture to the dish while providing a dose of healthy fats and nutrients.

Here are two delicious recipes that feature avocado as a key ingredient:

Avocado Toast with Poached Egg:

Ingredients:

- 2 slices whole-grain bread
- 1 ripe avocado
- 2 large eggs
- Salt and pepper to taste
- Optional toppings: red pepper flakes, sliced tomatoes, microgreens, or crumbled feta cheese

Instructions:

1. Toast the slices of whole-grain bread until golden and crispy.
2. While the bread is toasting, halve the avocado, remove the pit, and scoop the flesh into a small bowl. Mash the avocado with a fork until smooth.
3. Poach the eggs: Bring a pot of water to a gentle simmer. Crack each egg into a small cup or ramekin. Carefully slide each egg into the simmering water. Cook for about 3-4 minutes until the whites are set but the yolks are still runny.
4. Spread the mashed avocado evenly onto the toasted bread slices. Season with salt and pepper to taste.
5. Carefully remove the poached eggs from the water using a slotted spoon and place one egg on top of each slice of avocado toast.

6. Sprinkle with additional toppings if desired, such as red pepper flakes, sliced tomatoes, microgreens, or crumbled feta cheese.
7. Serve immediately, enjoying the creamy avocado and perfectly poached egg combination on crunchy toast.

Avocado and Black Bean Salad:

Ingredients:

- 2 ripe avocados, diced
- 1 can (15 ounces) black beans, rinsed and drained
- 1 cup cherry tomatoes, halved
- 1/2 red onion, finely chopped
- 1/4 cup fresh cilantro, chopped
- Juice of 1 lime
- 2 tablespoons extra virgin olive oil
- Salt and pepper to taste

Instructions:

1. In a large mixing bowl, combine the diced avocado, black beans, cherry tomatoes, chopped red onion, and chopped cilantro.
2. In a small bowl, whisk together the lime juice and extra virgin olive oil to make the dressing. Season with salt and pepper to taste.
3. Pour the dressing over the avocado and black bean mixture. Gently toss until everything is evenly coated.
4. Taste and adjust seasoning if necessary.
5. Serve immediately as a refreshing and nutritious salad, or chill in the refrigerator for 30 minutes to allow the flavors to meld together before serving.

These recipes showcase the versatility of avocados and how they can be incorporated into both savory breakfasts and salads for a delicious and nutritious meal. Enjoy!

Ancient Mesoamerican Culinary and Medicinal Uses:

Historical evidence suggests that the Aztecs and other Mesoamerican civilizations cultivated and consumed avocados.

Benefits: Avocados were used not only as a nutritious food source but also for their potential medicinal properties. The fruit was believed to have aphrodisiac effects, and its consumption was associated with vitality and energy.

Traditional Mexican Healing Applications:

In Mexican traditional medicine, various parts of the avocado tree, including the leaves, bark, and seeds, were used for medicinal purposes.

Benefits: Avocado leaves were employed to make infusions believed to treat ailments such as diarrhea, dysentery, and abdominal pain. The leaves were also thought to have anti-inflammatory properties.

Conclusion: Avocado's allure extends far beyond its delicious taste and creamy texture. As we celebrate this green gold, we recognize its significant contributions to heart health, weight management, and overall well-being. Whether enjoyed in classic guacamole, on toast, or as a salad topping, avocados continue to captivate the culinary world while promoting a healthier, happier lifestyle. So, let's savor the goodness of avocados and reap the benefits of this remarkable fruit.

If you have specific health concerns, allergies, or conditions, it's advisable to consult with a healthcare professional or a registered dietitian before making significant changes to your diet.

Back to Table of Contents

Banana (Green)

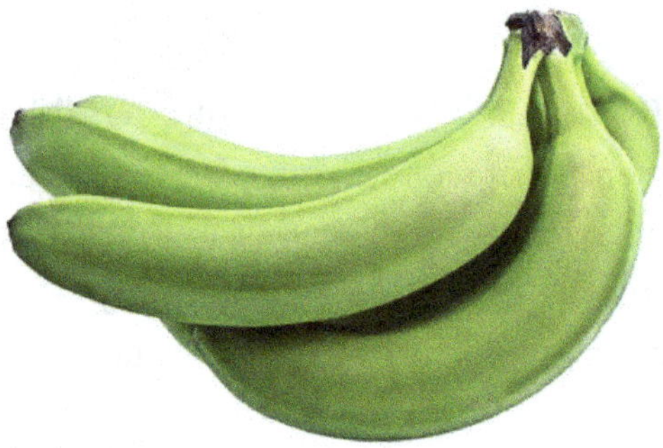

The Health Benefits and Versatile Uses of Green Bananas

Green bananas, often overlooked in comparison to their ripe, yellow counterparts, are a nutritional powerhouse with numerous health benefits. While many people are familiar with the sweet taste of ripe bananas, the green variety offers a unique set of advantages and versatile uses that deserve recognition. In this article, we will explore the various benefits of green bananas and the creative ways in which they can be incorporated into your diet.

Nutritional Content:

Green bananas are an excellent source of essential nutrients, including dietary fiber, vitamins, and minerals. They are rich in resistant starch, a type of starch that acts similarly to soluble fiber, promoting a healthy digestive system. Additionally, green bananas contain essential vitamins such as vitamin C, vitamin B6, and potassium, all of which play crucial roles in supporting overall well-being.

Dietary Fiber:

- **Benefits:**
  - ***Supports Digestive Health:*** Green bananas are rich in dietary fiber, promoting regular bowel movements and preventing constipation.
  - ***Helps Maintain Healthy Weight:*** Fiber contributes to a feeling of fullness, aiding in weight management by reducing overall calorie intake.

Resistant Starch:

- **Benefits:**
  - ***Blood Sugar Regulation:*** Resistant starch in green bananas has a lower impact on blood sugar levels, making them a suitable option for individuals managing diabetes.

- ***Supports Gut Health:*** Acts as a prebiotic, nourishing beneficial gut bacteria and promoting a healthy gut microbiome.

Vitamin C:

- **Benefits:**
    - ***Immune System Support***: Vitamin C is essential for the proper functioning of the immune system, helping the body defend against infections and illnesses.
    - ***Collagen Synthesis:*** Contributes to the synthesis of collagen, a protein important for skin, blood vessels, and connective tissues.

Potassium:

- **Benefits:**
    - ***Regulates Blood Pressure:*** Potassium helps balance sodium levels in the body, playing a crucial role in maintaining healthy blood pressure.
    - ***Muscle and Nerve Function:*** Supports proper muscle and nerve function, contributing to overall cardiovascular health.

Magnesium:

- **Benefits:**
- ***Bone Health:*** Magnesium is essential for bone formation and helps in the absorption of calcium, contributing to overall bone health.

- ***Energy Production: It*** plays a role in the conversion of food into energy, supporting various metabolic processes in the body.

Copper:

- **Benefits:**
- ***Iron Absorption:*** Copper aids in the absorption of iron from the digestive tract, supporting the formation of red blood cells and preventing anemia.

- ***Antioxidant Activity:*** Copper acts as an antioxidant, helping neutralize free radicals and protecting cells from oxidative stress.

Digestive Health:

One of the key benefits of green bananas lies in their impact on digestive health. The high levels of resistant starch act as a prebiotic, nourishing the beneficial bacteria in the gut. This promotes a healthy gut microbiome, leading to improved digestion and a reduced risk of digestive issues such as constipation.

Blood Sugar Control:

Green bananas have a lower glycemic index compared to ripe bananas, making them a favorable choice for individuals looking to manage their blood sugar levels. The resistant starch in green bananas may help regulate blood sugar and insulin levels, making them a suitable option for those with diabetes or those aiming to prevent spikes in blood sugar.

Weight Management:

The fiber content in green bananas contributes to a feeling of fullness, which can aid in weight management. Including green bananas in your diet may help control appetite and reduce overall calorie intake, supporting weight loss efforts.

Nutritional Content

The nutritional content of 1 medium-sized green banana (approximately 7-8 inches or 118 grams) typically includes:

- Carbohydrates: Approximately 31 grams
- Protein: Approximately 1.3 grams
- Fiber: Approximately 3.1 grams
- Fat: Approximately 0.4 grams
- Sugar: Approximately 4 grams

These values may vary slightly depending on the size of the banana and its exact stage of ripeness. Green bananas tend to have slightly higher starch content and lower sugar content compared to ripe bananas.

Versatile Culinary Uses:

Green bananas are incredibly versatile in the kitchen and can be used in various culinary applications. Here are some creative ways to incorporate green bananas into your meals:

1. Green Banana Chips: Slice green bananas thinly and bake or fry them to create a healthy and crunchy snack.
2. Green Banana Smoothies: Add green bananas to your favorite smoothie recipes for a nutritious and energizing boost.
3. Green Banana Curry: Use green bananas in savory dishes, such as curries or stews, for a unique and delicious flavor.
4. Green Banana Flour: Ground green bananas can be used to make gluten-free flour, suitable for baking.

Here are a few green banana recipes:

Green Banana Chips:

- **Ingredients:**
  - Green bananas (unripe)
  - Olive oil
  - Salt
- **Instructions:**

1. Preheat your oven to 350°F (175°C).
2. Peel the green bananas and slice them thinly.
3. Toss the banana slices with olive oil and spread them in a single layer on a baking sheet.

4. Sprinkle salt over the slices for seasoning.
5. Bake in the preheated oven for 15-20 minutes or until the chips are golden brown and crispy.

Allow the chips to cool before serving. Enjoy as a healthy snack or side dish!

Green Banana Smoothie:

- **Ingredients:**
  - 2 green bananas (peeled and sliced)
  - 1 cup spinach leaves (fresh or frozen)
  - 1/2 cup Greek yogurt
  - 1/2 cup almond milk
  - 1 tablespoon honey or maple syrup (optional, for sweetness)
  - Ice cubes (optional)
- **Instructions:**

1. Combine green banana slices, spinach, Greek yogurt, almond milk, and sweetener (if using) in a blender.
2. Blend until smooth and creamy. Add ice cubes if you prefer a colder consistency.
3. Pour the smoothie into a glass and garnish with additional banana slices or a sprinkle of chia seeds if desired.
4. Refreshing and nutritious, this green banana smoothie makes for a perfect breakfast or a post-workout energy boost.

Jamaican Green Banana Porridge:

Ingredients:

- 4 green bananas (unripe)
- 1 cup coconut milk
- 3 cups water
- 1/2 cup condensed milk (adjust to taste)
- 1/2 teaspoon vanilla extract
- 1/4 teaspoon ground cinnamon
- Pinch of salt
- Grated nutmeg for garnish (optional)

Instructions:

1. **Prepare the Green Bananas:**
   - Peel the green bananas and cut them into small pieces.
2. **Boil the Green Bananas:**
   - In a large pot, bring 3 cups of water to a boil.
   - Add the green banana pieces to the boiling water and cook until they are soft and easily pierced with a fork (about 15-20 minutes).
3. **Blend the Green Bananas:**

- Once the green bananas are cooked, carefully drain the water, reserving a small amount.
- Transfer the boiled green bananas to a blender or food processor.
- Add 1 cup of coconut milk and blend until you get a smooth consistency. Add reserved water if needed.

4. **Cook the Porridge:**
    - Pour the blended green banana mixture back into the pot.
    - Place the pot over medium heat and add condensed milk, vanilla extract, ground cinnamon, and a pinch of salt.
    - Stir continuously to prevent lumps and ensure even cooking.
5. **Simmer and Serve:**
    - Allow the porridge to simmer on low heat for an additional 10-15 minutes, stirring frequently until it reaches your desired thickness.
    - Taste the porridge and adjust sweetness by adding more condensed milk if needed.
6. **Garnish and Serve:**
    - Once the porridge reaches the desired consistency, remove it from heat.
    - Serve the Jamaican Green Banana Porridge hot, garnished with a sprinkle of grated nutmeg if desired.

This hearty and delicious Jamaican Green Banana Porridge is a comforting breakfast option that showcases the unique flavor and texture of green bananas. Enjoy it as is or customize with your favorite toppings such as sliced almonds, fresh berries, or a drizzle of honey.

Feel free to customize these recipes based on your preferences and explore the versatility of green bananas in both savory and sweet dishes.

Conclusion: Green bananas are a nutritious and versatile addition to your diet, offering a range of health benefits and culinary possibilities. Whether you're looking to improve digestive health, manage blood sugar levels, or simply diversify your meals, green bananas are a valuable and often underestimated ingredient. Consider incorporating green bananas into your regular diet to experience their many advantages and enhance your overall well-being.

If you have specific health concerns, allergies, or conditions, it's advisable to consult with a healthcare professional or a registered dietitian before making significant changes to your diet.

Back to Table of Contents

Banana (Ripe)

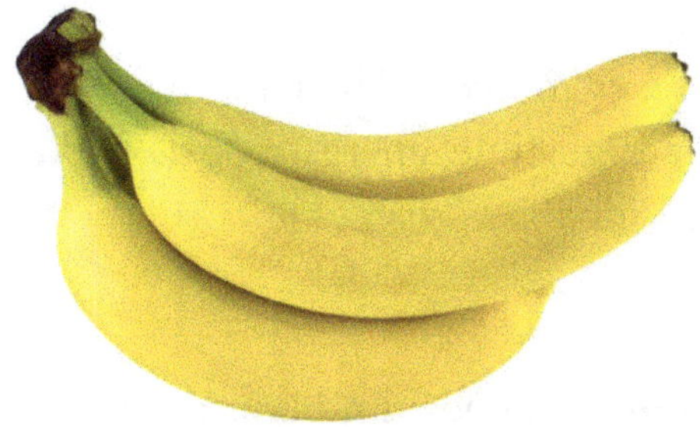

The Sweet Goodness of Ripe Bananas: Benefits and Versatile Uses

Ripe bananas, with their sweet and creamy flesh, are a beloved fruit enjoyed by people of all ages around the world. Beyond their delicious taste, ripe bananas offer a range of health benefits and can be used in various culinary applications. In this article, we will explore the nutritional advantages of ripe bananas and the versatile ways in which they can be incorporated into your diet.

Nutritional Content:

Ripe bananas are a nutritional powerhouse, packed with essential vitamins, minerals, and natural sugars. While the green variety is known for its resistant starch, ripe bananas shine with increased levels of antioxidants and easy-to-digest sugars. Here are some key nutrients found in ripe bananas:

Potassium:

- **Benefits:**
    - ***Supports Heart Health***: Potassium is crucial for maintaining a healthy heart by regulating blood pressure and supporting proper muscle and nerve function.
    - ***Electrolyte Balance:*** Helps maintain electrolyte balance in the body, contributing to overall well-being.

Vitamin C:

- **Benefits:**
    - ***Immune System Boost:*** Vitamin C is an antioxidant that supports the immune system, helping the body defend against infections and illnesses.
    - ***Collagen Production:*** Contributes to the synthesis of collagen, promoting healthy skin and connective tissues.

Dietary Fiber:

- **Benefits:**
    - ***Digestive Health:*** The fiber content aids in digestion, preventing constipation and promoting a healthy gut.

- ***Satiety:*** Contributes to a feeling of fullness, supporting weight management by reducing overeating.

Natural Sugars:

- **Benefits:**
    - ***Quick Energy Source:*** The natural sugars in ripe bananas provide a quick and easily digestible energy boost, making them an excellent snack for active individuals.

Magnesium:

- **Benefits:**

Bone Health: Magnesium plays a role in bone formation and helps in the absorption of calcium, promoting strong and healthy bones.

Energy Production: Contributes to the body's energy production and metabolism.

Copper:

- **Benefits:**

Iron Absorption: Copper aids in the absorption of iron, supporting the formation of red blood cells and preventing anemia.

Antioxidant Activity: Acts as an antioxidant, helping neutralize free radicals and protect cells from oxidative stress.

Incorporating ripe bananas into your diet provides these essential vitamins and minerals, promoting cardiovascular health, bone health, and supporting vital physiological functions in the body.

Nutritional Content

The nutritional content of 1 medium-sized ripe banana (approximately 7-8 inches or 118 grams) typically includes:

- Carbohydrates: Approximately 27 grams
- Protein: Approximately 1.3 grams
- Fiber: Approximately 3.1 grams
- Fat: Approximately 0.4 grams
- Sugar: Approximately 14 - 15 grams

These values may vary slightly depending on the size and ripeness of the banana.

Versatile Culinary Uses:

Ripe bananas are incredibly versatile in the kitchen and can be used in a variety of dishes. Here are some creative ways to incorporate ripe bananas into your meals:

Smoothies and Shakes:

- Blend ripe bananas with yogurt, milk, and your favorite fruits for a delicious and nutritious smoothie.

Baking and Desserts:

- Ripe bananas add natural sweetness and moisture to baked goods like banana bread, muffins, and pancakes.

Frozen Treats:

- Freeze ripe banana slices and blend them into a creamy, dairy-free banana ice cream.

Cereal and Yogurt Toppings:

- Slice ripe bananas and add them as a topping to your morning cereal or yogurt for added flavor and nutrition.

Here are a few common recipes:

1. **Classic Banana Bread:**
   - **Ingredients:**
     - 3 ripe bananas, mashed
     - 2 cups all-purpose flour
     - 1 teaspoon baking soda
     - 1/4 teaspoon salt
     - 1/2 cup unsalted butter, softened
     - 1 cup granulated sugar
     - 2 large eggs
     - 1 teaspoon vanilla extract
     - 1/2 cup plain yogurt or buttermilk
     - 1/2 cup chopped nuts or chocolate chips (optional)
   - **Instructions:**

   1. Preheat your oven to 350°F (175°C) and grease a 9x5-inch loaf pan.
   2. In a bowl, whisk together flour, baking soda, and salt.
   3. In a separate large bowl, cream together butter and sugar until light and fluffy. Add eggs one at a time, beating well after each addition.
   4. Stir in mashed bananas and vanilla extract.
   5. Gradually add the dry ingredients to the wet ingredients, alternating with yogurt or buttermilk. Mix until just combined.
   6. Fold in nuts or chocolate chips if desired.
   7. Pour the batter into the prepared loaf pan and bake for 60-70 minutes or until a toothpick inserted into the center comes out clean.
   8. Allow the banana bread to cool in the pan for 10 minutes before transferring it to a wire rack to cool completely.

2. **Banana Smoothie Bowl:**
   - **Ingredients:**
     - 2 ripe bananas, frozen
     - 1/2 cup Greek yogurt
     - 1/4 cup milk (dairy or plant-based)
     - 1 tablespoon almond butter or peanut butter

- Toppings: sliced fresh bananas, granola, chia seeds, shredded coconut, and a drizzle of honey

- **Instructions:**

1. In a blender, combine frozen bananas, Greek yogurt, milk, and almond butter.
2. Blend until smooth and creamy, adding more milk if needed to reach your desired consistency.
3. Pour the smoothie into a bowl.
4. Top with sliced fresh bananas, granola, chia seeds, shredded coconut, and a drizzle of honey.
5. Enjoy this nutritious and delicious banana smoothie bowl as a satisfying breakfast or a refreshing snack.

Jamaican Ripe Banana Fritters Recipe:

Ingredients:

- 3 ripe bananas, mashed
- 1 cup all-purpose flour
- 1 teaspoon baking powder
- 1/4 teaspoon salt
- 1/4 cup granulated sugar (adjust to taste)
- 1/2 teaspoon ground cinnamon
- 1/4 teaspoon nutmeg
- 1 teaspoon vanilla extract
- 1 large egg
- 1/4 cup milk (dairy or plant-based)
- Vegetable oil for frying
- Powdered sugar for dusting (optional)

Instructions:

1. **Prepare the Batter:**
    - In a large bowl, combine the mashed ripe bananas, flour, baking powder, salt, sugar, ground cinnamon, nutmeg, and vanilla extract.
2. **Add Wet Ingredients:**
    - In a separate bowl, beat the egg and then add it to the banana mixture.
    - Pour in the milk and mix well until all ingredients are thoroughly combined. The batter should be thick and smooth.
3. **Heat the Oil:**
    - In a frying pan, heat enough vegetable oil over medium heat to cover the bottom of the pan.
4. **Fry the Banana Fritters:**
    - Once the oil is hot, use a spoon to drop portions of the batter into the pan. Ensure that each fritter has enough space to spread without touching each other.

- Fry until the edges are golden brown, and then flip the fritters to cook the other side. This should take about 2-3 minutes per side.

5. **Drain Excess Oil:**
    - Place the cooked banana fritters on a plate lined with paper towels to drain any excess oil.
6. **Repeat and Keep Warm:**
    - Continue frying the remaining batter in batches until all the fritters are cooked. You may need to add more oil as needed.
    - To keep the fritters warm, you can place them in a preheated oven (around 200°F or 95°C) while you finish frying the rest.
7. **Serve and Enjoy:**
    - Dust the banana fritters with powdered sugar if desired.
    - Serve warm and enjoy these delicious Jamaican banana fritters as a delightful snack or dessert.

This Jamaican Banana Fritters recipe captures the essence of Caribbean flavors with the natural sweetness of ripe bananas and warm spices. It's a simple and delightful treat that can be enjoyed on its own or with a sprinkle of powdered sugar for an extra touch of sweetness.

Conclusion: Ripe bananas are not only a tasty treat but also a nutritious addition to a well-balanced diet. Whether you enjoy them on their own, in smoothies, or as a key ingredient in various recipes, ripe bananas offer a delightful way to satisfy your sweet tooth while providing essential nutrients. Embrace the versatility of ripe bananas and explore the countless ways to incorporate them into your culinary repertoire for a delicious and healthful experience.

Back to Table of Contents

Barley

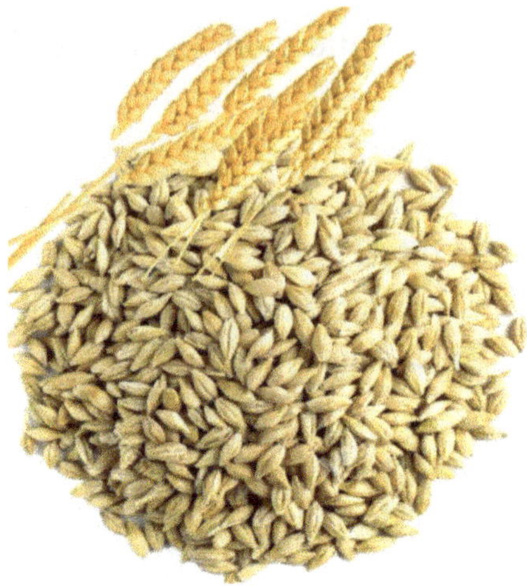

A Nutrient-Rich Ancient Grain with Health Benefits and Culinary Versatility

Barley, one of the oldest cultivated grains, has been a dietary staple for thousands of years, offering a host of nutritional benefits and culinary versatility. Rich in fiber, vitamins, and minerals, barley has earned its place as a wholesome and nutritious addition to a balanced diet. In this article, we'll explore the benefits, uses, and potential health advantages of incorporating barley into your meals.

Nutritional Profile:

Dietary Fiber:

Barley is an excellent source of both soluble and insoluble fiber. Fiber supports digestive health, helps maintain regular bowel movements, and may contribute to weight management by promoting a feeling of fullness.

Soluble Fiber:

- Barley is particularly rich in soluble fiber, primarily in the form of beta-glucans. Soluble fiber dissolves in water to form a gel-like substance, which helps lower cholesterol levels by binding to cholesterol molecules and removing them from the body. This type of fiber also contributes to better blood sugar control, making it beneficial for individuals with diabetes or those aiming to regulate their blood glucose levels.

Insoluble Fiber:

- The insoluble fiber in barley comes from its outer layer, particularly the bran. Insoluble fiber adds bulk to stool and aids in promoting regular bowel movements, preventing constipation, and supporting overall digestive health. It also provides a feeling of fullness, making it a valuable component in weight management or weight loss diets.

Vitamins and Minerals:

- Barley contains essential vitamins and minerals, including B-vitamins (such as niacin, thiamine, and folate), iron, magnesium, phosphorus, and selenium. These nutrients play critical roles in energy metabolism, immune function, and overall well-being.

Essential Vitamins in Barley:

Niacin (Vitamin B3):

- **Benefits:** Niacin plays a key role in energy metabolism, supporting the conversion of carbohydrates, fats, and proteins into usable energy. It also contributes to maintaining healthy skin, nerves, and digestive system.

Thiamine (Vitamin B1):

- **Benefits:** Thiamine is essential for energy metabolism, aiding in the conversion of carbohydrates into energy. It also supports proper nerve function and is crucial for the synthesis of neurotransmitters.

Folate (Vitamin B9):

- **Benefits:** Folate is crucial for DNA synthesis and repair, making it essential during periods of rapid cell division and growth. Adequate folate intake is particularly important for pregnant women to prevent neural tube defects in developing fetuses.

Riboflavin (Vitamin B2):

- **Benefits:** Riboflavin is involved in energy production, supporting the metabolism of fats, drugs, and steroids. It also plays a role in maintaining healthy skin, eyes, and nerve functions.

Essential Minerals in Barley:

Manganese:

- **Benefits:** Manganese is involved in the formation of connective tissues, bone metabolism, and the metabolism of amino acids, cholesterol, and carbohydrates. It also acts as an antioxidant, protecting cells from damage.

Magnesium:

- **Benefits:** Magnesium plays a crucial role in muscle and nerve function, bone health, and energy metabolism. It contributes to the regulation of blood pressure and supports the immune system.

Phosphorus:

- **Benefits:** Phosphorus is a structural component of DNA, RNA, and ATP (adenosine triphosphate), the primary energy carrier in cells. It is essential for bone health, kidney function, and the metabolism of macronutrients.

Iron:

- **Benefits:** Iron is vital for the formation of hemoglobin, the oxygen-carrying component of red blood cells. Adequate iron intake is essential for preventing iron-deficiency anemia and supporting overall energy levels.

Antioxidants:

Barley is rich in antioxidants, including tocotrienols and phenolic compounds. Antioxidants help neutralize harmful free radicals in the body, protecting cells from oxidative stress and potentially reducing the risk of chronic diseases.

Beta-Glucans:

- **Benefits:** Beta-glucans are a type of soluble fiber found in barley that possesses antioxidant properties. These compounds help neutralize free radicals in the body, reducing oxidative stress. Additionally, beta-glucans have been linked to various health benefits, including supporting heart health by lowering cholesterol levels and promoting immune function.

Phenolic Compounds:

- **Benefits:** Barley contains phenolic compounds, including ferulic acid and caffeic acid, which contribute to its antioxidant capacity. These compounds help protect cells from oxidative damage caused by free radicals. Antioxidants play a crucial role in reducing inflammation and lowering the risk of chronic diseases, such as cardiovascular diseases and certain types of cancer.

Caffeic Acid:

- **Benefits:** Caffeic acid is another phenolic compound found in barley, known for its antioxidant and anti-inflammatory properties. It contributes to the overall antioxidant defense system, helping combat oxidative stress and its associated health risks.

Quercetin:

- Benefits: Quercetin is a flavonoid antioxidant present in barley. It has been linked to various health benefits, including anti-inflammatory and anti-cancer properties. Quercetin helps neutralize free radicals, supporting cellular health and reducing the risk of oxidative damage.

Health Benefits:

Heart Health:

- The beta-glucans in barley have been linked to heart health benefits. These soluble fibers help lower cholesterol levels, reducing the risk of cardiovascular diseases. Barley's fiber content also supports healthy blood pressure.

Blood Sugar Regulation:

- Barley has a low glycemic index, meaning it has a gradual impact on blood sugar levels. This characteristic can be particularly beneficial for individuals with diabetes or those aiming to manage their blood sugar.

Weight Management:

- The fiber and protein content in barley contribute to a feeling of satiety, making it a valuable component of weight management or weight loss diets. Its nutritional density ensures you get essential nutrients without excessive caloric intake.

Nutritional Content

The nutritional content of 1 cup (about 157 grams) of cooked barley typically includes:

- Carbohydrates: Approximately 44-45 grams
- Protein: Approximately 3.5-4 grams
- Fiber: Approximately 6 grams
- Fat: Approximately 0.5 grams

These values can vary slightly depending on factors such as the specific variety of barley and how it's prepared.

Culinary Uses:

Soups and Stews:

- Barley is often used to add texture and heartiness to soups and stews. Its chewy texture absorbs flavors well, making it a perfect addition to hearty winter dishes.

Salads:

- Barley salads, featuring cooked barley mixed with fresh vegetables, herbs, and dressings, are a refreshing and nutritious option for warm weather. The grains provide a satisfying chewiness to salads.

Side Dishes:

- Barley can be prepared as a flavorful side dish, similar to rice or couscous. Seasoned with herbs and spices, it complements a variety of main courses.

Breakfast Bowls:

- Cooked barley can be incorporated into breakfast bowls with yogurt, fruits, and nuts, providing a wholesome and filling start to the day.

Here are two delicious recipes featuring barley:

Mushroom Barley Soup:

Ingredients:

- 1 cup pearl barley
- 8 cups vegetable or mushroom broth
- 2 tablespoons olive oil
- 1 onion, diced
- 2 carrots, sliced

- 2 celery stalks, sliced
- 3 cloves garlic, minced
- 8 oz mushrooms, sliced
- 1 teaspoon dried thyme
- 1 bay leaf
- Salt and pepper to taste
- Fresh parsley, chopped (for garnish)

Instructions:

1. In a pot, heat olive oil over medium heat. Add diced onions, carrots, and celery. Sauté until the vegetables are softened.
2. Add minced garlic and sliced mushrooms to the pot. Cook until the mushrooms release their moisture and start to brown.
3. Rinse the pearl barley under cold water. Add the barley to the pot along with dried thyme and stir to combine.
4. Pour in the vegetable or mushroom broth and add the bay leaf. Bring the soup to a boil, then reduce the heat to low, cover, and simmer for about 45-50 minutes or until the barley is tender.
5. Season the soup with salt and pepper to taste. Remove the bay leaf before serving.
6. Ladle the soup into bowls, garnish with fresh parsley, and enjoy a hearty bowl of mushroom barley soup.

Barley and Roasted Vegetable Salad:

Ingredients:

- 1 cup pearl barley
- 3 cups mixed vegetables (zucchini, bell peppers, cherry tomatoes, red onion, etc.), chopped
- 3 tablespoons olive oil
- 2 cloves garlic, minced
- 1 teaspoon dried oregano
- Salt and pepper to taste
- 1/4 cup feta cheese, crumbled
- Fresh basil, chopped (for garnish)

Instructions:

1. Preheat the oven to 400°F (200°C).
2. Rinse the pearl barley under cold water. Cook the barley according to package instructions.
3. In a large bowl, toss the chopped vegetables with olive oil, minced garlic, dried oregano, salt, and pepper.
4. Spread the seasoned vegetables on a baking sheet in a single layer. Roast in the preheated oven for about 25-30 minutes or until the vegetables are tender and slightly caramelized.
5. Once the barley and roasted vegetables are ready, combine them in a large bowl. Mix well.
6. Sprinkle crumbled feta cheese over the salad and garnish with fresh chopped basil.

7. Serve the barley and roasted vegetable salad at room temperature or chilled. Enjoy a nutritious and flavorful salad!

Feel free to customize these recipes based on your preferences and dietary requirements. Enjoy the wholesome goodness of barley in these delightful dishes!

Historical uses:

Barley has a rich history of cultivation and use, that dates back thousands of years. Here are two historical uses of barley and their associated benefits:

Ancient Grains and Staple Food:

- **Historical Use:** Barley is one of the oldest cultivated grains, with evidence of its cultivation dating back to ancient civilizations in Mesopotamia, Egypt, and Asia. It was a staple food in these regions and played a crucial role in the diet of early agricultural societies.
- **Benefits:** Barley's historical use as a staple food provided ancient civilizations with a reliable source of nutrition. It served as a dietary foundation, supplying essential nutrients, energy, and sustenance to communities. The versatility of barley allowed it to be used in various culinary applications, including bread, porridge, and fermented beverages.

Medicinal and Healing Properties:

- **Historical Use:** Throughout history, barley has been recognized for its medicinal properties. Ancient civilizations, including the Greeks and Romans, used barley for its healing attributes. Barley water, made by boiling barley in water, was a common remedy for various ailments.
- **Benefits:** Barley water was traditionally consumed for its potential health benefits, including soothing digestive issues, promoting hydration, and supporting overall wellness. The beverage was often recommended for its mild, comforting nature, making it suitable for individuals with digestive discomfort or those in need of rehydration.

Barley's historical uses as both a staple food and a medicinal remedy underscore its importance in human history. Today, barley continues to be valued for its nutritional richness and versatility, with modern applications extending to various culinary dishes, beverages, and even as a key ingredient in health foods.

Conclusion:

Barley, with its impressive nutrient profile and versatility in the kitchen, offers a range of health benefits and culinary possibilities. While Barley are generally safe and healthy to consume as part of a balanced diet. As with any food, moderation is key. If you have specific health concerns, allergies, or conditions, it's advisable to consult with a healthcare professional or a registered dietitian before making significant changes to your diet.

Whether enjoyed in soups, salads, or as a side dish, barley stands out as a whole grain that brings both nutritional value and delightful flavors to the table. By incorporating barley into your diet, you can savor its rich history and contribute to your overall health and well-being.

Back to Table of Contents

Basil

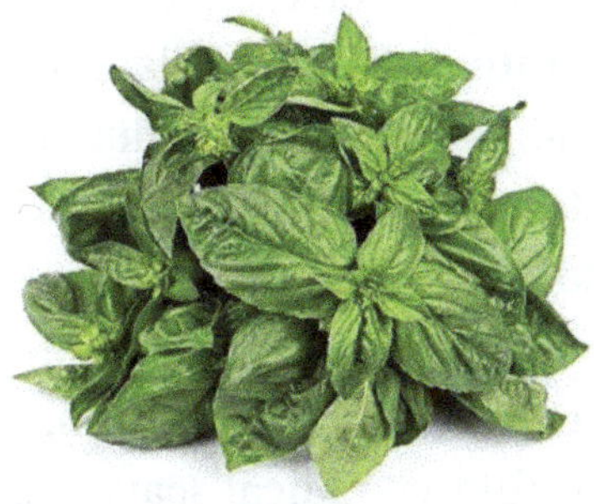

A Culinary Herb with Health Benefits and Endless Culinary Uses

Basil, a fragrant herb known for its distinctive aroma and flavorful leaves, has long been a staple in kitchens around the world. Beyond its culinary appeal, basil boasts an array of health benefits, making it a versatile herb that goes far beyond simple seasoning. In this article, we'll explore the numerous benefits and diverse uses of basil, celebrating its place as both a culinary delight and a source of well-being.

Culinary Marvel:

Rich Flavor Profile:

- Basil's vibrant and aromatic leaves add a unique depth of flavor to a variety of dishes. Whether it's the classic sweet basil, spicy Thai basil, or the citrusy notes of lemon basil, each variety lends its own character to culinary creations.

Versatile Ingredient:

- Basil is incredibly versatile and can be used fresh or dried in an array of recipes. From salads and sauces to soups, stews, and main dishes, basil's adaptability makes it an essential herb in diverse cuisines.

Key Component in Pesto:

- One of the most iconic uses of basil is in pesto sauce. A combination of fresh basil, garlic, pine nuts, Parmesan cheese, and olive oil creates a vibrant and flavorful sauce that can elevate pasta, sandwiches, and more.

Health Benefits:

Antioxidant Properties:

Basil is rich in antioxidants, including flavonoids and polyphenols, which help combat oxidative stress in the body. Antioxidants contribute to overall health by neutralizing free radicals and reducing inflammation.

Flavonoids, including Orientin and Vicenin:

- **Benefits:**
    - **Antioxidant Action:** Orientin and vicenin are flavonoids found in basil that exhibit strong antioxidant properties. These compounds help neutralize free radicals in the body, protecting cells from oxidative stress and damage.
    - **Anti-Inflammatory Effects:** Flavonoids, in general, have been linked to anti-inflammatory effects. By reducing inflammation, they may contribute to the prevention of chronic diseases and support overall well-being.

Polyphenols, such as Rosmarinic Acid:

- **Benefits:**
    - **Free Radical Scavenging:** Rosmarinic acid, a polyphenol abundant in basil, acts as a powerful free radical scavenger. It helps eliminate reactive oxygen species, reducing oxidative stress and preventing cellular damage.
    - **Anti-Inflammatory Properties:** Rosmarinic acid has been associated with anti-inflammatory effects, which may be beneficial in conditions related to inflammation, including arthritis and other inflammatory disorders.

Beta-Carotene:

- **Benefits:**
    - **Vitamin A Source:** Beta-carotene, present in basil, is a precursor to vitamin A. Vitamin A is essential for maintaining healthy vision, supporting immune function, and promoting skin health.
    - **Antioxidant Defense:** As a provitamin A compound, beta-carotene contributes to the antioxidant defense system in the body. It helps protect cells and tissues from oxidative damage.

Anti-Inflammatory Effects:

- Certain compounds in basil, such as eugenol, exhibit anti-inflammatory properties. Regular consumption of basil may help alleviate inflammation and support conditions related to inflammation, promoting overall well-being.

Nutrient-Rich:

- Basil is a good source of essential nutrients, including vitamin K, vitamin A, vitamin C, calcium, and iron. These nutrients play vital roles in bone health, immune function, and overall metabolic processes.

Adaptogenic Properties:

- Basil is considered an adaptogen, a substance that may help the body adapt to stress and restore balance. The compounds in basil are thought to have a calming effect on the nervous system, contributing to stress relief.

Nutritional Content

In 1 cup (about 21 grams) of fresh basil leaves, the approximate nutritional content is as follows:

- Carbohydrates: Approximately 1.4 grams
- Protein: Approximately 1.3 grams
- Fiber: Approximately 0.6 grams
- Fat: Approximately 0.2 grams

Please note that these values are approximate and can vary slightly based on factors such as the exact variety of basil and how it is harvested and prepared.

Versatile Uses:

Caprese Salad:

- Create a classic Caprese salad by layering fresh basil leaves with ripe tomatoes and mozzarella cheese. Drizzle with extra-virgin olive oil, balsamic glaze, and sprinkle with salt and pepper for a refreshing and visually appealing dish.

Basil Infused Beverages:

- Infuse beverages like water, lemonade, or iced tea with basil for a refreshing twist. Add a few basil leaves to your favorite drink to enjoy its subtle, herbal flavor.

Tomato Basil Pasta:

- Prepare a simple yet flavorful tomato basil pasta by sautéing fresh tomatoes, garlic, and basil in olive oil. Toss with cooked pasta and finish with a sprinkle of Parmesan cheese for a quick and delicious meal.

Here are two delicious recipes that highlight the aromatic flavor of basil:

Caprese Salad with Basil Pesto Drizzle:

Ingredients:

- Fresh basil leaves
- Ripe tomatoes, sliced
- Fresh mozzarella cheese, sliced
- Extra-virgin olive oil
- Balsamic glaze
- Salt and pepper to taste
- Pine nuts (optional)
- Fresh basil pesto (homemade or store-bought)

Instructions:

1. Arrange slices of ripe tomatoes and fresh mozzarella cheese on a serving platter.
2. Tuck fresh basil leaves between the tomato and mozzarella slices.
3. Drizzle extra-virgin olive oil and balsamic glaze over the salad.
4. Season with salt and pepper to taste.
5. Optionally, sprinkle pine nuts over the salad for added crunch.
6. Finish by drizzling fresh basil pesto over the entire salad.
7. Serve immediately and enjoy this refreshing and flavorful Caprese Salad.

Tomato Basil Pasta:

Ingredients:

- Pasta of your choice
- Fresh tomatoes, diced
- Garlic, minced
- Fresh basil leaves, torn
- Extra-virgin olive oil
- Salt and black pepper to taste
- Grated Parmesan cheese

Instructions:

1. Cook the pasta according to package instructions. Reserve a cup of pasta water before draining.
2. In a pan, heat extra-virgin olive oil over medium heat. Add minced garlic and sauté until fragrant.
3. Add diced tomatoes to the pan and cook until they start to soften.
4. Toss in torn fresh basil leaves and continue cooking for a few minutes.
5. Season with salt and black pepper to taste.
6. Add the cooked pasta to the pan and toss to combine, adding a bit of reserved pasta water if needed.
7. Serve the tomato basil pasta hot, garnished with grated Parmesan cheese.

Enjoy this simple and flavorful pasta dish that showcases the essence of basil.

These recipes demonstrate the versatility of basil in both salads and pasta, adding a burst of freshness and herbal flavor to your meals. Feel free to adjust the quantities and ingredients based on your preferences.

Conclusion:

Basil's aromatic allure and culinary versatility make it a kitchen favorite, but its health benefits add an extra layer of appreciation. Whether you're savoring its flavor in a homemade pesto or enjoying the calming effects of a basil-infused tea, this herb is a true culinary and wellness companion. However, if you have any underlying health conditions, are pregnant, nursing, or taking medications, it's always a good idea to consult with a healthcare professional before making significant changes to your diet. Embrace the many dimensions of basil in your kitchen and discover the joy it brings to both your palate and your overall well-being.

Back to Table of Contents

Bay Leaves

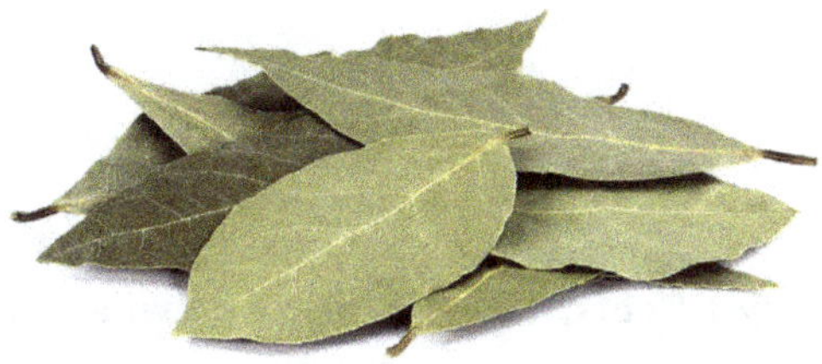

A Culinary Marvel with Health Benefits and Versatile Uses

Bay leaves, with their aromatic fragrance and distinctive flavor, are not just a staple in the culinary world but also harbor a range of health benefits. Derived from the bay laurel tree (Laurus nobilis), these leaves have been utilized for centuries in various cuisines and traditional remedies. In this article, we'll explore the benefits and versatile uses of bay leaves, showcasing their significance beyond their role as a flavorful seasoning.

Culinary Marvel:

Flavor Enhancer:

- Bay leaves are renowned for their ability to enhance the flavor of dishes. Whether used in soups, stews, sauces, or rice, the leaves impart a subtle, earthy taste that adds depth to the overall culinary experience.

Aromatic Presence:

- The aromatic oils present in bay leaves release a pleasant fragrance when exposed to heat, contributing to the overall aroma of cooked dishes. They are often used to infuse liquids, providing a fragrant backdrop to various recipes.

Staple in Spice Blends:

- Bay leaves are a key ingredient in many spice blends, such as bouquet garni and herbes de Provence. Their inclusion in these blends adds complexity to the flavor profile of a wide range of savory dishes.

Health Benefits:

Digestive Aid:

- Bay leaves contain compounds that have been associated with digestive benefits. They may help soothe indigestion, reduce bloating, and alleviate other digestive discomforts.

Anti-Inflammatory Properties:

- The presence of certain phytonutrients in bay leaves contributes to their anti-inflammatory properties. Consuming bay leaves may help reduce inflammation in the body, supporting overall health.

Bay leaves contain certain compounds that have been traditionally associated with potential anti-inflammatory properties, which may contribute to addressing joint pain. Some notable compounds in bay leaves are:

Cineole (Eucalyptol):

Benefits:

- **Anti-Inflammatory Effects:** Cineole, also known as eucalyptol, is a compound found in bay leaves known for its anti-inflammatory properties. It may help reduce inflammation, making it potentially beneficial for conditions involving joint pain or arthritis.
- **Analgesic (Pain-Relieving) Properties: Cineole** has been studied for its analgesic effects, suggesting that it may help alleviate pain. This property makes it relevant in addressing joint discomfort.

Linalool:

Benefits:

- **Anti-Inflammatory and Analgesic Properties:** Linalool, another compound present in bay leaves, has been associated with anti-inflammatory and analgesic effects. It may contribute to reducing inflammation and providing relief from pain, including joint pain.
- **Relaxant Effects:** Linalool is also known for its calming and relaxant properties, which can be beneficial for individuals experiencing muscle tension or joint discomfort.

Blood Sugar Regulation:

- Some studies suggest that compounds in bay leaves may help regulate blood sugar levels. While more research is needed, incorporating bay leaves into a balanced diet may have potential benefits for individuals managing blood sugar.

Rich in Antioxidants:

- Bay leaves contain antioxidants that help neutralize free radicals, reducing oxidative stress in the body. Antioxidants play a crucial role in supporting overall health and may contribute to disease prevention.

Versatile Uses:

Cooking Infusions:

- Bay leaves can be added to simmering liquids, such as soups, stews, and sauces, to infuse them with flavor. Remember to remove the bay leaves before serving, as they are generally not consumed whole.

Marinades and Pickling:

- Bay leaves are a fantastic addition to marinades for meats and pickling solutions for vegetables. Their aromatic qualities complement the preservation process, enhancing the overall taste.

Rice and Grain Dishes:

- Adding a bay leaf to rice or other grain dishes during cooking can impart a subtle, fragrant note. This simple addition elevates the dish without overwhelming the palate.

Herbal Teas:

- Bay leaves can be used to prepare herbal teas. Infuse dried bay leaves in hot water, allowing the natural oils and flavors to create a soothing and aromatic beverage.

Here are two classic recipes that feature the aromatic flavor of bay leaves:

Spaghetti Bolognese:

Ingredients:

- 1 lb ground beef
- 1 onion, finely chopped
- 2 carrots, grated
- 2 celery stalks, finely chopped
- 3 cloves garlic, minced
- 1 can (28 oz) crushed tomatoes
- 1/2 cup red wine (optional)
- 2 bay leaves
- 1 teaspoon dried oregano
- 1 teaspoon dried basil
- Salt and black pepper to taste
- Olive oil for cooking
- 1 lb spaghetti

Instructions:

1. In a large pot, heat olive oil over medium heat. Add chopped onion, grated carrots, and chopped celery. Cook until vegetables are softened.
2. Add minced garlic and ground beef. Cook until the beef is browned.
3. Pour in crushed tomatoes and red wine (if using). Stir in dried oregano, dried basil, bay leaves, salt, and black pepper.
4. Simmer the sauce for at least 30-40 minutes to allow the flavors to meld. Add more salt and pepper if needed.
5. Cook spaghetti according to package instructions. Drain.
6. Serve the Bolognese sauce over cooked spaghetti. Don't forget to remove the bay leaves before serving.

Classic Chicken Soup:

Ingredients:

- 1 whole chicken (about 4 lbs), giblets removed
- 1 onion, quartered
- 2 carrots, peeled and sliced
- 2 celery stalks, sliced
- 3 cloves garlic, smashed
- 2 bay leaves
- 1 teaspoon dried thyme
- Salt and black pepper to taste
- 8 cups water
- 1 cup egg noodles

Instructions:

1. Place the whole chicken in a large pot. Add quartered onion, sliced carrots, sliced celery, smashed garlic, bay leaves, dried thyme, salt, and black pepper.
2. Pour in 8 cups of water, or enough to cover the chicken and vegetables.
3. Bring the pot to a boil, then reduce the heat to simmer. Skim off any foam that rises to the surface.
4. Simmer for about 1.5 to 2 hours until the chicken is cooked through and the flavors have melded.
5. Remove the chicken from the pot and shred the meat. Discard bones and return shredded chicken to the pot.
6. Add egg noodles and cook until tender.
7. Adjust salt and pepper to taste and serve the comforting chicken soup with the aromatic essence of bay leaves.

These recipes showcase the versatility of bay leaves in enhancing the flavor of both meat-based and vegetable-based dishes. Remember to remove bay leaves before serving to prevent any bitterness. It's advisable to consult with healthcare professionals for personalized advice and guidance.

Historical Uses:

Medieval and Renaissance Medicine:

- During the medieval and Renaissance periods, bay leaves were a common ingredient in medicinal concoctions. They were believed to have various health benefits, including aiding digestion and alleviating respiratory issues. Bay leaves were often used in herbal remedies to create infusions or ointments for treating ailments such as indigestion, coughs, and joint pain. Their aromatic properties were also thought to have a positive impact on mental well-being.

Culinary Uses in Traditional Folk Medicine:

- Bay leaves have a rich history of use in traditional folk medicine, where they were believed to have digestive and anti-inflammatory properties. Infusions made from bay leaves were consumed to ease digestive discomforts and promote overall well-being. Additionally, bay leaves were included in various culinary preparations to enhance the flavor of dishes while potentially providing mild health benefits.

Conclusion:

Bay leaves are more than just a seasoning; they are a culinary marvel with a rich history and a range of health benefits. From enhancing the flavor of dishes to contributing to digestive health and beyond, bay leaves have rightfully earned their place in kitchens around the world. So, the next time you reach for these humble leaves, appreciate not just their aromatic contribution but also the potential benefits they bring to your culinary creations and well-being.

Back to Table of Contents

Beet Greens

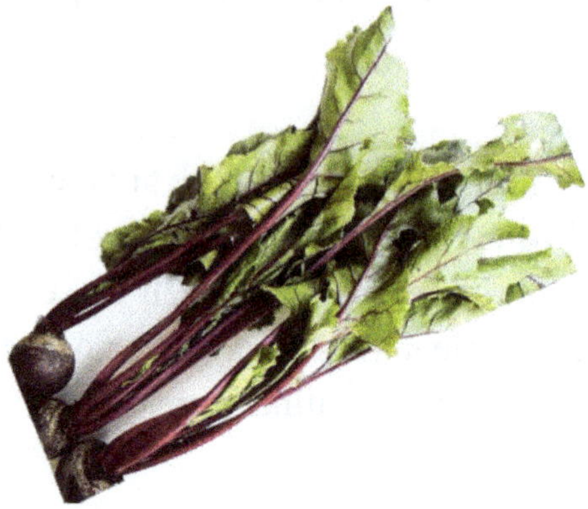

A Nutrient-Rich Gem Unveiled for Health and Culinary Delight

While beets often steal the spotlight with their vibrant color and earthy sweetness, the greens that crown these root vegetables are a nutritional powerhouse often overlooked. Beet greens, with their rich flavor and impressive nutrient profile, are not only delicious but also offer a myriad of health benefits. In this article, we'll explore the various advantages and creative uses that make beet greens a valuable addition to your diet.

Nutrient-Rich Composition:

Beet greens are a nutritional treasure trove, providing a wealth of essential vitamins, minerals, and antioxidants. Here's a closer look at the key components that make beet greens a nutritional gem:

Vitamins:

Vitamin K:

- Beet greens are particularly rich in vitamin K, which is essential for blood clotting and bone health.

Vitamin A:

- Beet greens contain beta-carotene, a precursor to vitamin A, which is important for vision, immune function, and skin health.

Vitamin C:

- A good source of vitamin C, beet greens provide this powerful antioxidant that supports the immune system and collagen synthesis.

Folate (Vitamin B9):

- Beet greens are rich in folate, a B-vitamin vital for DNA synthesis and cell division.

Vitamin E:

- While present in smaller amounts compared to some other vitamins, beet greens contribute to vitamin E intake, providing fat-soluble antioxidant benefits.

Vitamin B6 (Pyridoxine):

- Beet greens contain vitamin B6, which is important for the metabolism of amino acids and the synthesis of neurotransmitters.

Riboflavin (Vitamin B2):

- Beet greens provide riboflavin, a B-vitamin involved in energy production and the metabolism of fats.

Thiamine (Vitamin B1):

- Thiamine is found in beet greens and is essential for energy metabolism and nerve cell function.

Niacin (Vitamin B3):

- Beet greens contain niacin, a B-vitamin important for energy metabolism and the health of the nervous system.

Including beet greens in your diet can contribute to meeting your daily vitamin needs and provide a wide range of health benefits associated with these essential nutrients. As with any food, it's important to consume a variety of nutrient-rich foods to ensure a balanced intake of vitamins and other essential nutrients.

Minerals:

Beet greens are rich in various minerals, contributing to their nutritional value. Here is a list of minerals found in beet greens:

Calcium:

- Beet greens provide calcium, which is crucial for bone health, nerve function, and muscle contraction.

Iron:

- Iron is present in beet greens and is essential for the formation of hemoglobin, the protein responsible for carrying oxygen in the blood.

Potassium:

- Beet greens are a good source of potassium, an electrolyte that helps regulate fluid balance, nerve signals, and muscle contractions.

Magnesium:

- Magnesium in beet greens supports muscle and nerve function, regulates blood pressure, and contributes to bone health.

Phosphorus:

- Phosphorus is present in beet greens and is essential for bone and teeth formation, DNA synthesis, and energy metabolism.

Manganese:

- Manganese is a trace mineral found in beet greens, contributing to bone formation, blood clotting, and reducing inflammation.

Copper:

- Beet greens contain copper, which is essential for the formation of red blood cells, maintenance of healthy bones and nerves, and immune system function.

Zinc:

- Turnip greens contain zinc, a trace mineral that plays a role in immune function, wound healing, and DNA synthesis.

Including beet greens in your diet can help ensure a diverse intake of minerals, supporting various physiological functions and promoting overall health. As with any food, it's important to consume a variety of nutrient-rich foods to ensure a broad spectrum of minerals and other essential nutrients.

Antioxidants:

Beet greens contain various antioxidants, including beta-carotene, lutein, and zeaxanthin, which help combat oxidative stress and reduce inflammation.

Beta-Carotene:

- A precursor to vitamin A, beta-carotene is a powerful antioxidant found in beet greens. It contributes to eye health and overall antioxidant defense.

Lutein:

- Beet greens are rich in lutein, a carotenoid known for its role in maintaining eye health and preventing age-related macular degeneration.

Zeaxanthin:

- Zeaxanthin, another carotenoid found in beet greens, works alongside lutein to support eye health and protect against oxidative damage.

Quercetin:

- Quercetin is a flavonoid with antioxidant and anti-inflammatory properties. It is found in beet greens and may help reduce inflammation and lower the risk of chronic diseases.

Kaempferol:

- Kaempferol is a flavonoid present in beet greens, contributing to their antioxidant and anti-inflammatory effects.

Vitamin E:

- While present in smaller amounts compared to some other antioxidants, beet greens contribute to vitamin E intake, providing fat-soluble antioxidant benefits.

Selenium:

- Beet greens contain selenium, a trace mineral with antioxidant properties that work in conjunction with other antioxidants to protect cells from oxidative stress.

Including beet greens in your diet can help enhance your intake of these antioxidants, supporting overall health and potentially reducing the risk of chronic diseases associated with oxidative damage. As always, incorporating a variety of antioxidant-rich foods into your diet is essential for optimal health benefits.

Dietary Fiber:

- A rich source of dietary fiber, beet greens promote digestive health, regulate blood sugar levels, and contribute to a feeling of fullness.

Health Benefits:

Heart Health:

- The potassium, magnesium, and dietary fiber in beet greens contribute to heart health by regulating blood pressure, reducing cholesterol levels, and supporting overall cardiovascular function.

Bone Health:

- The combination of vitamin K and calcium in beet greens supports bone health, aiding in bone density and strength.

Anti-Inflammatory Properties:

- The antioxidants in beet greens help combat inflammation, potentially reducing the risk of chronic diseases.

Vision Support:

- Lutein and zeaxanthin in beet greens play a role in maintaining eye health and may reduce the risk of age-related macular degeneration.

Nutritional Content

In 1 cup (approximately 38 grams) of cooked beet greens, the approximate nutritional content is as follows:

- Carbohydrates: Approximately 3.7 grams
- Protein: Approximately 2.2 grams
- Fiber: Approximately 2.2 grams
- Fat: Approximately 0.2 grams

These values may vary slightly depending on factors such as the specific cooking method and the maturity of the beet greens.

Culinary Uses:

Sautéed Beet Greens:

- Sauté beet greens with garlic and olive oil for a quick and flavorful side dish.

Beet Green Pesto:

- Create a vibrant pesto by blending beet greens with nuts, garlic, Parmesan cheese, and olive oil. Use it as a pasta sauce or a spread.

Smoothies:

- Add beet greens to your favorite smoothie for a nutrient-packed boost. Pair them with fruits for a delicious and vibrant blend.

Salads:

- Incorporate raw or lightly steamed beet greens into salads for added color, flavor, and nutritional value.

Beet greens are not only nutritious but also versatile in the kitchen. Here are two delicious recipes that make the most of beet greens:

Sautéed Beet Greens with Garlic and Lemon:

Ingredients:

- 1 bunch of fresh beet greens, washed and chopped
- 2 tablespoons olive oil
- 3 cloves garlic, minced
- 1 tablespoon lemon juice
- Salt and pepper to taste
- Red pepper flakes (optional)

Instructions:

1. Heat olive oil in a large pan over medium heat.
2. Add minced garlic and sauté for 1-2 minutes until fragrant.
3. Add chopped beet greens to the pan and toss to coat them with the garlic-infused oil.
4. Sauté the greens for 3-5 minutes or until they are wilted and tender.
5. Drizzle lemon juice over the greens and season with salt and pepper to taste.
6. Optional: Add a pinch of red pepper flakes for a hint of heat.
7. Toss the greens once more to evenly distribute the flavors.
8. Serve the sautéed beet greens as a side dish or over rice for a simple and nutritious meal.

Beet Greens and Feta Tart:

Ingredients:

- 1 sheet of puff pastry, thawed
- 1 bunch of fresh beet greens, washed and chopped
- 1 cup crumbled feta cheese
- 1/4 cup pine nuts
- 2 tablespoons olive oil
- Salt and pepper to taste
- 1 egg (for egg wash)

Instructions:

1. Preheat the oven to the temperature specified on the puff pastry package.
2. Roll out the puff pastry on a baking sheet lined with parchment paper.
3. In a pan, sauté the chopped beet greens in olive oil until wilted. Season with salt and pepper.
4. Spread the sautéed beet greens evenly over the puff pastry.
5. Sprinkle crumbled feta cheese and pine nuts over the beet greens.
6. Fold the edges of the puff pastry slightly to create a rustic tart.

7. Beat the egg and brush it over the edges of the puff pastry for a golden finish.
8. Bake in the preheated oven according to the puff pastry package instructions or until the tart is golden brown and puffed.
9. Allow the tart to cool slightly before slicing and serving.

These recipes showcase the delicious and nutritious qualities of beet greens, whether sautéed as a side dish or used as a flavorful topping in a savory tart. Enjoy the vibrant flavors and health benefits that beet greens bring to your table!

Conclusion:

Beet greens, often relegated to the sidelines, are a nutritional powerhouse that deserves a prime spot on your plate. Whether sautéed, blended into pesto, tossed into salads, or added to smoothies, beet greens offer a delicious and nutritious way to enhance your culinary creations. If you have specific health concerns, allergies, or conditions, it's advisable to consult with a healthcare professional or a registered dietitian before making significant changes to your diet.

Embrace the vibrant flavors and health benefits that beet greens bring to your meals and let this often-overlooked green shine in both your kitchen and your well-balanced diet.

Back to Table of Contents

Beet Root

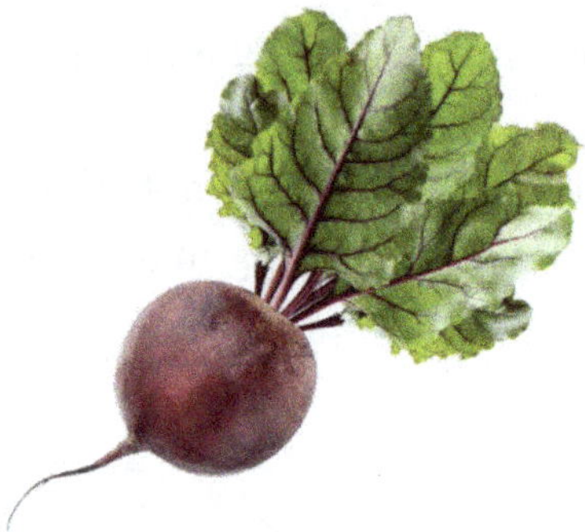

The Nutritional Powerhouse: Exploring the Benefits and Uses of Beets

Beets, with their vibrant hues and earthy flavor, have emerged as nutritional powerhouses that offer a plethora of health benefits. These versatile root vegetables are not only delicious but also packed with essential nutrients that contribute to overall well-being. In this article, we delve into the myriad benefits and diverse uses of beets.

Nutrient-Rich Profile:

One of the key reasons behind the growing popularity of beets is their impressive nutritional content. Rich in vitamins, minerals, and antioxidants, beets provide a nutrient boost that supports various aspects of health. They are a good source of folate, potassium, vitamin C, and fiber, making them a valuable addition to a balanced diet.

Folate:

- ***Benefit:*** Folate, also known as vitamin B9, plays a crucial role in DNA synthesis and repair. It is especially important during periods of rapid cell division and growth, making it essential for pregnant women to prevent neural tube defects in developing fetuses. Folate also supports overall cell function and contributes to a healthy cardiovascular system.

Potassium:

- ***Benefit:*** Beets are rich in potassium, a crucial mineral for maintaining proper electrolyte balance, helps regulate blood pressure, supports cardiovascular health, and plays a role in muscle and nerve function. Adequate potassium intake is associated with a lower risk of hypertension and cardiovascular diseases.

  By balancing sodium levels in the body, potassium supports proper fluid balance and helps prevent the negative effects of high blood pressure on the heart and arteries.

Manganese:

- ***Benefit:*** Manganese is an essential trace mineral found in beets that plays a role in bone formation, blood clotting, and reducing inflammation. It is a cofactor for various enzymes involved in metabolism and antioxidant defense. Manganese also contributes to the formation of connective tissues and supports overall bone health.

Iron:

- ***Benefit:*** Beets contain iron, a vital mineral necessary for the production of hemoglobin, the protein responsible for transporting oxygen in the blood. Iron is crucial for preventing iron-deficiency anemia, fatigue, and supporting overall energy levels. While the iron in beets is non-heme iron (plant-based), consuming vitamin C-rich foods alongside beets can enhance iron absorption.

Magnesium:

- ***Benefit:*** Magnesium is involved in over 300 biochemical reactions in the body, and beets provide a modest amount of this essential mineral. Magnesium supports muscle and nerve function, helps regulate blood sugar levels, and contributes to bone health. It also plays a role in energy metabolism and supports the body's stress response. Consuming magnesium-rich foods like beets is essential for maintaining overall health and well-being.

Vitamin C:

- ***Benefit:*** Vitamin C is a powerful antioxidant that helps protect cells from damage caused by free radicals. It plays a crucial role in collagen synthesis, promoting skin health and wound healing. Additionally, vitamin C enhances the absorption of non-heme iron (plant-based iron) from foods, supporting the body's ability to maintain healthy iron levels.

Dietary Fiber:

- ***Benefit:*** Beets are an excellent source of dietary fiber, which is essential for digestive health. Fiber adds bulk to stool, promoting regular bowel movements and preventing constipation. It also supports the growth of beneficial gut bacteria, contributing to a healthy and balanced gut microbiome. A high-fiber diet is associated with a lower risk of various digestive issues, including colorectal cancer.

Heart Health:

Beets have been associated with heart health, thanks to their high potassium content. Potassium plays a crucial role in regulating blood pressure, and including beets in your diet may contribute to cardiovascular well-being. Additionally, the nitrates found in beets are converted into nitric oxide in the body, which helps dilate blood vessels, improving blood flow and reducing the risk of heart-related issues.

Enhanced Exercise Performance:

The nitrate content in beets has been linked to improved exercise performance. Athletes and fitness enthusiasts often turn to beet juice or beet supplements to enhance endurance and stamina. The increased nitric oxide levels support efficient oxygen delivery to muscles, reducing fatigue and enhancing overall physical performance.

Digestive Health:

Beets are an excellent source of dietary fiber, promoting digestive health. Fiber aids in regular bowel movements, preventing constipation and supporting a healthy gut. Including beets in your diet can contribute to a well-functioning digestive system and may help prevent digestive issues.

Detoxification and Liver Support:

The betalains present in beets are potent antioxidants known for their detoxifying properties. These compounds support the body's natural detoxification processes, particularly in the liver. Regular consumption of beets may help flush out toxins and promote liver health.

Nutritional Content

In 1 cup (approximately 136 grams) of cooked beetroot, the approximate nutritional content is as follows:

- Carbohydrates: Approximately 13 grams
- Protein: Approximately 2.5 grams
- Fiber: Approximately 3.8 grams
- Fat: Approximately 0.2 grams

Please note that these values are approximate and can vary slightly based on factors such as the size of the beetroot and how it is prepared.

Versatile Culinary Uses:

Beyond their health benefits, beets are incredibly versatile in the kitchen. They can be enjoyed in various forms, such as roasted, boiled, steamed, or raw. Beets add vibrant color and a sweet, earthy flavor to salads, soups, and side dishes. They can also be juiced for a refreshing and nutrient-packed beverage.

Roasted Beets:

- ***Preparation:*** Preheat the oven to 400°F (200°C). Wash and peel the beets, then cut them into cubes or wedges. Toss the beets with olive oil, salt, and pepper. Spread them in a single layer on a baking sheet and roast for about 30-40 minutes or until tender. Roasted beets develop a sweet and caramelized flavor, making them a delightful side dish or salad ingredient.

Beet Salad:

- ***Preparation:*** Grate or thinly slice raw beets and combine them with your favorite salad greens. Add ingredients like goat cheese, walnuts, and a light vinaigrette for a refreshing beet salad. You can also roast or steam beets before adding them to the salad for a different texture and flavor profile. This salad is not only nutritious but also visually appealing with the vibrant colors of the beets.

Beet Soup (Borscht):

- ***Preparation:*** Borscht is a traditional Eastern European soup that prominently features beets. To prepare, sauté onions, carrots, and celery in a pot. Add diced beets, vegetable or beef broth, and season with salt, pepper, and herbs like dill. Simmer until the beets are tender, and flavors meld together. Borscht can be served hot or cold and is often garnished with sour cream for added richness.

Pickled Beets:

- ***Preparation:*** Pickling beets is a great way to preserve them and enhance their tangy flavor. Boil whole or sliced beets until tender. In a separate pot, combine vinegar, sugar, salt, and spices (such as cloves or cinnamon). Place the beets in sterilized jars and pour the pickling liquid over them. Seal the jars and refrigerate for a few days to allow the flavors to develop. Pickled beets make a tasty addition to salads, sandwiches, or as a side dish.

Beet Juice:

- **Preparation:** To make refreshing beet juice, start by washing and peeling the beets. Cut them into smaller pieces for easier blending. Use a juicer or a high-powered blender to extract the juice from the beets. You may also add other complementary ingredients like apples, carrots, lime or ginger for added flavor. Strain the juice to remove any pulp if desired. Serve the beet juice over ice for a cool and hydrating beverage. This vibrant drink not only quenches your thirst but also provides a nutrient-packed boost, thanks to the goodness of beets.

Conclusion:

Incorporating beets into your diet can be a flavorful and health-conscious choice. Whether you savor them for their nutritional benefits or appreciate their versatility in the kitchen, beets stand out as a valuable addition to a well-balanced and wholesome lifestyle. From supporting heart health to enhancing exercise performance, the humble beet has earned its place as a nutritional powerhouse that deserves a spot on your plate.

If you have specific health concerns, allergies, or conditions, it's advisable to consult with a healthcare professional or a registered dietitian before making significant changes to your diet.

Back to Table of Contents

Bell Peppers

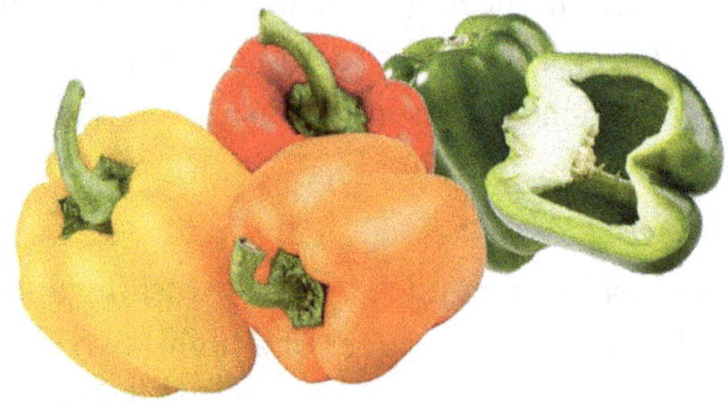

The Vibrant and Nutrient-Packed Bell Pepper: Benefits and Uses

Bell peppers, with their vibrant colors and crisp texture, are not just a feast for the eyes but also a nutritional powerhouse. Belonging to the Capsicum annuum species, bell peppers come in various colors, including green, red, yellow, and orange. These versatile vegetables offer a wide array of health benefits and culinary uses, making them a staple in kitchens around the world.

Nutritional Profile:

Bell peppers are rich in essential nutrients, making them a valuable addition to a healthy diet. They are an excellent source of vitamin C, providing more than twice the daily recommended intake in just one cup of chopped peppers. Additionally, bell peppers are low in calories but high in fiber, vitamins A and K, and various antioxidants. The combination of these nutrients contributes to the numerous health benefits associated with bell pepper consumption.

Health Benefits:

High in Vitamin C:

Bell peppers are renowned for their exceptionally high vitamin C content, which plays a crucial role in boosting the immune system, promoting skin health, and supporting overall well-being.

Vitamin C:

- **Benefits:**
    - Boosts the immune system.
    - Promotes healthy skin by aiding collagen synthesis.
    - Acts as an antioxidant, protecting cells from damage.
    - Supports the absorption of iron from plant-based foods.

Vitamin A:

- **Benefits:**
    - Essential for maintaining healthy vision.
    - Supports immune function.

- Contributes to the health of skin and mucous membranes.
- Plays a role in the proper functioning of the heart, lungs, and kidneys.

Vitamin K:

- **Benefits:**
  - Essential for blood clotting, preventing excessive bleeding.
  - Supports bone health by aiding in calcium absorption and bone mineralization.
  - Contributes to heart health by preventing arterial calcification.

Vitamin B6 (Pyridoxine):

- **Benefits:**
  - Supports brain development and function.
  - Aids in the production of neurotransmitters, such as serotonin and norepinephrine.
  - Plays a role in the metabolism of proteins, carbohydrates, and fats.
  - Supports the immune system.

Minerals:

Potassium:

- **Benefits:**
  - Helps regulate fluid balance in the body.
  - Supports proper muscle and nerve function.
  - Plays a role in maintaining healthy blood pressure.
  - Aids in the balance of electrolytes.

Magnesium:

- **Benefits:**
  - Supports muscle and nerve function.
  - Contributes to bone health by aiding in calcium absorption.
  - Plays a role in energy metabolism.
  - Helps regulate blood sugar levels.

Manganese:

- **Benefits:**
  - Acts as a cofactor for various enzymes involved in metabolism.
  - Contributes to the formation of connective tissues, bones, and blood clotting factors.
  - Plays a role in antioxidant defense.

Rich in Antioxidants:

The vibrant colors of bell peppers signify the presence of potent antioxidants, such as carotenoids and flavonoids. These antioxidants help neutralize free radicals in the body, reducing the risk of chronic diseases.

Here are some antioxidants found in bell peppers and their benefits:

Capsanthin:

- **Benefits:**
    - Acts as a powerful antioxidant, protecting cells from oxidative stress.
    - Contributes to the vibrant red color of red bell peppers.
    - May have potential anti-inflammatory properties.

Quercetin:

- **Benefits:**
    - Exhibits anti-inflammatory and antioxidant properties.
    - Supports cardiovascular health by helping to lower blood pressure and reduce inflammation.
    - May have anti-allergic and anti-cancer effects.

Luteolin:

- **Benefits:**
    - Acts as an antioxidant with potential anti-inflammatory properties.
    - May have neuroprotective effects, supporting brain health.
    - Exhibits anti-cancer properties and may inhibit the growth of certain cancer cells.

Heart Health:

The fiber, potassium, and folate found in bell peppers contribute to heart health by supporting healthy blood pressure levels and reducing the risk of cardiovascular diseases.

Eye Health:

Bell peppers are a good source of zeaxanthin and lutein, antioxidants known to promote eye health by protecting against age-related macular degeneration and other vision issues.

Weight Management:

With their low-calorie and high-fiber content, bell peppers can be a valuable ally in weight management. The fiber helps promote satiety, making it easier to maintain a healthy weight.

Nutritional Content

In 1 cup (approximately 149 grams) of raw bell pepper, the approximate nutritional content is as follows:

- Carbohydrates: Approximately 9 grams
- Protein: Approximately 1 gram
- Fiber: Approximately 3 grams
- Fat: Approximately 0.5 grams

Please note that these values are approximate and can vary slightly based on factors such as the specific variety of bell pepper and its size.

Culinary Uses:

Raw Snack: Enjoy bell peppers in their raw form as a crunchy and flavorful snack. Simply slice them into strips and dip them in hummus or your favorite healthy dip.

Salads and Salsas: Bell peppers add color, crunch, and a sweet flavor to salads and salsas. Mix them with other fresh vegetables, greens, and a light dressing for a nutritious and delicious meal.

Stir-Fries and Sautes: Incorporate bell peppers into stir-fries and sautés to enhance the taste and nutritional content of your dishes. Their versatility allows them to pair well with a variety of proteins and other vegetables.

Stuffed Peppers: Create a wholesome meal by stuffing bell peppers with a mixture of lean protein, whole grains, and flavorful spices. Baking or grilling stuffed peppers results in a satisfying and nutritious dish.

Roasted or Grilled: Roasting or grilling bell peppers intensifies their natural sweetness and imparts a smoky flavor. Use them as a side dish, in sandwiches, or as a topping for pizzas and pastas.

Here are two delicious and versatile recipes that make excellent use of bell peppers:

Stuffed Bell Peppers

Ingredients:

- 4 large bell peppers (any color)
- 1 pound lean ground turkey or beef
- 1 cup cooked quinoa or rice
- 1 cup black beans, drained and rinsed
- 1 cup corn kernels (fresh or frozen)
- 1 cup diced tomatoes
- 1 cup shredded cheese (cheddar or Mexican blend)
- 1 tablespoon olive oil
- 1 teaspoon cumin
- 1 teaspoon chili powder
- 1 teaspoon garlic powder
- Salt and pepper to taste
- Fresh cilantro for garnish

Instructions:

1. Preheat the oven to 375°F (190°C).
2. Cut the tops off the bell peppers and remove the seeds and membranes.
3. In a skillet, heat olive oil over medium heat. Add ground turkey or beef, and cook until browned.
4. Add cumin, chili powder, garlic powder, salt, and pepper to the meat.

5. In a large bowl, combine the cooked meat, cooked quinoa or rice, black beans, corn, diced tomatoes, and half of the shredded cheese. Mix well.
6. Stuff each bell pepper with the mixture and place them in a baking dish.
7. Top each stuffed pepper with the remaining cheese.
8. Bake in the preheated oven for 25-30 minutes or until the peppers are tender.
9. Garnish with fresh cilantro before serving.

Bell Pepper and Chickpea Salad

Ingredients:

- 2 bell peppers (mix of colors), diced
- 1 can (15 oz) chickpeas, drained and rinsed
- 1 cucumber, diced
- 1 cup cherry tomatoes, halved
- 1/2 red onion, finely chopped
- 1/4 cup feta cheese, crumbled
- 1/4 cup Kalamata olives, sliced
- 2 tablespoons extra-virgin olive oil
- 1 tablespoon red wine vinegar
- 1 teaspoon dried oregano
- Salt and pepper to taste
- Fresh parsley for garnish

Instructions:

1. In a large bowl, combine diced bell peppers, chickpeas, cucumber, cherry tomatoes, red onion, feta cheese, and Kalamata olives.
2. In a small bowl, whisk together olive oil, red wine vinegar, dried oregano, salt, and pepper to create the dressing.
3. Pour the dressing over the salad and toss until all ingredients are well coated.
4. Refrigerate the salad for at least 30 minutes to let the flavors meld.
5. Garnish with fresh parsley before serving.

These recipes showcase the versatility of bell peppers, whether used as a vessel for a hearty stuffing or as a colorful addition to a refreshing salad. Enjoy these dishes as a main course or a side, and feel free to customize the ingredients to suit your taste preferences.

Conclusion:

Bell peppers are more than just a colorful addition to your plate – they are a nutritional powerhouse offering a wide array of health benefits. With their high vitamin C content, antioxidants, and versatility in the kitchen, bell peppers are a fantastic choice for those looking to enhance both the flavor and nutrition of their meals. Additionally, individuals with known allergies or sensitivities should exercise caution and seek guidance from a medical professional. Whether enjoyed raw as a snack, tossed in salads, or incorporated into various cooked dishes, bell peppers are a delicious and nutritious option that can easily become a staple in a balanced and wholesome diet.

Back to Table of Contents

Bergamot

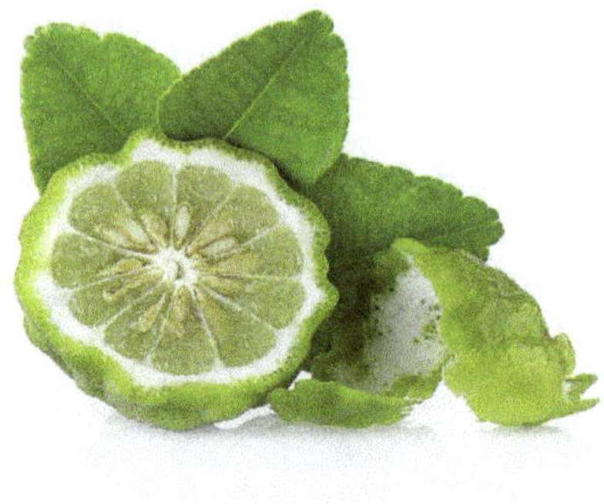

The Versatile Bergamot Plant: Benefits and Uses

The Bergamot plant, scientifically known as Citrus bergamia, is a fragrant and versatile plant that has been cherished for centuries for its various benefits and uses. Native to Southeast Asia, Bergamot is now cultivated in several regions around the world, with Italy being a prominent producer. This article explores the numerous advantages and applications of the Bergamot plant.

Aromatic Delight:

One of the most well-known features of the Bergamot plant is its distinctive citrusy fragrance. The essential oil extracted from Bergamot is widely used in the perfume industry, adding a refreshing and uplifting scent to many popular fragrances. The oil's unique aroma also makes it a key ingredient in aromatherapy, promoting relaxation and stress relief.

Culinary Marvel:

Beyond its aromatic properties, Bergamot is also valued in the culinary world. The peel of the Bergamot fruit is used to extract an oil that is a crucial component in the production of Earl Grey tea. The oil imparts a distinct citrus flavor to the tea, creating a delightful and popular beverage enjoyed worldwide.

Bergamot Tea:

- *Process:* Dried or fresh bergamot peel can be used to make flavorful and aromatic tea. Simply steep the peel in hot water, and you can add other herbs or tea leaves for a customized blend.
- *Usage:* Bergamot tea is known for its pleasant citrusy aroma and potential health benefits. It can be enjoyed hot or iced, and some people add honey or sweeteners for added flavor.

Bergamot Zest:

- *Process:* The zest of bergamot, which is the outer colored part of the peel, can be grated or peeled from the fruit.
- *Usage:* Bergamot zest is a versatile ingredient used in both sweet and savory dishes. It adds a distinctive citrus flavor to recipes such as desserts, salads, marinades, and sauces.

Bergamot Essential Oil:

- *Process:* Bergamot essential oil is extracted from the peel of the fruit. It is important to use food-grade, pure essential oil for culinary purposes.
- *Usage:* A drop or two of bergamot essential oil can be added to recipes for a concentrated citrus flavor. It is commonly used in baking, dressings, and beverages. Note that essential oils are potent, so a small amount goes a long way.

Bergamot Marmalade:

- *Process:* The peel of bergamot can be used to make marmalade by cooking it with sugar and water.
- *Usage:* Bergamot marmalade is a delightful spread that can be enjoyed on toast, pastries, or used as a topping for desserts. Its tangy and citrusy flavor adds a unique twist to traditional marmalades.

These preparation methods showcase the versatility of bergamot in culinary applications, allowing it to be used in various forms to enhance the flavor of a wide range of dishes and beverages. Whether you prefer the zest, tea, essential oil, or marmalade, bergamot brings a delightful citrusy aroma and taste to your culinary creations.

Health Benefits:

Bergamot is rich in beneficial compounds that contribute to its numerous health benefits. The plant contains flavonoids, polyphenols, and essential oils that have antioxidant and anti-inflammatory properties. These properties make Bergamot a potential ally in promoting cardiovascular health, reducing cholesterol levels, and supporting overall well-being.

Bergamot Essential Oil (BEO):

- *Compound:* Bergamot essential oil contains compounds such as limonene, linalool, and citral.
- *Benefits:*
    - **Aromatherapy:** The aroma of bergamot essential oil is known for its calming and uplifting effects, making it a popular choice in aromatherapy for stress reduction.
    - **Antioxidant Properties:** Limonene, a major component of bergamot essential oil, exhibits antioxidant properties, which may help neutralize free radicals in the body.

Flavonoids:

- *Compound:* Bergamot is rich in flavonoids, including neoeriocitrin, naringin, and rutin.
- *Benefits:*
  - **Cardiovascular Health:** Flavonoids have been associated with cardiovascular benefits, including potential improvements in blood vessel function and reduction of oxidative stress.

Bergamottin:

- *Compound:* Bergamottin is a furanocoumarin compound found in bergamot.
- *Benefits:*
  - **Cholesterol Regulation:** Some studies suggest that bergamottin may have cholesterol-lowering properties, making it potentially beneficial for heart health.

Polyphenols:

- *Compound:* Bergamot contains various polyphenols, including hesperidin.
- *Benefits:*
  - **Antioxidant and Anti-Inflammatory Effects:** Polyphenols, including hesperidin, possess antioxidant and anti-inflammatory properties, which may contribute to overall health by reducing oxidative stress and inflammation.

Skin Care Wonder:

The essential oil extracted from Bergamot is a common ingredient in skincare products due to its antibacterial and antifungal properties. It is known to help with acne-prone skin, balance oil production, and promote a clear complexion. Additionally, Bergamot oil is often used in massage oils and creams for its soothing effects on the skin.

Stress Relief and Anxiety Reduction:

Bergamot essential oil is renowned for its ability to alleviate stress and anxiety. Aromatherapists often use Bergamot oil to create a calming atmosphere, helping individuals relax and unwind. Its uplifting scent is believed to positively impact mood and emotional well-being.

Natural Insect Repellent:

Bergamot oil is a natural insect repellent, making it an eco-friendly alternative to chemical-based repellents. Its pleasant fragrance masks human scent, deterring mosquitoes and other insects. This makes Bergamot an excellent addition to natural insect repellent formulations.

Conclusion: The Bergamot plant is a true gem with a wide range of benefits and uses. From its aromatic allure to its contributions in the culinary, health, and skincare realms, Bergamot continues to captivate and enrich our lives. Whether enjoyed in a cup of Earl Grey tea, diffused in an aromatherapy session, or applied to the skin for its skincare benefits. Additionally, individual responses may vary, and it's advisable to consult with healthcare professionals before making significant changes to one's diet or lifestyle based on specific compounds in foods. Bergamot remains a versatile and cherished plant with a long history of global appreciation.

Back to Table of Contents

Bissy / Kola Nuts

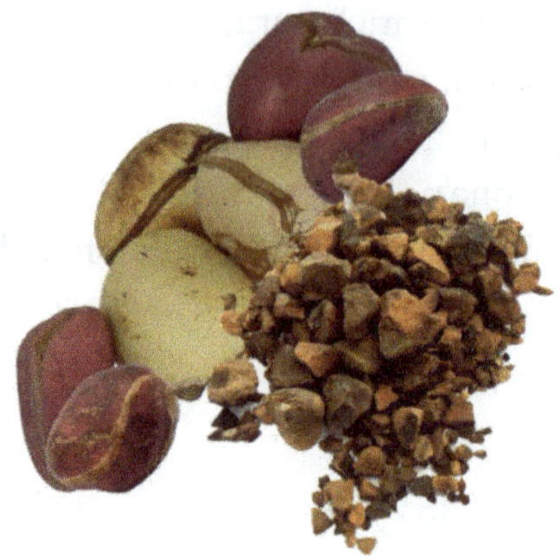

Exploring the Health Benefits and Cultural Significance of Kola Nuts (Bissy)

Kola nuts, commonly known as Bissy, have a rich history and cultural significance in various parts of the world, particularly in West Africa. These nuts come from the evergreen kola tree (Cola spp.) and have been utilized for centuries due to their unique flavor, stimulating properties, and numerous health benefits. In this article, we will delve into the nutritional content, health advantages, and cultural uses of Kola nuts.

Nutritional Profile:

Kola nuts are packed with essential nutrients that contribute to their popularity as a dietary supplement. These nuts contain caffeine, theobromine, tannins, and various phytochemicals. The combination of these compounds gives Kola nuts their stimulating effects, making them a natural source of energy.

Caffeine:

- **Benefits:** Caffeine is a natural stimulant that can enhance alertness, improve mood, and boost energy levels. It stimulates the central nervous system, promoting wakefulness and reducing the perception of fatigue. Additionally, caffeine may improve cognitive functions such as concentration and memory.

Theobromine:

- **Benefits:** Theobromine is a stimulant that belongs to the same family as caffeine. It has a milder stimulating effect and is known for its vasodilatory properties, which can help in improving blood flow. Theobromine may also have mild diuretic effects and is believed to contribute to the overall mood-enhancing properties of Kola nuts.

Tannins:

- **Benefits:** Tannins are polyphenolic compounds with antioxidant properties. They help neutralize free radicals in the body, protecting cells from oxidative stress. In addition to their antioxidant effects, tannins may have anti-inflammatory properties and are often associated with digestive benefits, such as reducing inflammation in the gastrointestinal tract.

- **Alleviation of Poisoning:** Tannins are known for their astringent properties, which may contribute to the binding and precipitation of certain toxic substances. In cases of poisoning, tannins are believed to help by binding to toxins and preventing their absorption or facilitating their elimination from the body.

Phytochemicals:

- **Benefits:** Kola nuts contain various phytochemicals, including alkaloids and flavonoids. These compounds contribute to the overall antioxidant and anti-inflammatory effects of Kola nuts. Phytochemicals play a role in supporting the body's immune system and may have protective effects against certain chronic diseases.

Health Benefits:

Energy Boost: The caffeine content in Kola nuts provides a natural energy boost, making them a popular choice in traditional medicine for combating fatigue and enhancing alertness.

Weight Management: The stimulating properties of Kola nuts may aid in weight management by increasing metabolic rate and promoting the breakdown of fats. However, moderation is key, as excessive consumption may lead to undesirable side effects.

Antioxidant Properties: Kola nuts are rich in tannins, which exhibit antioxidant properties. Antioxidants help neutralize free radicals in the body, protecting cells from damage and reducing the risk of chronic diseases.

Digestive Aid: Traditionally, Kola nuts have been used to alleviate digestive issues. The tannins present in the nuts may have anti-inflammatory effects on the digestive tract.

Culinary Uses:

Chewing:

- In many cultures, especially in West Africa, it is common to chew Kola nuts directly. The nuts are often broken into smaller pieces, and individuals chew them to extract the stimulating compounds, including caffeine. Chewing Kola nuts is a traditional practice and is often associated with social gatherings.

Powdered Form:

- Kola nuts can be ground into a fine powder, which can then be incorporated into various culinary dishes or used as a supplement. The powdered form allows for versatile usage, such as adding it to smoothies, energy bars, or even using it as a seasoning in certain recipes. This method provides a convenient way to include Kola nuts in the diet.

Infusion/Tea:

- Kola nuts can be used to prepare a beverage by infusing them in hot water. The infusion, often referred to as Kola nut tea, is made by steeping crushed or powdered Kola nuts in hot water. The resulting beverage is then strained and can be consumed as a warm or cold drink. This method allows for a milder consumption of the stimulating compounds found in Kola nuts.

While there may not be a standardized recipe for Jamaican Bissy tea, the preparation often involves a simple infusion of crushed or powdered Bissy nuts in hot water.

Here is my basic recipe for making Jamaican Bissy tea:

Jamaican Bissy Tea

Ingredients:

- 1 to 2 pieces of Bissy nuts (Kola Nuts), crushed or powdered.
- 2 cups of water
- Optional: Sweetener (sugar, honey, evaporated milk or sweet milk) to taste, vanilla, nutmeg and cinnamon leaf or powder.

Instructions:

1. **Prepare the Bissy Nuts:**
    - If using whole Bissy nuts, crush them into smaller pieces using a mortar and pestle or another suitable tool. Alternatively, if you have powdered Bissy, measure out the desired amount.
2. **Boil Water:**
    - In a pot or kettle, bring 2 cups of water to a boil. (With cinnamon leaf if desire).
3. **Add Bissy Nuts:**
    - Once the water is boiling, add the crushed or powdered Bissy nuts to the pot. Stir to ensure that the Bissy is well-distributed in the water.
4. **Steep:**
    - Reduce the heat to a simmer and let the Bissy nuts steep in the hot water for about 10 to 15 minutes. This allows the bioactive compounds in the nuts to infuse into the water.
    - If desired, add evaporated milk, nutmeg and vanilla extract.
5. **Strain:**
    - After steeping, strain the Bissy tea to remove any solid particles. You can use a fine mesh strainer or cheesecloth for this step.
6. **Optional Sweetening:**
    - If desired, add sweetener such as sugar, sweet milk or honey to taste. Stir well to dissolve the sweetener.
7. **Serve:**

- Pour the Bissy tea into cups and serve it hot. Alternatively, you can let it cool and serve it over ice for a refreshing cold beverage.

It's important to note that the taste of Bissy tea can be somewhat bitter, and the addition of sweetener can help balance the flavor. Additionally, individual preferences may vary, so you can adjust the quantity of Bissy nuts and steeping time according to your taste preferences.

Cultural Uses:

Social and Ceremonial: Kola nuts hold immense cultural significance in many African societies. They are often presented as a gesture of hospitality during social gatherings and ceremonies. Breaking and sharing Kola nuts symbolize unity, friendship, and mutual respect.

Traditional Medicine: In traditional medicine practices, Kola nuts are used to treat various ailments, including headaches, migraines, and respiratory conditions. The stimulating properties are believed to improve mental clarity and focus.

Rituals and Spirituality: In some cultures, Kola nuts are used in religious and spiritual ceremonies. The nuts are considered sacred and are believed to have divine qualities.

Conclusion:

Kola nuts, known as Bissy, are not only a flavorful addition to traditional cuisines but also a source of various health benefits. From providing a natural energy boost to being deeply ingrained in cultural practices, these nuts have stood the test of time. However, it's essential to consume them in moderation to reap the benefits without experiencing adverse effects. As with any natural remedy, consulting with a healthcare professional is recommended, particularly for individuals with pre-existing health conditions or sensitivities. As we continue to explore the world of natural remedies, Kola nuts remain a fascinating and multifaceted element in the tapestry of global traditions and well-being.

Back to Table of Contents

Black Beans

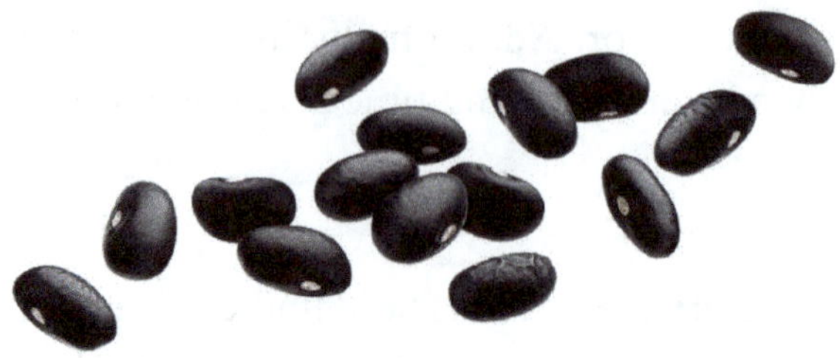

A Nutrient-Rich Superfood with Health Benefits

Black beans, a staple in many cuisines worldwide, are not only delicious but also pack a nutritional punch. These legumes, also known as turtle beans, boast a rich flavor and a velvety texture that makes them a versatile ingredient in a variety of dishes. Beyond their culinary appeal, black beans offer a myriad of health benefits, making them a valuable addition to a balanced and nutritious diet. In this article, we'll explore the benefits and diverse uses of black beans, shedding light on why they've earned a reputation as a superfood.

Nutritional Powerhouse:

Black beans are a nutritional powerhouse, providing a range of essential nutrients that contribute to overall well-being. Key nutritional components of black beans include:

Protein:

- Black beans are an excellent source of plant-based protein, making them an essential component for vegetarians and vegans. Protein is crucial for muscle repair, immune function, and the overall growth and maintenance of the body.

Dietary Fiber:

- Rich in dietary fiber, black beans support digestive health by promoting regular bowel movements, preventing constipation, and fostering a healthy gut microbiome. The combination of soluble and insoluble fiber in black beans contributes to heart health and blood sugar regulation.

Complex Carbohydrates:

- Black beans provide complex carbohydrates, offering a steady release of energy. They have a low glycemic index, making them a suitable choice for individuals looking to manage blood sugar levels.

Vitamins and Minerals:

Black beans contain essential vitamins such as folate, vitamin B6, thiamine, and minerals including iron, magnesium, phosphorus, and potassium. These nutrients play vital roles in various bodily functions, including blood formation, energy metabolism, and bone health.

Essential Vitamins in Black Beans:

Folate (Vitamin B9):

- **Benefits:** Folate is essential for DNA synthesis and repair. Adequate folate intake is crucial during periods of rapid cell division, such as pregnancy, and it helps prevent neural tube defects in developing fetuses.

Thiamine (Vitamin B1):

- **Benefits:** Thiamine is vital for energy metabolism, playing a key role in converting carbohydrates into energy. It also supports proper nerve function and is essential for the synthesis of neurotransmitters.

Vitamin B6:

- **Benefits:** Vitamin B6 is involved in over 100 enzymatic reactions in the body, including the metabolism of amino acids and the production of neurotransmitters. It plays a role in immune function, cognitive development, and the regulation of mood.

Niacin (Vitamin B3):

- **Benefits:** Niacin is crucial for energy metabolism, DNA repair, and the production of various enzymes. It contributes to maintaining healthy skin, nerves, and the digestive system.

Essential Minerals in Black Beans:

Iron:

- **Benefits:** Iron is essential for the formation of hemoglobin, the oxygen-carrying component of red blood cells. Adequate iron intake is crucial for preventing iron-deficiency anemia and supporting overall energy levels.

Magnesium:

- **Benefits:** Magnesium is involved in various physiological processes, including muscle and nerve function, bone health, and energy metabolism. It contributes to the regulation of blood pressure and supports the immune system.

Phosphorus:

- **Benefits:** Phosphorus is a structural component of DNA, RNA, and ATP (adenosine triphosphate), the primary energy carrier in cells. It is essential for bone health, kidney function, and the metabolism of macronutrients.

Potassium:

- **Benefits:** Potassium plays a crucial role in maintaining proper fluid balance, nerve impulses, and muscle contractions. It also supports heart health by helping to regulate blood pressure.

Health Benefits:

Heart Health:

- The high fiber content, potassium, and magnesium in black beans contribute to heart health. Fiber helps lower cholesterol levels, potassium helps regulate blood pressure, and magnesium supports overall cardiovascular function.

Blood Sugar Regulation:

- The fiber and low glycemic index of black beans make them an excellent choice for individuals aiming to manage blood sugar levels. They provide a gradual release of glucose, promoting stable energy levels.

Weight Management:

- The combination of protein and fiber in black beans promotes a feeling of fullness, aiding in weight management. Including black beans in meals can help control appetite and reduce overall calorie intake.

Antioxidant Properties:

- Black beans are rich in antioxidants, including flavonoids and polyphenols, which help neutralize free radicals in the body. Antioxidants play a role in reducing oxidative stress and inflammation.

Nutritional Content

In 1 cup (about 172 grams) of cooked black beans, the approximate nutritional content is as follows:

- Carbohydrates: Approximately 40 grams
- Protein: Approximately 15 grams
- Fiber: Approximately 15 grams
- Fat: Approximately 1 gram

Please note that these values are approximate and can vary slightly depending on factors such as the cooking method and the specific variety of black beans.

Culinary Versatility:

Black beans are incredibly versatile in the kitchen, lending themselves to a variety of dishes. Some common culinary uses include:

Black Bean Soup:

- A hearty and nutritious soup featuring black beans, vegetables, and savory spices.

Black Bean Salad:

- A refreshing salad combining black beans with colorful vegetables, herbs, and a zesty dressing.

Black Bean Burritos or Tacos:

- A flavorful and protein-packed filling for burritos or tacos, combining black beans with spices, salsa, and other toppings.

Black Bean Brownies:

- A healthier twist on classic brownies, incorporating black beans for added moisture and protein.

Here are two delicious and nutritious recipes featuring black beans:

Black Bean and Vegetable Quinoa Bowl:

Ingredients:

- 1 cup cooked quinoa
- 1 can (15 ounces) black beans, drained and rinsed
- 1 cup cherry tomatoes, halved
- 1 avocado, diced
- 1 cup corn kernels (fresh or frozen, thawed)
- 1 red bell pepper, diced
- 1/4 cup red onion, finely chopped
- Fresh cilantro, chopped (for garnish)

For the Lime Cilantro Dressing:

- 3 tablespoons extra-virgin olive oil
- 2 tablespoons fresh lime juice
- 1 tablespoon fresh cilantro, finely chopped
- 1 teaspoon honey or maple syrup
- Salt and pepper to taste

Instructions:

1. In a large bowl, combine cooked quinoa, black beans, cherry tomatoes, avocado, corn, red bell pepper, and red onion.
2. In a small bowl, whisk together the ingredients for the lime cilantro dressing: olive oil, lime juice, chopped cilantro, honey or maple syrup, salt, and pepper.
3. Pour the dressing over the quinoa and black bean mixture, tossing gently to coat all ingredients evenly.
4. Garnish with fresh chopped cilantro.
5. Serve the black bean and vegetable quinoa bowl as a nutritious and satisfying meal.

Spicy Black Bean Soup:

Ingredients:

- 2 cans (15 ounces each) black beans, drained and rinsed
- 1 onion, finely chopped
- 3 cloves garlic, minced
- 1 jalapeño, seeds removed and finely chopped
- 1 red bell pepper, diced

- 1 carrot, diced
- 1 teaspoon ground cumin
- 1 teaspoon chili powder
- 1/2 teaspoon smoked paprika
- 4 cups vegetable or chicken broth
- Salt and pepper to taste
- Fresh cilantro, chopped (for garnish)
- Lime wedges (for serving)

Optional Toppings:

- Sour cream or Greek yogurt
- Shredded cheese
- Avocado slices

Instructions:

1. In a large pot, sauté the chopped onion, garlic, and jalapeño in a bit of olive oil until softened.
2. Add the diced red bell pepper and carrot to the pot and cook for a few minutes.
3. Stir in the ground cumin, chili powder, and smoked paprika, allowing the spices to toast for about a minute.
4. Add the black beans and vegetable or chicken broth to the pot. Bring the soup to a simmer.
5. Season with salt and pepper to taste.
6. Simmer the soup for 20-25 minutes to allow the flavors to meld.
7. Serve the spicy black bean soup hot, garnished with fresh chopped cilantro and lime wedges. Add optional toppings as desired.

These recipes showcase the versatility of black beans, whether in a vibrant bowl or a warming soup. Black beans not only add a hearty texture to dishes but also provide a healthy dose of protein and fiber.

Conclusion:

Incorporating black beans into your diet is a tasty and health-conscious choice. Whether enjoyed in soups, salads, or as a main dish, black beans offer a nutrient-dense and delicious addition to meals. While black beans are generally safe and healthy to consume as part of a balanced diet. As with any food, moderation is key. If you have specific health concerns, allergies, or conditions, it's advisable to consult with a healthcare professional or a registered dietitian before making significant changes to your diet.

With their robust nutritional profile and culinary versatility, black beans stand as a testament to the idea that wholesome foods can be both good for you and a delight for your taste buds.

Back to Table of Contents

Blackberry

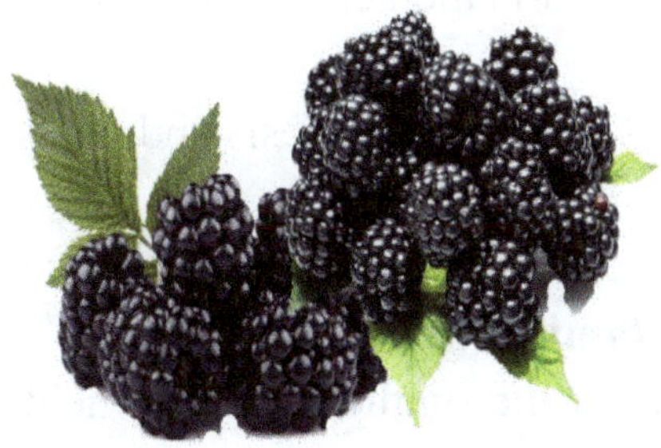

The Berry Bounty: Health Benefits and Culinary Wonders of Blackberries

Blackberries, with their deep, rich color and succulent sweetness, are more than just a delightful addition to your summer fruit bowl. These berries are a powerhouse of nutrition, offering a wide array of health benefits and culinary possibilities. In this article, we'll explore the nutritional wonders of blackberries and delve into their versatile uses in the kitchen.

Nutritional Marvels:

Blackberries are not only delicious but also packed with essential vitamins, minerals, and antioxidants. Here are some key components of the nutritional profile of blackberries:

Antioxidants:

- Blackberries are rich in antioxidants, including anthocyanins, quercetin, and vitamin C. These compounds help combat oxidative stress, reduce inflammation, and protect against chronic diseases.

Vitamin C:

- An important immune-boosting vitamin, vitamin C in blackberries supports the body's defense system and contributes to skin health.

Dietary Fiber:

- Blackberries are a great source of dietary fiber, promoting digestive health, regulating blood sugar levels, and aiding in weight management.

Vitamin K:

- Essential for blood clotting and bone health, vitamin K is found in blackberries in significant amounts.

Vitamin A:

- **Benefits:** Essential for vision health, supports immune function, maintains healthy skin.

Vitamin E:

- **Benefits:** Acts as an antioxidant, supports skin health, protects cells from damage.

Vitamin B6 (Pyridoxine):

- **Benefits:** Important for brain development and function, helps the body convert food into energy, supports the nervous system.

Folate (Vitamin B9):

- **Benefits:** Important for DNA synthesis and repair, aids in red blood cell formation.

Niacin (Vitamin B3):

- **Benefits:** Supports energy metabolism, helps maintain skin health.

Pantothenic Acid (Vitamin B5):

- **Benefits:** Essential for the synthesis of fatty acids, supports energy metabolism.

Riboflavin (Vitamin B2):

- **Benefits:** Supports energy metabolism, promotes healthy skin and eyes.

Thiamine (Vitamin B1):

- **Benefits:** Important for energy metabolism, supports nerve function.

Manganese:

- **Benefits:** Contributes to bone formation, supports metabolism, acts as an antioxidant.

Copper:

- **Benefits:** Supports the formation of red blood cells, aids in iron absorption.

Potassium:

- **Benefits:** Helps regulate blood pressure, supports heart and muscle function, aids in fluid balance.

Magnesium:

- **Benefits:** Important for muscle and nerve function, supports bone health.

Phosphorus:

- **Benefits:** Essential for bone and teeth health, involved in energy metabolism.

Zinc:

- **Benefits:** Supports immune function, involved in wound healing, essential for DNA synthesis.

Iron:

- **Benefits:** Important for oxygen transport in the blood, supports energy metabolism.

Calcium:

- **Benefits:** Important for bone and teeth health, supports muscle and nerve function.

Selenium:

- **Benefits:** Acts as an antioxidant, supports the immune system.

These antioxidants, vitamins and minerals make blackberries a nutrient-dense fruit, offering a range of health benefits as part of a balanced and varied diet.

Health Benefits:

Blackberries offer a wide range of health benefits due to their rich nutritional profile. Here are some of the key health benefits associated with consuming blackberries:

Antioxidant Protection:

- Blackberries are rich in antioxidants, including anthocyanins, quercetin, and vitamin C. These compounds help neutralize free radicals, reducing oxidative stress and lowering the risk of chronic diseases.

Heart Health:

- The fiber, potassium, and anthocyanins in blackberries contribute to heart health by supporting healthy blood pressure, reducing inflammation, and improving overall cardiovascular function.

Improved Cognitive Function:

- Anthocyanins found in blackberries have been linked to improved cognitive function, potentially enhancing memory and reducing the risk of age-related cognitive decline.

Digestive Health:

- The high fiber content in blackberries promotes digestive health by preventing constipation, supporting regular bowel movements, and fostering a healthy gut microbiota.

Blood Sugar Regulation:

- The fiber and anthocyanins in blackberries may help regulate blood sugar levels, making them a suitable option for individuals managing diabetes or those aiming to maintain stable blood glucose levels.

Weight Management:

- The combination of fiber and low-calorie content in blackberries can contribute to weight management by promoting satiety and reducing overall calorie intake.

Skin Health:

- Antioxidants like vitamin C and anthocyanins contribute to healthy skin by protecting against free radical damage, promoting collagen production, and maintaining skin elasticity.

Anti-Inflammatory Properties:

- Compounds in blackberries have anti-inflammatory effects, potentially reducing inflammation and alleviating symptoms associated with inflammatory conditions.

Bone Health:

- Blackberries contain essential minerals such as manganese, which contributes to bone health by supporting bone formation and density.

Eye Health Support:

- Antioxidants like lutein and zeaxanthin found in blackberries may help protect against age-related macular degeneration (AMD) and support overall eye health.

Cancer Prevention:

- Some studies suggest that the antioxidants and phytochemicals in blackberries may have protective effects against certain types of cancers, although more research is needed to establish a conclusive link.

Immune System Support:

- The vitamin C content in blackberries boosts the immune system, supporting the body's defense against infections and illnesses.

Hydration:

- Blackberries have a high water content, contributing to overall hydration, which is essential for various bodily functions and skin health.

It's important to note that these health benefits are best realized when blackberries are part of a balanced and varied diet, along with other fruits, vegetables, whole grains, and nutrient-rich foods.

Nutritional Content

In 1 cup (approximately 144 grams) of raw blackberries, the approximate nutritional content is as follows:

- Carbohydrates: Approximately 14 grams
- Protein: Approximately 2 grams
- Fiber: Approximately 8 grams
- Fat: Approximately 0.5 grams

Please note that these values are approximate and can vary slightly based on factors such as the size and variety of the blackberries.

Versatile Culinary Uses:

Blackberries are not only enjoyed fresh but can be incorporated into a variety of culinary creations. Here are some creative ways to use blackberries in the kitchen:

Fresh Snacking:

- Enjoy blackberries as a quick and delicious snack on their own or paired with other berries and fruits.

Smoothies and Juices:

- Blend blackberries into smoothies or juices for a burst of flavor and a nutritional boost.

Desserts:

- From blackberry pies and cobblers to jams and sorbets, these berries add a sweet and tangy touch to a range of desserts.

Salads:

- Toss blackberries into salads for a burst of color, sweetness, and added nutritional value.

Here are two delicious recipes that showcase the sweet and tangy flavors of blackberries:

Blackberry Mint Lemonade:

Ingredients:

- 2 cups fresh blackberries
- 1 cup fresh mint leaves
- 1 cup freshly squeezed lemon juice (about 4-6 lemons)
- 1/2 cup honey or to taste
- 4 cups cold water
- Ice cubes
- Fresh blackberries and mint sprigs for garnish

Instructions:

1. In a blender, combine blackberries, mint leaves, and honey. Blend until smooth.
2. Strain the blackberry-mint mixture through a fine-mesh sieve or cheesecloth into a large pitcher to remove seeds and pulp.
3. Add freshly squeezed lemon juice to the pitcher.
4. Pour in cold water and stir well to combine.
5. Taste the lemonade and adjust sweetness with more honey if needed.
6. Chill the lemonade in the refrigerator for at least 1-2 hours.
7. Serve the blackberry mint lemonade over ice cubes, garnished with fresh blackberries and mint sprigs.
8. Enjoy a refreshing and vibrant Blackberry Mint Lemonade on a warm day.

Blackberry and Almond Overnight Oats:

Ingredients:

- 1/2 cup rolled oats
- 1/2 cup almond milk (or any milk of your choice)
- 1/4 cup Greek yogurt
- 1/2 cup fresh blackberries
- 1 tablespoon almond butter
- 1 tablespoon chia seeds
- 1 teaspoon honey or maple syrup (optional)
- Sliced almonds for topping

Instructions:

1. In a jar or container, combine rolled oats, almond milk, Greek yogurt, almond butter, chia seeds, and honey (if using).

2. Stir the ingredients well, ensuring oats are fully submerged in the liquid.
3. Gently fold in fresh blackberries.
4. Seal the jar or container and refrigerate overnight or for at least 4 hours to allow the oats to absorb the liquid.
5. Before serving, give the overnight oats a good stir.
6. Top with additional blackberries and a sprinkle of sliced almonds.
7. Enjoy a nutritious and convenient breakfast with Blackberry and Almond Overnight Oats.

These recipes showcase the versatility of blackberries, whether blended into a refreshing beverage or incorporated into a wholesome and convenient overnight oats dish. Enjoy the burst of flavor and nutritional benefits these recipes bring to your table!

Conclusion:

In conclusion, blackberries are a delicious and nutritious addition to your diet, offering a plethora of health benefits and culinary possibilities. Whether enjoyed fresh, blended into smoothies, or featured in a delectable dessert, blackberries are a versatile fruit that can elevate both the taste and nutritional value of your meals. If you have specific health concerns, allergies, or conditions, it's advisable to consult with a healthcare professional or a registered dietitian before making significant changes to your diet.

Embrace the goodness of blackberries as you explore creative ways to incorporate them into your culinary adventures.

Back to Table of Contents

Blueberry

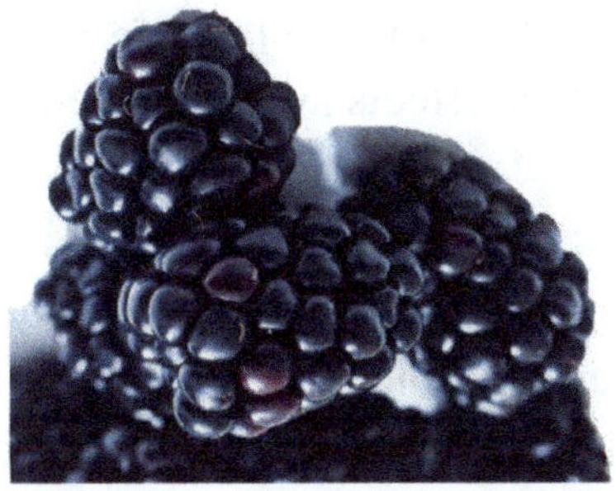

Exploring the Nutritional Powerhouse: Blueberries

Blueberries, with their vibrant hue and burst of flavor, are more than just a tasty treat—they're a nutritional powerhouse packed with health benefits. These small, round berries belong to the Vaccinium genus and are native to North America, where they have been cherished by indigenous peoples for centuries. From their impressive antioxidant content to their versatile culinary uses, blueberries offer a myriad of reasons to incorporate them into your diet. Let's dive into the benefits and uses of these delicious berries.

Nutritional Profile:

Blueberries are renowned for their exceptional nutritional content, making them a superfood worthy of attention. Here's a glimpse into the impressive array of nutrients found in blueberries:

Antioxidants:

Blueberries are rich in antioxidants, particularly flavonoids such as anthocyanins, quercetin, and kaempferol. These compounds help neutralize free radicals, reduce oxidative stress, and protect cells from damage.

Anthocyanins:

- **Benefits:** Anthocyanins are powerful antioxidants responsible for the vibrant blue color of blueberries. They help neutralize free radicals, reduce oxidative stress, and protect cells from damage. Anthocyanins have been associated with improved heart health, cognitive function, and vision.

Quercetin:

- **Benefits:** Quercetin is a flavonoid antioxidant found in blueberries that has anti-inflammatory and immune-boosting properties. It helps reduce inflammation, support cardiovascular health, and may have anticancer effects. Quercetin also supports respiratory health and may alleviate allergy symptoms.

Kaempferol:

- **Benefits:** Kaempferol is a flavonoid antioxidant found in blueberries that has anti-inflammatory and neuroprotective properties. It helps reduce inflammation, protect against oxidative damage in the brain, and support cognitive function. Kaempferol may also have anticancer effects and promote heart health.

Vitamin C:

- **Benefits:** Vitamin C is a water-soluble antioxidant found in blueberries that helps protect cells from oxidative damage, boost immune function, and support collagen synthesis. It plays a crucial role in skin health, wound healing, and iron absorption. Vitamin C may also reduce the risk of chronic diseases such as heart disease and cancer.

Vitamin E:

- **Benefits:** Vitamin E is a fat-soluble antioxidant found in blueberries that helps protect cell membranes from oxidative damage caused by free radicals. It supports immune function, skin health, and may have anti-aging effects. Vitamin E also plays a role in cardiovascular health and may reduce the risk of certain diseases.

Resveratrol:

- **Benefits:** Resveratrol is a polyphenol antioxidant found in blueberries that has anti-inflammatory and cardioprotective effects. It helps reduce inflammation, improve blood vessel function, and lower LDL (bad) cholesterol levels. Resveratrol may also support brain health and protect against age-related decline in cognitive function.

These antioxidants found in blueberries work synergistically to combat oxidative stress, reduce inflammation, and promote overall health and wellbeing. Incorporating blueberries into your diet can help boost your antioxidant intake and support optimal health.

Vitamins:

Blueberries are a good source of vitamins C and K, as well as several B vitamins like folate and vitamin B6. These vitamins play essential roles in immune function, blood clotting, and energy metabolism.

Vitamin K:

- **Benefits:** Vitamin K plays a crucial role in blood clotting, bone metabolism, and cardiovascular health. It helps regulate calcium levels in the body, supports bone mineralization, and may reduce the risk of fractures and osteoporosis. Vitamin K also contributes to healthy blood vessel function and may have anti-inflammatory effects.

Vitamin B6 (Pyridoxine):

- **Benefits:** Vitamin B6 is involved in more than 100 enzyme reactions in the body, including protein metabolism, neurotransmitter synthesis, and immune function. It supports brain health, mood regulation, and may reduce the risk of heart disease.

Vitamin B6 also plays a role in hormone regulation and may alleviate symptoms of premenstrual syndrome (PMS).

Folate (Vitamin B9):

- **Benefits:** Folate is essential for DNA synthesis, red blood cell formation, and fetal development during pregnancy. It supports brain health, cardiovascular health, and may reduce the risk of neural tube defects in infants. Folate also plays a role in mood regulation and may reduce the risk of depression.

Pantothenic Acid (Vitamin B5):

- **Benefits:** Pantothenic acid is involved in the synthesis of coenzyme A, which is essential for energy metabolism, hormone synthesis, and fatty acid synthesis. It supports adrenal function, stress management, and may improve skin health. Pantothenic acid also plays a role in wound healing and may reduce the risk of skin conditions such as acne.

Incorporating blueberries into your diet can help ensure you're getting a wide range of essential vitamins that support overall health and wellbeing. Whether eaten fresh, blended into smoothies, or added to baked goods, blueberries are a delicious and nutritious addition to any meal or snack.

Minerals:

Blueberries contain important minerals such as manganese, which supports bone health and antioxidant defense, and potassium, which helps regulate blood pressure and muscle function.

Manganese:

- **Benefits:** Manganese is important for bone health, metabolism, and antioxidant defense. It supports bone formation, collagen synthesis, and may reduce inflammation. Manganese also plays a role in carbohydrate metabolism, cholesterol synthesis, and neurotransmitter production.

Potassium:

- **Benefits:** Potassium is essential for heart health, muscle function, and fluid balance. It helps regulate blood pressure, nerve transmission, and muscle contractions. Potassium also supports kidney function, electrolyte balance, and may reduce the risk of stroke and heart disease.

Copper:

- **Benefits:** Copper is important for energy metabolism, connective tissue formation, and antioxidant defense. It supports iron absorption, collagen synthesis, and may reduce inflammation. Copper also plays a role in nerve function, immune function, and may protect against cardiovascular disease.

Zinc:

- **Benefits:** Zinc is essential for immune function, wound healing, and DNA synthesis. It supports growth and development, hormone regulation, and may reduce the duration and severity of colds. Zinc also plays a role in taste perception, insulin sensitivity, and may protect against age-related macular degeneration.

Incorporating blueberries into your diet can help ensure you're getting a wide range of essential minerals that support overall health and wellbeing. Whether eaten fresh, blended into smoothies, or added to yogurt, blueberries are a delicious and nutritious addition to any meal or snack.

Dietary Fiber:

Blueberries are high in dietary fiber, both soluble and insoluble, which supports digestive health, promotes satiety, and helps regulate blood sugar levels.

Low in Calories:

Despite their sweet flavor, blueberries are relatively low in calories, making them a guilt-free addition to meals and snacks.

Health Benefits:

Incorporating blueberries into your diet can offer numerous health benefits. Here are some of the key advantages:

Heart Health: The antioxidants in blueberries help lower LDL (bad) cholesterol levels, reduce inflammation, and improve blood vessel function, promoting heart health and reducing the risk of cardiovascular disease.

Brain Health: Blueberries have been shown to improve cognitive function, enhance memory, and protect against age-related decline in brain function. The antioxidants in blueberries may help prevent oxidative damage and inflammation in the brain.

Eye Health: The antioxidants lutein and zeaxanthin found in blueberries support eye health by protecting against age-related macular degeneration and reducing the risk of cataracts.

Blood Sugar Control: The fiber and antioxidants in blueberries help stabilize blood sugar levels, improve insulin sensitivity, and reduce the risk of type 2 diabetes.

Anti-Inflammatory Effects: Blueberries have potent anti-inflammatory properties, which may help reduce the risk of chronic diseases such as cancer, arthritis, and neurodegenerative disorders.

Nutritional Content

In 1 cup (approximately 148 grams) of raw blueberries, the approximate nutritional content is as follows:

- Carbohydrates: Approximately 21 grams
- Protein: Approximately 1 gram
- Fiber: Approximately 4 grams
- Fat: Approximately 0.5 grams

Please note that these values are approximate and can vary slightly based on factors such as the size and variety of the blueberries.

Culinary Uses:

Blueberries are incredibly versatile and can be enjoyed in a variety of ways. Here are some delicious ways to incorporate blueberries into your meals and snacks:

Fresh: Enjoy blueberries as a refreshing snack on their own or mixed into yogurt, oatmeal, or cereal for a nutritious breakfast.

Smoothies: Blend blueberries with other fruits, leafy greens, and a liquid base such as almond milk or coconut water to create a delicious and nutritious smoothie.

Baked Goods: Add blueberries to muffins, pancakes, waffles, or quick breads for a burst of flavor and added nutrition.

Salads: Toss blueberries into green salads or fruit salads for a pop of color and sweetness.

Sauces and Compotes: Cook down blueberries with a bit of sweetener to make a versatile sauce or compote that can be drizzled over desserts, yogurt, or grilled meats.

Here are two delicious recipes featuring blueberries:

Blueberry Oatmeal Breakfast Muffins:

Ingredients:

- 1 1/2 cups rolled oats
- 1 cup whole wheat flour
- 1/2 cup brown sugar or coconut sugar
- 1 teaspoon baking powder
- 1/2 teaspoon baking soda
- 1/2 teaspoon ground cinnamon
- 1/4 teaspoon salt
- 1 cup plain Greek yogurt
- 1/4 cup unsweetened applesauce
- 1/4 cup milk (dairy or non-dairy)
- 2 tablespoons coconut oil, melted
- 1 teaspoon vanilla extract
- 1 large egg
- 1 cup fresh blueberries

Instructions:

1. Preheat the oven to 375°F (190°C). Grease a muffin tin or line with muffin liners.
2. In a large mixing bowl, combine the rolled oats, whole wheat flour, brown sugar, baking powder, baking soda, cinnamon, and salt.
3. In a separate bowl, whisk together the Greek yogurt, applesauce, milk, coconut oil, vanilla extract, and egg until smooth.

4. Pour the wet ingredients into the dry ingredients and stir until just combined. Gently fold in the blueberries.
5. Divide the batter evenly among the muffin cups, filling each about 3/4 full.
6. Bake in the preheated oven for 18-20 minutes, or until the muffins are golden brown and a toothpick inserted into the center comes out clean.
7. Allow the muffins to cool in the tin for 5 minutes, then transfer to a wire rack to cool completely.
8. Enjoy these wholesome blueberry oatmeal breakfast muffins as a nutritious grab-and-go breakfast or snack.

Spinach and Blueberry Salad with Balsamic Vinaigrette:

Ingredients:

- 6 cups fresh baby spinach leaves
- 1 cup fresh blueberries
- 1/4 cup sliced almonds, toasted
- 1/4 cup crumbled feta cheese (optional)
- 2 tablespoons balsamic vinegar
- 1 tablespoon extra virgin olive oil
- 1 teaspoon honey or maple syrup
- Salt and pepper to taste

Instructions:

1. In a large salad bowl, combine the baby spinach leaves, fresh blueberries, toasted almonds, and crumbled feta cheese (if using).
2. In a small bowl, whisk together the balsamic vinegar, olive oil, honey or maple syrup, salt, and pepper to make the dressing.
3. Drizzle the dressing over the salad and toss gently to coat the ingredients evenly.
4. Serve the spinach and blueberry salad immediately as a refreshing and nutritious side dish or light meal.

These recipes showcase the versatility of blueberries in both sweet and savory dishes, allowing you to enjoy their delicious flavor and nutritional benefits in a variety of culinary creations

In Conclusion:

Blueberries are not only delicious but also incredibly nutritious, offering a wide range of health benefits. Whether eaten fresh, blended into smoothies, or baked into goodies, blueberries are a versatile ingredient that can be enjoyed in countless ways. So next time you're looking for a healthy and delicious snack or addition to your meals, reach for some vibrant blueberries and reap the rewards of their nutritional goodness.

If you have specific health concerns, allergies, or conditions, it's advisable to consult with a healthcare professional or a registered dietitian before making significant changes to your diet.

Bok Choy

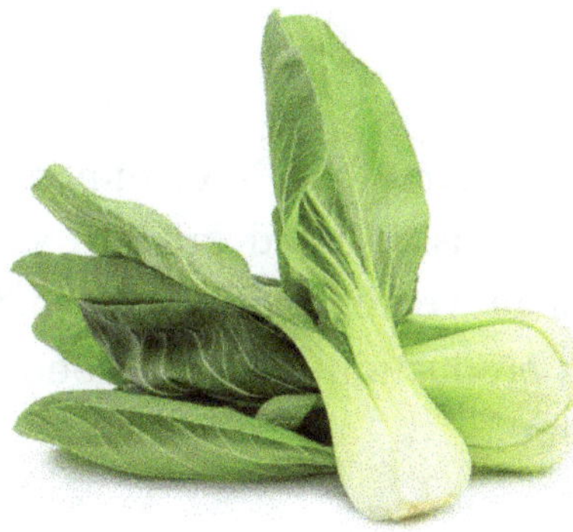

A Nutrient-Packed Cruciferous Marvel with Culinary Versatility

Bok choy, also known as Chinese cabbage or pak choi, is a leafy green vegetable that has become a staple in many cuisines worldwide. With its mild flavor, crisp texture, and impressive nutritional profile, bok choy is not only a culinary delight but also a powerhouse of health benefits. In this article, we will explore the various advantages and versatile uses of this cruciferous marvel.

Nutritional Powerhouse:

Bok choy is celebrated for its rich array of nutrients, making it a valuable addition to a balanced diet. Packed with vitamins, minerals, and antioxidants, bok choy offers the following nutritional benefits:

Vitamins and Minerals:

Bok choy is a great source of vitamins A, C, and K. These vitamins play crucial roles in supporting immune function, promoting skin health, and contributing to proper blood clotting. Additionally, bok choy provides essential minerals such as calcium, potassium, and folate.

Vitamin A:

- **Benefits:** Vitamin A is crucial for maintaining healthy vision, skin, and mucous membranes. It plays a key role in immune function, supporting the body's defense against infections. Additionally, vitamin A is involved in cell differentiation and may contribute to the prevention of age-related macular degeneration.

Vitamin C:

- **Benefits:** Known for its antioxidant properties, vitamin C is essential for the synthesis of collagen, a structural protein in skin, blood vessels, and bones. It promotes wound healing, supports the immune system, and may contribute to reducing the risk of chronic diseases by neutralizing free radicals.

Vitamin K:

- **Benefits:** Vitamin K is crucial for blood clotting and bone health. It plays a key role in synthesizing proteins necessary for proper blood coagulation. Additionally, vitamin K is involved in bone mineralization, contributing to maintaining strong and healthy bones.

Folate (Vitamin B9):

- **Benefits:** Folate is essential for DNA synthesis and cell division. It is particularly important during periods of rapid growth, such as pregnancy. Adequate folate intake is crucial for preventing neural tube defects in developing fetuses. Folate also supports the production of red blood cells and contributes to overall cardiovascular health.

Calcium:

- **Benefits:** Calcium is essential for the formation and maintenance of strong bones and teeth. Adequate calcium intake supports bone density and can help prevent conditions such as osteoporosis. Calcium is also involved in muscle contraction, blood clotting, and nerve function.

Potassium:

- **Benefits:** Potassium plays a crucial role in regulating fluid balance, nerve signals, and muscle contractions. It helps maintain healthy blood pressure by counteracting the effects of sodium. Adequate potassium intake is associated with a reduced risk of stroke and cardiovascular diseases.

Phosphorus:

- **Benefits:** Phosphorus is a key component of DNA, RNA, and ATP (adenosine triphosphate), the primary energy carrier in cells. It is essential for bone and teeth formation, kidney function, and the maintenance of the body's pH balance. Phosphorus also plays a role in the activation of various enzymes.

Magnesium:

- Benefits: Magnesium is involved in over 300 enzymatic reactions in the body, contributing to energy metabolism, muscle and nerve function, and the synthesis of DNA and proteins. Adequate magnesium intake is associated with maintaining healthy blood pressure, bone density, and cardiovascular health.

Antioxidant Properties:

The presence of antioxidants, including beta-carotene and selenium, in bok choy helps combat oxidative stress in the body. Antioxidants play a vital role in neutralizing free radicals, contributing to overall cellular health and potentially reducing the risk of chronic diseases.

Beta-Carotene:

- **Benefits:** Bok choy contains beta-carotene, a carotenoid with antioxidant properties. Beta-carotene is a precursor to vitamin A, an essential nutrient for vision, immune function, and skin health. As an antioxidant, beta-carotene helps combat oxidative stress, reducing the risk of age-related macular degeneration and supporting overall cellular health.

Selenium:

- **Benefits:** Selenium is a trace element with antioxidant properties found in bok choy. It is a component of selenoproteins, which play a role in protecting cells from oxidative damage. Selenium is essential for thyroid function, immune system support, and may have potential anti-cancer effects by inhibiting the growth of malignant cells.

Low in Calories, High in Fiber:

- Bok choy is a low-calorie vegetable that is rich in dietary fiber. This combination makes it an excellent choice for those looking to maintain a healthy weight and support digestive health. Fiber aids in digestion, helps regulate blood sugar levels, and contributes to a feeling of fullness.

Health Benefits:

Heart Health:

- The high potassium content in bok choy supports cardiovascular health by helping regulate blood pressure. Additionally, the presence of folate contributes to the reduction of homocysteine levels, a factor associated with a lower risk of heart disease.

Bone Health:

- Bok choy is an excellent source of calcium and vitamin K, both of which are essential for maintaining strong and healthy bones. Adequate calcium intake supports bone density, while vitamin K is involved in bone mineralization and may reduce the risk of fractures.

Cancer Prevention:

- As a cruciferous vegetable, bok choy contains glucosinolates, compounds known for their potential anti-cancer properties. These compounds may help reduce the risk of certain cancers by promoting detoxification and inhibiting the growth of cancer cells.

Nutritional Content

In 1 cup (approximately 156 grams) of cooked bok choy, the approximate nutritional content is as follows:

- Carbohydrates: Approximately 2.7 grams
- Protein: Approximately 1.5 grams
- Fiber: Approximately 2.8 grams

- Fat: Approximately 0.2 grams

Please note that these values are approximate and can vary slightly based on factors such as the cooking method and the specific variety of bok choy.

Culinary Versatility:

Bok choy's versatility in the kitchen extends to various cooking methods, allowing it to shine in a variety of dishes. Here are some popular culinary uses:

Stir-Fries and Sautés:

- Bok choy's crisp texture and mild flavor make it a perfect addition to stir-fries and sautés. Quickly cook it with other vegetables, protein, and your favorite sauces for a nutritious and flavorful dish.

Soups and Stews:

- Bok choy adds a nutritious element to soups and stews. Its leaves and stalks can be chopped and added towards the end of the cooking process, maintaining a satisfying crunch.

Raw in Salads:

- Bok choy can be enjoyed raw in salads, providing a refreshing and slightly peppery flavor. Its sturdy leaves make it an excellent choice for salads with robust dressings.

Tips on Growing Bok Choy

The time it takes for bok choy to grow from seed to harvest depends on various factors including the variety of bok choy, growing conditions, and desired size at harvest.

However, on average, bok choy typically takes about 45 to 60 days to reach maturity when grown from seed.

Keep in mind that bok choy is a cool-season crop, so it tends to grow best in cooler temperatures, ideally between 45°F and 75°F (7°C to 24°C). Additionally, bok choy can be harvested at different stages of maturity, from baby bok choy to full-sized heads, so the time to maturity can vary based on your desired harvest size.

Conclusion:

Bok choy's combination of delightful taste, versatility in the kitchen, and impressive health benefits makes it a standout vegetable in the world of nutrition. Whether stir-fried, added to soups, or enjoyed fresh in salads, bok choy deserves its place on the table as a nutrient-packed cruciferous marvel that contributes to overall well-being. Embrace the culinary possibilities and health advantages of bok choy, making it a vibrant and delicious addition to your meals.

Back to Table of Contents

Brazil Nuts

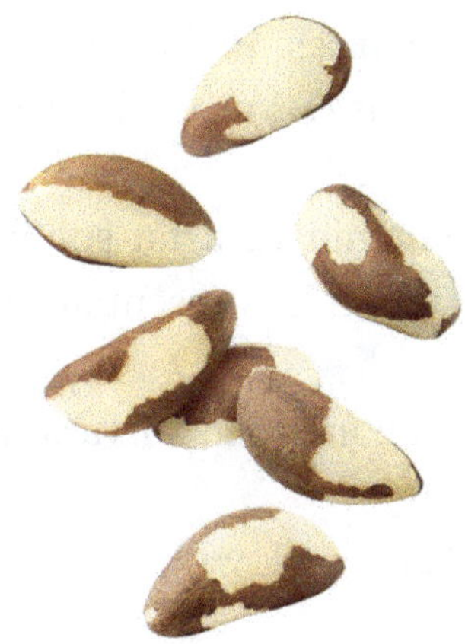

Nature's Bounty Packed in a Nutshell

Hailing from the lush rainforests of the Amazon basin, Brazil nuts are more than just a tasty snack; they are a nutritional powerhouse with a unique flavor and a host of health benefits. Renowned for their large size and rich, creamy taste, Brazil nuts are more than just a culinary delight; they offer a diverse array of nutrients that contribute to overall well-being. In this article, we'll explore the numerous benefits and versatile uses that make Brazil nuts an essential addition to a wholesome diet.

Nutrient-Rich Composition:

Brazil nuts boast a remarkable nutritional profile, offering an abundance of essential nutrients in every bite. Here's a closer look at the key nutrients found in these delectable nuts:

Selenium:

- Brazil nuts are the unrivaled champions when it comes to selenium content. Selenium is a vital mineral with antioxidant properties that support the immune system, thyroid function, and overall cellular health. Just a few Brazil nuts can meet or exceed the daily recommended intake of selenium.

Healthy Fats:

- These nuts are rich in monounsaturated and polyunsaturated fats, including omega-6 fatty acids. Healthy fats are essential for cardiovascular health, supporting proper cholesterol levels and reducing the risk of heart disease.

Protein:

- Brazil nuts provide a source of plant-based protein, making them a valuable addition to vegetarian and vegan diets. Protein is crucial for muscle repair, immune function, and overall body maintenance.

Fiber:

- Fiber is abundant in Brazil nuts, aiding in digestion, promoting a feeling of fullness, and supporting gut health.

Vitamins:

Brazil nuts contain various vitamins, including vitamin E, which is a potent antioxidant, and B-complex vitamins such as thiamine (B1) and niacin (B3), contributing to energy metabolism.

Vitamin E:

- Brazil nuts contain vitamin E, a fat-soluble antioxidant that protects cells from oxidative damage. Vitamin E is essential for skin health and immune function.

B Vitamins:

- Brazil nuts contain small amounts of various B-complex vitamins, including:
    - Thiamine (B1)
    - Riboflavin (B2)
    - Niacin (B3)
    - Pantothenic acid (B5)

While Brazil nuts contribute some vitamins, their standout nutritional feature is the exceptionally high content of selenium, a mineral with antioxidant properties.

Health Benefits:

Antioxidant Defense:

- The high selenium content in Brazil nuts provides robust antioxidant defense, protecting cells from oxidative stress and reducing inflammation in the body.

Thyroid Support:

- Selenium is crucial for proper thyroid function, and Brazil nuts can play a role in supporting a healthy thyroid gland.

Heart Health:

- The combination of healthy fats, selenium, and other nutrients supports cardiovascular health, helping to lower bad cholesterol levels and reduce the risk of heart disease.

Immune System Boost:

- Selenium is known to enhance immune function, and incorporating Brazil nuts into the diet can contribute to a resilient immune system.

Nutritional Content

In 1 cup (approximately 133 grams) of Brazil nuts, the approximate nutritional content is as follows:

- Carbohydrates: Approximately 12 grams
- Protein: Approximately 19 grams
- Fiber: Approximately 10 grams
- Fat: Approximately 88 grams

Brazil nuts are notably high in fat, particularly healthy unsaturated fats like monounsaturated and polyunsaturated fats. They are also a good source of protein and fiber, while containing fewer carbohydrates. These values are approximate and can vary slightly based on factors such as the size and specific variety of Brazil nuts.

Culinary Uses:

Snacking:

- Enjoy Brazil nuts as a simple and satisfying snack. Their rich and creamy flavor makes them a delightful treat on their own.

Trail Mixes:

- Include Brazil nuts in homemade trail mixes with other nuts, seeds, and dried fruits for a nutrient-packed and energy-boosting snack.

Baking:

- Incorporate chopped Brazil nuts into baked goods like cookies, brownies, or granola for added texture and flavor.

Nut Butters:

- Blend Brazil nuts into a creamy nut butter to spread on toast, use as a dip, or add to smoothies.

Here are two delicious recipes that incorporate the unique flavor and nutritional benefits of Brazil nuts:

Brazil Nut Pesto

Ingredients:

- 1 cup Brazil nuts, toasted
- 2 cups fresh basil leaves
- 2 cloves garlic, minced
- 1/2 cup grated Parmesan cheese
- 1/2 cup extra-virgin olive oil
- Salt and pepper to taste
- Lemon juice (optional)

Instructions:

1. In a food processor, combine toasted Brazil nuts, fresh basil leaves, minced garlic, and grated Parmesan cheese.
2. Pulse the ingredients until coarsely chopped.
3. With the food processor running, gradually add the olive oil in a steady stream until the pesto reaches your desired consistency.
4. Season with salt and pepper to taste. Add a squeeze of lemon juice for a citrusy kick if desired.

5. Serve the Brazil nut pesto over pasta, spread it on bread, or use it as a flavorful topping for grilled vegetables.

Chocolate-Dipped Brazil Nut Clusters

Ingredients:

- 1 cup Brazil nuts
- 1 cup dark chocolate chips
- 1 tablespoon coconut oil
- Sea salt for sprinkling (optional)

Instructions:

1. Line a baking sheet with parchment paper.
2. In a heatproof bowl, melt the dark chocolate chips and coconut oil together using a double boiler or in the microwave, stirring until smooth.
3. Add Brazil nuts to the melted chocolate, making sure each nut is well coated.
4. Using a spoon, drop clusters of chocolate-covered Brazil nuts onto the prepared baking sheet.
5. Optionally, sprinkle a pinch of sea salt over each cluster for a sweet and salty contrast.
6. Place the baking sheet in the refrigerator for about 30 minutes or until the chocolate hardens.
7. Once the chocolate is set, transfer the clusters to an airtight container and store in the refrigerator until ready to enjoy.

These recipes showcase the versatility of Brazil nuts, whether blended into a vibrant pesto or used to create irresistible chocolate-dipped clusters. Incorporate these nutrient-rich nuts into your culinary creations for a delightful combination of taste and health benefits.

Caution: Moderation is Key:

- While Brazil nuts offer numerous health benefits, it's important to consume them in moderation due to their extremely high selenium content. Excessive selenium intake can lead to selenium toxicity, which may have adverse effects on health. A few Brazil nuts per day are sufficient to meet recommended selenium levels.

In **conclusion**, Brazil nuts stand as a testament to the bounty of nature, offering not only a unique and delicious taste but also a wealth of nutrients that promote overall health. Whether enjoyed as a snack or incorporated into various culinary creations, Brazil nuts can be a flavorful and nutritious addition to a well-balanced diet. If you have specific health concerns, allergies, or conditions, it's advisable to consult with a healthcare professional or a registered dietitian before making significant changes to your diet.

Embrace the goodness of Brazil nuts and savor the benefits they bring in each delightful bite.

Back to Table of Contents

Broad Beans

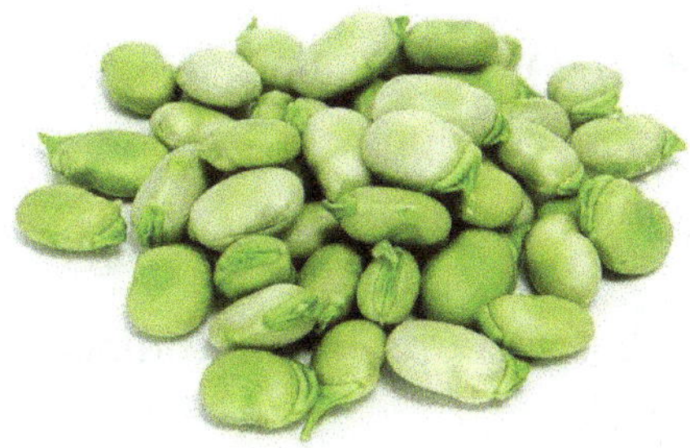

A Nutrient-Rich Gem in the World of Legumes

Broad beans, also known as fava beans, have been a culinary delight and nutritional powerhouse for thousands of years. These vibrant green legumes, native to North Africa and Southwest Asia, have earned their place on plates around the world. In this article, we will explore the benefits and diverse uses of broad beans, shedding light on their nutritional richness and culinary versatility.

Nutritional Profilc:

Broad beans are celebrated for their impressive nutritional content, offering a range of essential vitamins, minerals, and other health-promoting compounds. Here's a glimpse of the nutritional profile of broad beans:

Protein:

- Broad beans are an excellent source of plant-based protein, making them a valuable addition to vegetarian and vegan diets.

Dietary Fiber:

- Rich in dietary fiber, broad beans contribute to digestive health, regulate blood sugar levels, and support weight management.

Vitamins:

Broad beans contain various vitamins, including vitamin K, vitamin B1 (thiamine), vitamin B2 (riboflavin), vitamin B3 (niacin), vitamin B6, vitamin C, and folate (vitamin B9).

Vitamin K:

- Essential for blood clotting and bone health.

Vitamin B1 (Thiamine):

- Crucial for energy metabolism and the proper functioning of the nervous system.

Vitamin B2 (Riboflavin):

- Plays a key role in energy production, cell growth, and the maintenance of healthy skin.

Vitamin B3 (Niacin):

- Essential for DNA repair, energy metabolism, and the proper functioning of the nervous system.

Vitamin B6 (Pyridoxine):

- Important for brain development, the production of neurotransmitters, and the metabolism of amino acids.

Vitamin C:

- An antioxidant that supports immune function, helps the body absorb iron, and promotes healthy skin.

Folate (Vitamin B9):

- Important for DNA synthesis and cell division. Adequate folate intake is particularly important during pregnancy for fetal development.

Pantothenic Acid (Vitamin B5):

- Involved in the synthesis of fatty acids, amino acids, and other important molecules.

It's important to note that while broad beans contain a variety of vitamins, the specific nutrient content can vary based on factors such as the variety of beans, growing conditions, and preparation methods. Including broad beans in a balanced and diverse diet can contribute to meeting your daily vitamin requirements and supporting overall health.

Minerals:

Abundant in essential minerals such as iron, potassium, magnesium, phosphorus, and zinc, broad beans contribute to bone health, blood pressure regulation, and overall well-being.

Iron:

- Essential for the formation of hemoglobin, which carries oxygen in the blood.

Potassium:

- Important for maintaining proper heart and muscle function, regulating fluid balance, and supporting overall cardiovascular health.

Magnesium:

- Crucial for muscle and nerve function, energy metabolism, and bone health.

Phosphorus:

- Vital for bone and teeth health, energy production, and the synthesis of DNA and RNA.

Zinc:

- Important for immune function, wound healing, and DNA synthesis.

Calcium:

- Essential for bone and teeth health, blood clotting, and muscle function.

Copper:

- Involved in the formation of red blood cells, maintenance of bones and nerves, and the immune system.

Manganese:

- Plays a role in bone formation, blood clotting, and reducing inflammation.

Sodium:

- While sodium is typically present in smaller amounts, it is important for maintaining fluid balance and nerve function.

Selenium:

- An antioxidant that supports thyroid function and immune system health.

Phytosterols:

- Plant compounds with potential health benefits, including cholesterol-lowering properties.

It's important to note that the specific mineral content of broad beans can vary based on factors such as the variety of beans, growing conditions, and preparation methods. Including broad beans in a well-balanced diet can contribute to meeting your daily mineral requirements and promoting overall health.

Antioxidants:

Broad beans contain antioxidants, including flavonoids and polyphenols, which help neutralize free radicals and reduce oxidative stress in the body.

Quercetin:

- A flavonoid with antioxidant and anti-inflammatory properties.

Kaempferol:

- Another flavonoid that exhibits antioxidant effects and has potential health benefits.

Catechins:

- A type of flavonoid with antioxidant properties commonly found in tea, chocolate, and certain fruits and vegetables.

Epicatechin:

- A flavonoid with antioxidant activity found in various plant foods.

Lutein:

- A carotenoid with antioxidant properties known for its role in supporting eye health.

Zeaxanthin:

- Another carotenoid found in broad beans that contributes to their antioxidant capacity and eye health benefits.

Vitamin C:

- An essential antioxidant that helps protect cells from oxidative stress, supports the immune system, and aids in collagen formation.

Vitamin E:

- A fat-soluble antioxidant that protects cell membranes from oxidative damage.

Phenolic Compounds:

- Broad beans contain various phenolic compounds, including hydroxybenzoic acids and hydroxycinnamic acids, which contribute to their overall antioxidant profile.

Antioxidants play a crucial role in neutralizing free radicals and reducing oxidative stress, which, in turn, may contribute to the prevention of chronic diseases and support overall health. Including a variety of antioxidant-rich foods, such as broad beans, in your diet can contribute to a well-rounded and health-promoting nutritional intake.

Health Benefits:

Heart Health:

- The combination of fiber, potassium, and antioxidants in broad beans supports cardiovascular health by helping to lower cholesterol levels and regulate blood pressure.

Blood Sugar Regulation:

- The fiber content in broad beans aids in slowing down the absorption of sugars, contributing to better blood sugar control.

Bone Health:

- Rich in minerals like calcium, phosphorus, and magnesium, broad beans support bone health and help prevent conditions such as osteoporosis.

Weight Management:

- The high protein and fiber content in broad beans promotes satiety, making them a satisfying and nutritious option for those aiming to manage their weight.

Nutritional Content

In 1 cup (approximately 170 grams) of boiled broad beans (also known as fava beans), the approximate nutritional content is as follows:

- Carbohydrates: Approximately 34 grams
- Protein: Approximately 12 grams
- Fiber: Approximately 9 grams
- Fat: Approximately 1 gram

Please note that these values are approximate and can vary slightly based on factors such as the cooking method and the specific variety of broad beans.

Culinary Uses:

Broad beans' versatility in the kitchen makes them suitable for a variety of culinary creations. Here are some popular ways to enjoy broad beans:

Fresh and Raw:

- Young, tender broad beans can be enjoyed fresh and raw in salads, adding a crisp texture and a nutty flavor.

Cooked:

- Broad beans can be boiled, steamed, or sautéed and served as a standalone side dish or incorporated into various recipes.

Purees and Dips:

- Create creamy purees or dips by blending cooked broad beans with garlic, olive oil, and herbs for a delicious spread.

Stews and Soups:

- Add broad beans to stews, soups, and casseroles for a hearty and nutritious boost.

Roasted Snack:

- Roast broad beans with a sprinkle of salt and enjoy them as a crunchy and protein-packed snack.

Broad beans, also known as fava beans, can add a delightful and nutritious element to various dishes. ***Here are two recipes, including the Jamaican Oxtail with Broad Beans:***

Jamaican Oxtail with Broad Beans:

Ingredients:

- 2.5 to 3 pounds oxtail, cut into segments
- 2 cups broad beans (fava beans), shelled and peeled
- 2 tablespoons vegetable oil
- 1 large onion, chopped
- 4 cloves garlic, minced
- 2 teaspoons thyme, dried
- 2 teaspoons allspice
- 2 scallions, chopped
- 2 carrots, diced
- 2 potatoes, peeled and diced
- 2 cups beef broth
- 1 cup coconut milk
- Salt and pepper to taste
- Scotch bonnet pepper (optional, for heat)
- Lime wedges for serving

Instructions:

1. **Preparation:**
    - Season oxtail with salt, pepper, and allspice. (Grace oxtail seasoning: optional) Let it marinate for at least 30 minutes or overnight for enhanced flavor.
2. **Brown the Oxtail:**
    - Heat vegetable oil in a large, heavy pot over medium-high heat. Brown the oxtail on all sides until well-seared. Remove oxtail and set aside.
3. **Sauté Aromatics:**
    - In the same pot, sauté onions, garlic, thyme, and scallions until fragrant.

4. **Combine Ingredients:**
    - Return the oxtail to the pot. Add carrots, potatoes, broad beans, beef broth, and coconut milk. If using Scotch bonnet pepper, add it whole for flavor (remove before serving).
5. **Simmer:**
    - Bring the mixture to a boil, then reduce the heat to low. Cover and simmer for 2.5 to 3 hours or until the oxtail is tender.
6. **Adjust Seasoning:**
    - Season with salt and pepper to taste. Adjust the consistency by adding more broth if needed.
7. **Serve:**
    - Serve the Jamaican Oxtail with Broad Beans over rice or with traditional rice and peas. Garnish with lime wedges.
8. **Enjoy the rich and flavorful Jamaican Oxtail with the added goodness of broad beans!**

Broad Bean and Mint Hummus:

Ingredients:

- 2 cups cooked and peeled broad beans
- 1/4 cup fresh mint leaves
- 3 tablespoons tahini
- 2 cloves garlic, minced
- 1/4 cup fresh lemon juice
- 1/3 cup extra-virgin olive oil
- Salt and pepper to taste
- Toasted pita bread or vegetable sticks for serving

Instructions:

Prepare Broad Beans:
- Cook broad beans in boiling water for 3-5 minutes, then transfer to an ice bath to cool. Peel the outer skin from each bean.

Blend Ingredients:
- In a food processor, combine broad beans, mint leaves, tahini, minced garlic, and lemon juice. Blend until smooth.

Add Olive Oil:
- With the food processor running, gradually add the olive oil until the hummus reaches your desired consistency.

Season:
- Season the hummus with salt and pepper to taste. Adjust lemon juice or olive oil as needed.

Serve:

- Transfer the broad bean and mint hummus to a serving bowl. Drizzle with a bit of olive oil and garnish with additional mint leaves.

Enjoy this refreshing and vibrant Broad Bean and Mint Hummus with toasted pita or vegetable sticks!

These recipes showcase the versatility of broad beans in both hearty stews and light dips, allowing you to savor their unique flavor and reap their nutritional benefits.

Conclusion:

Broad beans, with their nutritional richness and culinary adaptability, stand as a testament to the abundance of health benefits found in legumes. Whether enjoyed fresh in salads, incorporated into main dishes, or blended into creamy dips, broad beans offer a spectrum of flavors and textures to please every palate. If you have specific health concerns, allergies, or conditions, it's advisable to consult with a healthcare professional or a registered dietitian before making significant changes to your diet.

As you savor the unique taste and reap the nutritional rewards of broad beans, you're not just indulging in a delicious legume – you're embracing a wholesome addition to your culinary repertoire and a nutrient-packed ally on your journey to overall well-being.

Back to Table of Contents

Broccoli

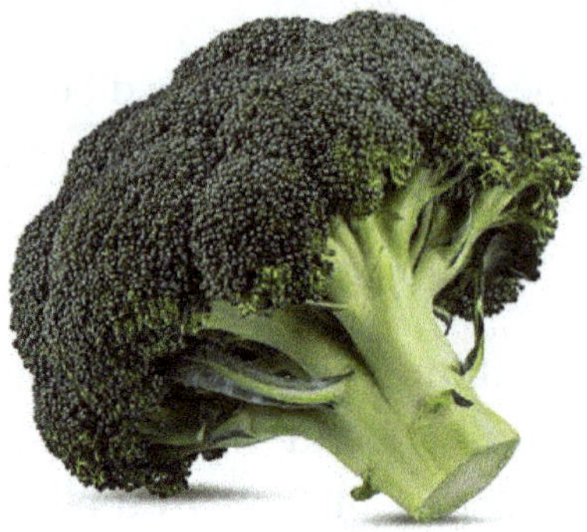

A Nutrient-Rich Cruciferous Gem for Health and Flavor

Broccoli, with its vibrant green florets and distinctively crunchy texture, is a nutritional powerhouse that has earned its reputation as a superfood. Packed with essential vitamins, minerals, and antioxidants, broccoli not only adds a burst of flavor to meals but also contributes to overall well-being. In this article, we explore the myriad benefits of broccoli and delve into its versatile uses in the kitchen.

Nutritional Benefits:

Rich in Vitamin C:

- Broccoli is a potent source of vitamin C, a crucial antioxidant that supports the immune system, aids in collagen formation for skin health, and promotes overall vitality.

High in Fiber:

- A fiber-rich vegetable, broccoli aids in digestion, promotes a feeling of fullness, and helps maintain stable blood sugar levels.

Abundance of Vitamin K:

- Broccoli is a notable source of vitamin K, essential for blood clotting and bone health. Adequate vitamin K intake contributes to maintaining strong and healthy bones.

Vitamin A and Folate Content:

- Broccoli provides significant amounts of vitamin A, vital for vision and immune function, and folate, important for DNA synthesis and cell **division.**

Calcium:

Benefits:

- Essential for the formation and maintenance of strong bones and teeth.
- Supports proper muscle function and nerve transmission.
- Plays a role in blood clotting and cellular signaling.

Potassium:

Benefits:

- Helps regulate blood pressure by balancing sodium levels.
- Supports proper fluid balance in the body.
- Aids in muscle contractions and nerve transmissions.

Magnesium:

Benefits:

- Important for muscle and nerve function.
- Contributes to bone health by aiding in the absorption of calcium.
- Plays a role in energy metabolism and protein synthesis.

Phosphorus:

Benefits:

- Essential for the formation and maintenance of healthy bones and teeth.
- Involved in the metabolism of macronutrients (carbohydrates, proteins, and fats).
- Contributes to the synthesis of DNA and RNA.

Health Benefits:

Anti-Cancer Properties:

- Broccoli belongs to the cruciferous vegetable family, known for its cancer-fighting compounds. Sulforaphane, a sulfur-containing compound in broccoli, has been studied for its potential anti-cancer properties.

Heart Health Support:

- The fiber, potassium, and antioxidants in broccoli contribute to heart health by lowering cholesterol levels, regulating blood pressure, and reducing oxidative stress.

Bone Health:

- Broccoli's rich vitamin K content plays a role in bone metabolism, promoting calcium absorption and contributing to bone density and strength.

Detoxification and Immune Support:

- Sulforaphane in broccoli supports the body's natural detoxification processes and enhances immune function, aiding in the defense against infections.

Nutritional Content

In 1 cup (approximately 156 grams) of cooked broccoli, the approximate nutritional content is as follows:

- Carbohydrates: Approximately 6 grams
- Protein: Approximately 4 grams
- Fiber: Approximately 2.4 grams
- Fat: Approximately 0.5 grams

Please note that these values are approximate and can vary slightly based on factors such as the cooking method and the specific variety of broccoli.

Culinary Versatility:

Steamed Broccoli:

- A simple and nutritious side dish, steamed broccoli retains its vibrant color and crunch while preserving its nutritional value.

Broccoli Salad:

- Toss blanched broccoli florets with cherry tomatoes, red onion, feta cheese, and a light vinaigrette for a refreshing salad.

Broccoli Stir-Fry:

- Combine broccoli with other colorful vegetables and your choice of protein for a quick and flavorful stir-fry.

Roasted Broccoli:

- Roasting broccoli with olive oil, garlic, and a sprinkle of parmesan creates a savory and caramelized side dish.

Broccoli's versatility makes it a great addition to various recipes. Here are a few delicious and easy-to-make recipes featuring broccoli:

Broccoli and Cheddar Stuffed Baked Potatoes:

Ingredients:

- 4 large russet potatoes
- 2 cups broccoli florets, steamed
- 1 cup shredded cheddar cheese
- 1/2 cup sour cream
- 2 tablespoons butter
- Salt and pepper to taste
- Chopped green onions for garnish (optional)

Instructions:

1. Preheat the oven to 400°F (200°C).
2. Wash and scrub the potatoes, then pierce them with a fork. Bake the potatoes directly on the oven rack for about 45-60 minutes or until tender.
3. While the potatoes are baking, steam the broccoli until just tender. Chop into small florets.
4. Once the potatoes are cooked, allow them to cool slightly. Cut a slit in the top of each potato and gently fluff the insides with a fork.
5. In a bowl, mix the steamed broccoli, shredded cheddar, sour cream, butter, salt, and pepper.
6. Spoon the broccoli and cheddar mixture into each baked potato.
7. Place the stuffed potatoes back in the oven for about 10 minutes or until the cheese is melted and bubbly.
8. Garnish with chopped green onions if desired and serve.

Garlic Parmesan Roasted Broccoli:

Ingredients:

- 4 cups broccoli florets
- 3 tablespoons olive oil
- 4 cloves garlic, minced
- 1/4 cup grated Parmesan cheese
- Salt and black pepper to taste
- Lemon wedges for serving (optional)

Instructions:

1. Preheat the oven to 425°F (220°C).
2. In a large bowl, toss the broccoli florets with olive oil, minced garlic, salt, and black pepper until evenly coated.
3. Spread the broccoli in a single layer on a baking sheet lined with parchment paper.
4. Roast in the preheated oven for about 20-25 minutes or until the edges are crispy and golden.
5. Remove from the oven and sprinkle grated Parmesan over the roasted broccoli.
6. Toss the broccoli to coat it evenly with the Parmesan.
7. Return the baking sheet to the oven for an additional 5 minutes or until the cheese is melted and bubbly.
8. Serve the garlic Parmesan roasted broccoli hot, with optional lemon wedges for squeezing over the top.

These recipes showcase the versatility of broccoli, whether stuffed into baked potatoes or roasted with flavorful garlic and Parmesan. Enjoy these nutritious and delicious dishes!

Tips on Growing Broccoli

Broccoli typically takes about 60 to 100 days to grow from seed to harvest, depending on the variety and growing conditions. Here's a general timeline:

1. **Seedling Stage**: Broccoli seeds are usually started indoors about 6 to 8 weeks before the last spring frost date. They are then transplanted outdoors when they have grown to about 4 to 6 inches tall, which typically takes about 3 to 4 weeks.
2. **Growth Stage**: Once transplanted, broccoli plants continue to grow and develop. They require consistent watering, adequate sunlight, and proper nutrition during this stage.
3. **Head Formation**: Depending on the variety, broccoli heads begin to form within 60 to 90 days after transplanting. This process may take longer for some varieties.
4. **Harvesting**: Broccoli heads are typically ready to harvest when they are firm, compact, and dark green in color. Harvesting usually occurs when the main head is fully developed but before the florets start to separate or open up. This can occur anywhere from 60 to 100 days after transplanting, depending on the variety and growing conditions.

It's important to note that broccoli is a cool-season crop and prefers cooler temperatures for optimal growth. Additionally, factors such as soil quality, watering, and pest management can also affect the growth rate of broccoli plants.

Conclusion:

Broccoli stands as a nutritional powerhouse, offering a spectrum of health benefits and culinary versatility. Incorporating this cruciferous gem into your diet not only enhances the flavor of your meals but also contributes to a well-rounded and healthful lifestyle. If you have specific health concerns or conditions, it's advisable to consult with a healthcare professional or a registered dietitian for personalized advice. Celebrate the goodness of broccoli as you explore its benefits and savor its delicious presence on your plate.

Back to Table of Contents

Brussels Sprouts

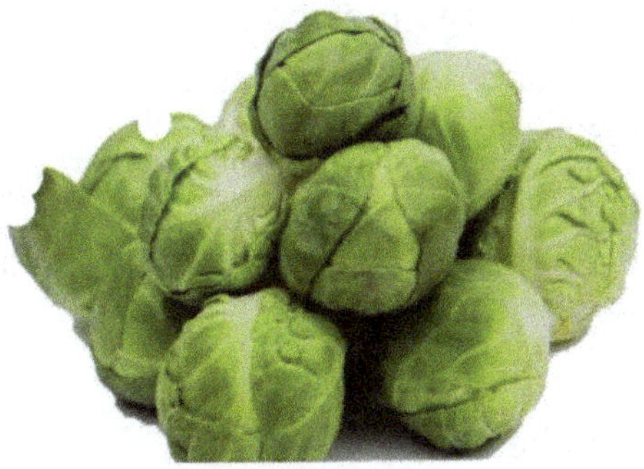

The Nutrient-Packed Gem: Unveiling the Benefits and Uses of Brussels Sprouts

Brussels sprouts, often overlooked in the world of vegetables, are miniature members of the cruciferous family, boasting a myriad of health benefits and culinary possibilities. These tiny, cabbage-like vegetables pack a powerful nutritional punch, making them a valuable addition to any well-balanced diet. Let's explore the benefits and creative uses that make Brussels sprouts a versatile and nutritious choice.

Nutrient Profile:

Brussels sprouts are nutrient-dense, offering an array of essential vitamins, minerals, and antioxidants. Here's a glimpse into their impressive nutritional profile:

Vitamin C (Ascorbic Acid):

- Acts as a powerful antioxidant, protecting cells from oxidative damage.
- Supports the immune system by enhancing the function of white blood cells.
- Promotes collagen synthesis for healthy skin.

Vitamin K:

- Essential for blood clotting, preventing excessive bleeding.
- Supports bone health by aiding in the regulation of calcium.

Vitamin A:

- Important for vision and eye health.
- Supports immune function.
- Contributes to skin health.

Folate (Vitamin B9)

- Essential for DNA synthesis and cell division.

- Crucial during pregnancy for fetal development.

Vitamin B6 (Pyridoxine):

- Supports brain development and function.
- Aids in the metabolism of amino acids and neurotransmitters.

Thiamine (Vitamin B1):

- Plays a role in energy metabolism.
- Essential for nerve function.

Riboflavin (Vitamin B2):

- Supports energy metabolism.
- Contributes to the health of the skin, eyes, and nervous system.

Niacin (Vitamin B3):

- Plays a role in energy metabolism.
- Supports skin health.

Vitamin E:

- Acts as an antioxidant, protecting cells from oxidative stress.
- Supports immune function.

Pantothenic Acid (Vitamin B5):

- Plays a role in energy metabolism.
- Contributes to the synthesis of fatty acids and cholesterol.

Fiber:

- Aids in digestion and promotes a feeling of fullness.
- Supports heart health and regulates blood sugar levels.

Antioxidants (including Glucosinolates):

- Combat oxidative stress and inflammation.
- May have potential cancer-fighting properties.

Minerals (such as Potassium and Manganese):

Potassium:

- **Benefits:**
    1. Regulates fluid balance in the body.
    2. Supports proper muscle and nerve function.
    3. Helps maintain healthy blood pressure.

Manganese:

- **Benefits:**
    1. Essential for bone health and development.
    2. Plays a role in collagen formation and wound healing.
    3. Acts as an antioxidant.

Phosphorus:

- **Benefits:**
    1. Essential for bone and teeth formation.
    2. Involved in energy metabolism.
    3. Plays a role in maintaining pH balance in the body.

Magnesium:

- **Benefits:**
    1. Supports muscle and nerve function.
    2. Contributes to bone health.
    3. Aids in energy metabolism.

Iron:

- **Benefits:**
    1. Essential for the formation of hemoglobin, which carries oxygen in the blood.
    2. Supports energy metabolism.

Calcium:

- **Benefits:**
    1. Important for bone and teeth health.
    2. Supports muscle function and nerve transmission.
    3. Plays a role in blood clotting.

Zinc:

- **Benefits:**
    1. Supports immune function.
    2. Plays a role in wound healing.
    3. Contributes to DNA synthesis.

Copper:

- **Benefits:**
    1. Supports the formation of red blood cells.
    2. Contributes to the maintenance of connective tissues and the nervous system.
    3. Acts as an antioxidant.

Selenium:

- **Benefits:**
    1. Acts as an antioxidant, protecting cells from oxidative damage.
    2. Supports the immune system.

Health Benefits:

Rich in Antioxidants:

Brussels sprouts are packed with antioxidants, including glucosinolates, which have been associated with reducing inflammation and may play a role in preventing certain cancers.

Heart Health:

The fiber, potassium, and other heart-healthy compounds in Brussels sprouts contribute to cardiovascular well-being by helping regulate blood pressure, cholesterol levels, and supporting overall heart function.

Bone Health:

The combination of vitamin K and other minerals in Brussels sprouts supports bone health, contributing to the prevention of osteoporosis and fractures.

Digestive Health: The fiber content aids in digestion, promotes regular bowel movements, and supports a healthy gut microbiome.

Weight Management: With a low calorie count and high fiber content, Brussels sprouts are an excellent addition to a weight management plan, promoting satiety and aiding in portion control.

Nutritional Content

In 1 cup (approximately 88 grams) of cooked Brussels sprouts, the approximate nutritional content is as follows:

- Carbohydrates: Approximately 8 grams
- Protein: Approximately 3 grams
- Fiber: Approximately 4 grams
- Fat: Approximately 0.4 grams

Please note that these values are approximate and can vary slightly based on factors such as the cooking method and the specific variety of Brussels sprouts.

Creative Culinary Uses:

Roasted Brussels Sprouts:

- Toss Brussels sprouts with olive oil, salt, and pepper.
- Roast in the oven until golden brown and crispy.
- Enhance with balsamic glaze, Parmesan cheese, or a sprinkle of nuts.

Brussels Sprouts Salad:

- Shred raw Brussels sprouts and mix with your favorite salad greens.
- Add diced apples, cranberries, and a light vinaigrette dressing for a refreshing salad.

Sautéed Brussels Sprouts:

- Sauté sliced Brussels sprouts with garlic, lemon zest, and a touch of olive oil.
- Finish with a sprinkle of fresh herbs or grated cheese.

Brussels Sprouts Slaw:

- Thinly slice Brussels sprouts and toss with shredded cabbage and carrots.
- Create a zesty slaw with a citrus-based dressing.

Brussels Sprouts and Bacon:

- Sauté Brussels sprouts with crispy bacon for a flavorful and savory side dish.

Here are two delicious recipes featuring Brussels sprouts:

Roasted Balsamic Brussels Sprouts:

Ingredients:

- 1 lb Brussels sprouts, trimmed and halved
- 2 tablespoons olive oil
- 2 tablespoons balsamic vinegar
- 2 cloves garlic, minced
- Salt and pepper to taste
- Optional: Parmesan cheese for topping

Instructions:

1. Preheat the oven to 400°F (200°C).
2. In a bowl, toss Brussels sprouts with olive oil, balsamic vinegar, minced garlic, salt, and pepper until evenly coated.
3. Spread the Brussels sprouts in a single layer on a baking sheet.
4. Roast in the preheated oven for 20-25 minutes or until the edges are crispy and golden brown.
5. Optional: Sprinkle freshly grated Parmesan cheese over the roasted Brussels sprouts before serving.

Brussels Sprouts and Quinoa Salad:

Ingredients:

- 1 cup quinoa, cooked according to package instructions
- 1 lb Brussels sprouts, trimmed and thinly sliced
- 1/2 cup dried cranberries
- 1/2 cup chopped pecans, toasted
- 1/4 cup feta cheese, crumbled
- 3 tablespoons olive oil
- 2 tablespoons balsamic vinegar
- Salt and pepper to taste

Instructions:

1. In a large bowl, combine cooked quinoa, sliced Brussels sprouts, dried cranberries, toasted pecans, and crumbled feta cheese.
2. In a small bowl, whisk together olive oil and balsamic vinegar to create the dressing.
3. Pour the dressing over the salad and toss until well combined.
4. Season with salt and pepper to taste.
5. Serve the Brussels sprouts and quinoa salad chilled or at room temperature.

These recipes showcase the versatility of Brussels sprouts, whether roasted to perfection or featured in a vibrant salad. Feel free to customize these recipes based on your preferences and enjoy the wonderful flavors and nutritional benefits of Brussels sprouts!

Tips on Growing Brussels Sprouts

Brussels sprouts typically take about 80 to 100 days to grow from seed to harvest. Here's a general timeline:

1. **Seedling Stage**: Brussels sprouts are usually started indoors about 12 to 14 weeks before the last spring frost date. They are then transplanted outdoors when they have grown to about 4 to 6 inches tall, which typically takes about 4 to 6 weeks.
2. **Growth Stage**: Once transplanted, Brussels sprout plants continue to grow and develop. They require consistent watering, adequate sunlight, and proper nutrition during this stage.
3. **Sprout Formation**: Brussels sprouts form along the stem of the plant, starting from the bottom and working their way up. This process can take several weeks, usually around 80 to 100 days after transplanting, depending on the variety and growing conditions.
4. **Harvesting**: Brussels sprouts are typically ready to harvest when the sprouts are firm, green, and about 1 to 1.5 inches in diameter. Harvesting usually occurs from the bottom of the stem upwards, as the lower sprouts mature first. This can occur around 80 to 100 days after transplanting, depending on the variety and growing conditions.

It's important to note that Brussels sprouts are a cool-season crop and prefer cooler temperatures for optimal growth. Additionally, factors such as soil quality, watering, and pest management can also affect the growth rate of Brussels sprout plants.

Cautions and Considerations:

While Brussels sprouts offer numerous health benefits, they contain compounds known as FODMAPs (fermentable oligosaccharides, disaccharides, monosaccharides, and polyols) that may cause digestive discomfort in some individuals. Cooking methods, such as roasting or steaming, can help mitigate this issue. If you have specific health concerns, allergies, or conditions, it's advisable to consult with a healthcare professional or a registered dietitian before making significant changes to your diet.

In **conclusion**, Brussels sprouts are a nutritional powerhouse that can be enjoyed in various culinary creations. Whether roasted to crispy perfection, tossed in a vibrant salad, or sautéed with complementary flavors, these tiny cruciferous wonders deserve a place on your plate. Embrace the versatility and reap the health benefits of Brussels sprouts as you embark on a journey to savor their delicious offerings.

Back to Table of Contents

Buckwheat

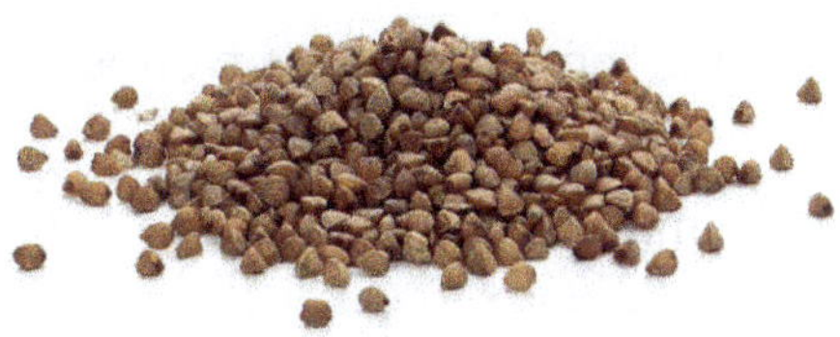

Unveiling the Marvels of Buckwheat: Nutrient-Rich and Versatile

Buckwheat, often associated with hearty pancakes, is much more than a beloved breakfast staple. This gluten-free pseudo-grain, despite its name, is not a type of wheat at all. The seeds of the buckwheat plant are used for culinary purposes and are prized for their unique nutritional profile and earthy flavor. Buckwheat seeds are small, triangular in shape, and usually a light to dark brown color. They can be consumed whole, cracked, or ground into flour, offering versatility in cooking and baking.

Buckwheat, scientifically known as Fagopyrum esculentum, has a rich history, impressive nutritional profile, and a wide range of culinary applications. Let's explore the benefits and uses of this versatile and nutrient-packed grain alternative.

Nutritional Powerhouse:

Buckwheat is a nutritional powerhouse, offering a variety of essential nutrients that contribute to overall well-being. Here are some key components of its nutritional profile:

Protein:

- Buckwheat is a notable plant-based source of high-quality protein, containing all essential amino acids. This makes it an excellent choice for those following vegetarian or vegan diets.

Fiber:

- Rich in both soluble and insoluble fiber, buckwheat supports digestive health, helps maintain blood sugar levels, and contributes to a feeling of fullness.

Minerals:

Buckwheat is a good source of minerals such as magnesium, manganese, phosphorus, and copper. These minerals play crucial roles in bone health, energy metabolism, and antioxidant defense.

Magnesium:

- Essential for muscle and nerve function, bone health, and energy metabolism.

Manganese:

- Plays a role in bone formation, blood clotting, and reducing inflammation.

Phosphorus:

- Important for bone and teeth health, as well as energy metabolism.

Copper:

- Necessary for the formation of red blood cells and the absorption of iron.

Iron:

- Vital for oxygen transport in the blood and overall energy metabolism.

Zinc:

- Supports immune function, wound healing, and DNA synthesis.

Potassium:

- Helps regulate fluid balance, supports proper muscle and nerve function, and contributes to heart health.

Selenium:

- Acts as an antioxidant, protecting cells from oxidative damage.

Calcium:

- Important for bone and teeth health, muscle function, and blood clotting.

Cobalt:

- While only present in trace amounts, cobalt is a component of vitamin B12, which is produced by certain bacteria and is found in small amounts in foods like buckwheat.

Zirconium:

- Present in trace amounts, zirconium is a naturally occurring element found in various minerals, including some grains like buckwheat.

It's important to note that the mineral content of buckwheat can vary based on factors such as growing conditions, soil composition, and processing methods. Including a variety of nutrient-rich foods in your diet is key to ensuring an adequate intake of essential minerals and other nutrients.

Vitamins:

Buckwheat contains various B-vitamins, including B1 (thiamine), B2 (riboflavin), B3 (niacin), B5 (pantothenic acid), B6 (pyridoxine), and folate. These vitamins are essential for energy production and overall cellular function.

Buckwheat is a nutrient-rich pseudo-grain that contains various vitamins essential for overall health. Here is a list of vitamins found in buckwheat:

Vitamin B1 (Thiamine):

- Essential for energy metabolism, nerve function, and maintaining a healthy cardiovascular system.

Vitamin B2 (Riboflavin):

- Plays a key role in energy production, supports cellular function, and is important for maintaining healthy skin and eyes.

Vitamin B3 (Niacin):

- Involved in energy metabolism, supports proper functioning of the nervous system, and plays a role in skin health.

Vitamin B5 (Pantothenic Acid):

- Necessary for the synthesis of fatty acids and energy production from carbohydrates.

Vitamin B6 (Pyridoxine):

- Important for amino acid metabolism, neurotransmitter synthesis, and immune function.

Folate (Vitamin B9):

- Essential for DNA synthesis, cell division, and the formation of red blood cells. It is particularly important during periods of rapid growth and development.

Vitamin E:

- An antioxidant that helps protect cells from oxidative damage. It also plays a role in immune function.

Vitamin K:

- Essential for blood clotting and bone health. It helps regulate calcium and supports overall cardiovascular health.

While these vitamins are present in buckwheat, it's important to note that the amounts can vary based on factors such as the variety of buckwheat, growing conditions, and processing methods. Including a variety of nutrient-dense foods in your diet is key to ensuring a well-rounded intake of essential vitamins and other nutrients. If you have specific dietary concerns or health conditions, consulting with a healthcare professional or a registered dietitian is recommended.

Antioxidants:

With its rich content of flavonoids and other antioxidants, buckwheat helps protect the body's cells from oxidative stress. Rutin, a specific flavonoid found in buckwheat, is known for its anti-inflammatory and antioxidant properties.

Rutin:

- Rutin is a flavonoid that is particularly abundant in buckwheat. It is known for its antioxidant and anti-inflammatory properties. Rutin has been associated with cardiovascular health benefits and may help protect blood vessels.

Quercetin:

- Another flavonoid, quercetin is found in buckwheat and exhibits antioxidant and anti-inflammatory effects. It has been linked to various health benefits, including immune system support and cardiovascular health.

Catechins:

- Catechins are a type of polyphenol that acts as antioxidants. They are present in buckwheat and contribute to its overall antioxidant capacity.

Vitamin E:

- While primarily known as a vitamin, vitamin E also functions as an antioxidant. Buckwheat contains vitamin E, contributing to its ability to protect cells from oxidative damage.

Beta-Carotene:

- Beta-carotene is a precursor to vitamin A and functions as a powerful antioxidant. While not as abundant as in some fruits and vegetables, buckwheat contains beta-carotene.

Phenolic Acids:

- Buckwheat contains various phenolic acids, including ferulic acid and caffeic acid, which contribute to its antioxidant activity.

Lignans:

- Lignans are phytochemicals found in plants, and buckwheat is a source of these compounds. They have been associated with antioxidant and potential anticancer effects.

The combination of these antioxidants helps protect cells from oxidative stress, reduce inflammation, and contribute to the overall health benefits of including buckwheat in the diet. Consuming a diverse range of antioxidant-rich foods is essential for supporting overall well-being.

Health Benefits:

Heart Health:

- Buckwheat has been linked to heart health due to its ability to lower cholesterol levels. The fiber, magnesium, and flavonoids in buckwheat contribute to cardiovascular well-being.

Blood Sugar Control:

- The complex carbohydrates and fiber in buckwheat contribute to stabilized blood sugar levels, making it a suitable option for individuals with diabetes or those seeking to manage blood glucose.

Digestive Health:

- The fiber in buckwheat promotes regular bowel movements and supports a healthy digestive system. It can be beneficial for preventing constipation and maintaining gut health.

Nutritional Content

In 1 cup (approximately 168 grams) of cooked buckwheat groats, the approximate nutritional content is as follows:

- Carbohydrates: Approximately 34 grams

- Protein: Approximately 6 grams
- Fiber: Approximately 5 grams
- Fat: Approximately 1 gram

Please note that these values are approximate and can vary slightly based on factors such as the cooking method and the specific variety of buckwheat.

Culinary Uses:

Buckwheat's nutty flavor and versatile nature make it a popular ingredient in a variety of dishes. Here are some common culinary uses:

Buckwheat Groats:

- Whole buckwheat groats can be cooked and used as a base for salads, pilafs, or as a side dish.

Flour:

- Buckwheat flour is a gluten-free alternative that can be used in baking, creating pancakes, bread, noodles, and other delicious treats.

Soba Noodles:

- Soba noodles, made from buckwheat flour, are a staple in Japanese cuisine. They can be enjoyed in soups, stir-fries, or chilled with dipping sauces.

Porridge:

- Buckwheat porridge, made by cooking buckwheat groats with water or plant-based milk, is a hearty and nutritious breakfast option.

Buckwheat Tea:

- Roasted buckwheat kernels can be used to make a flavorful and caffeine-free tea known as sobacha.

Buckwheat's nutty flavor and versatile nature make it a fantastic ingredient in a variety of recipes. ***Here are two delicious recipes featuring buckwheat:***

Buckwheat Pancakes:

Ingredients:

- 1 cup buckwheat flour
- 1 tablespoon sugar or sweetener of choice
- 1 teaspoon baking powder
- 1/2 teaspoon baking soda
- 1/4 teaspoon salt
- 1 cup plant-based milk (almond, soy, or oat)
- 1 tablespoon apple cider vinegar
- 1 flax egg (1 tablespoon ground flaxseed mixed with 3 tablespoons water)
- 1 tablespoon melted coconut oil or neutral oil
- Optional: Vanilla extract, berries, or sliced bananas for topping

Instructions:

1. In a mixing bowl, combine buckwheat flour, sugar, baking powder, baking soda, and salt.
2. In a separate bowl, mix plant-based milk with apple cider vinegar and let it sit for a few minutes to create "buttermilk."
3. Add the flax egg and melted coconut oil to the "buttermilk" and whisk until well combined.
4. Pour the wet ingredients into the dry ingredients and stir until just combined. Let the batter rest for a few minutes.
5. Heat a non-stick skillet or griddle over medium heat.
6. Pour 1/4 cup portions of batter onto the skillet to form pancakes.
7. Cook until bubbles form on the surface, then flip and cook until the other side is golden brown.
8. Repeat with the remaining batter.
9. Serve the buckwheat pancakes with your favorite toppings, such as berries, sliced bananas, or a drizzle of maple syrup.

Buckwheat Salad with Roasted Vegetables:

Ingredients:

- 1 cup raw buckwheat groats
- 2 cups water
- 1 red bell pepper, diced
- 1 zucchini, diced
- 1 cup cherry tomatoes, halved
- 1 red onion, finely sliced
- 3 tablespoons olive oil
- 2 tablespoons balsamic vinegar
- Salt and pepper to taste
- Fresh herbs (such as parsley or basil) for garnish

Instructions:

1. Rinse the buckwheat groats under cold water.
2. In a saucepan, combine the buckwheat groats and water. Bring to a boil, then reduce heat, cover, and simmer for 10-12 minutes or until the water is absorbed. Fluff with a fork and let it cool.
3. Preheat the oven to 400°F (200°C).
4. In a large bowl, toss the diced red bell pepper, zucchini, cherry tomatoes, and red onion with olive oil, balsamic vinegar, salt, and pepper.
5. Spread the vegetables on a baking sheet and roast in the preheated oven for about 20-25 minutes or until they are tender and slightly caramelized.
6. In a serving bowl, combine the cooked buckwheat groats with the roasted vegetables.
7. Garnish with fresh herbs and additional salt and pepper to taste.

8. Serve the buckwheat salad warm or at room temperature.

These recipes highlight the versatility of buckwheat, showcasing its use in both sweet and savory dishes. Enjoy the delicious and nutritious benefits of incorporating buckwheat into your culinary repertoire!

Conclusion:

Buckwheat's unique combination of nutrients, health benefits, and culinary versatility makes it a valuable addition to a well-balanced diet. Whether you're looking to enhance heart health, support digestion, or experiment with gluten-free cooking, buckwheat proves to be a versatile and nutrient-rich grain alternative. If you have specific health concerns, allergies, or conditions, it's advisable to consult with a healthcare professional or a registered dietitian before making significant changes to your diet.

Embrace the diverse uses of buckwheat in your kitchen and savor the nutritional benefits it brings to your plate.

Back to Table of Contents

Burdock

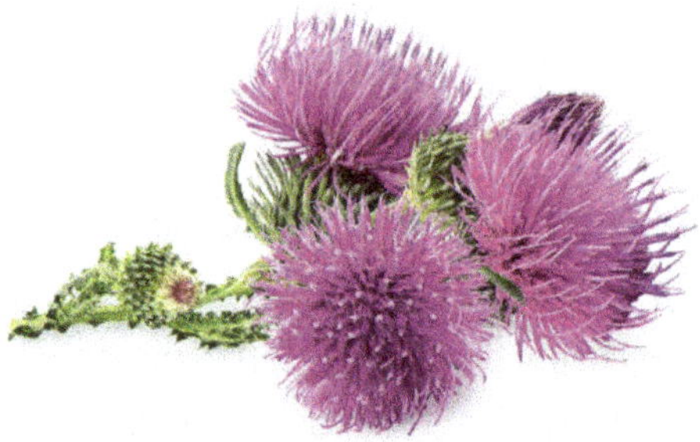

Unveiling the Bounty of Burdock: Benefits and Versatile Uses

Burdock, with its robust roots and distinctive, heart-shaped leaves, has long been celebrated in traditional medicine and culinary traditions around the world. This hardy plant, scientifically known as Arctium lappa, boasts a wealth of health-promoting properties and offers a wide range of uses, from supporting digestion to enhancing skin health. Let's embark on a journey to discover the remarkable benefits and versatile uses of burdock.

A Botanical Treasure: Understanding Burdock

Burdock is a biennial plant native to Europe and Asia but has since spread to other regions, including North America, where it is often considered a weed. The plant features large, coarse leaves and produces characteristic burrs that cling to clothing and animal fur, aiding in seed dispersal. However, it is the root of the burdock plant that holds the most medicinal and culinary value.

Burdock root is rich in various vitamins, minerals, and antioxidants, which contribute to its numerous health benefits. Here's a list of some of the key nutrients found in burdock root:

Vitamins:

Vitamin B1 (Thiamine): Important for energy metabolism and nerve function.

Vitamin B2 (Riboflavin): Involved in energy production and antioxidant defenses.

Vitamin B3 (Niacin): Supports energy metabolism and healthy skin.

Vitamin B5 (Pantothenic Acid): Essential for synthesizing and metabolizing fats, proteins, and carbohydrates.

Vitamin B6 (Pyridoxine): Necessary for amino acid metabolism, neurotransmitter synthesis, and immune function.

Vitamin B9 (Folate): Important for DNA synthesis, cell division, and red blood cell formation.

Vitamin C: A potent antioxidant that supports immune function and collagen synthesis.

Vitamin E: Fat-soluble antioxidant that protects cells from oxidative damage.

Minerals:

Iron: Essential for oxygen transport in the blood and energy metabolism.

Manganese: Important for bone health, collagen production, and antioxidant defenses.

Magnesium: Involved in over 300 enzymatic reactions in the body, including energy production and muscle function.

Potassium: Electrolyte essential for fluid balance, muscle function, and blood pressure regulation.

Phosphorus: Necessary for bone and teeth health, as well as energy metabolism.

Calcium: Crucial for bone health, muscle function, and nerve transmission.

Zinc: Supports immune function, wound healing, and DNA synthesis.

Copper: Essential for iron metabolism, connective tissue formation, and antioxidant defenses.

Antioxidants:

Phenolic Acids: Including caffeic acid, chlorogenic acid, and coumaric acid, which possess antioxidant and anti-inflammatory properties.

Flavonoids: Such as quercetin, kaempferol, and luteolin, which have antioxidant, anti-inflammatory, and immune-modulating effects.

Lignans: Plant compounds with antioxidant and estrogenic properties, which may have protective effects against certain chronic diseases.

Tannins: Polyphenolic compounds with antioxidant and astringent properties, which contribute to burdock's health benefits.

Anthraquinones: Compounds with antioxidant and antimicrobial properties, which may support digestive health and detoxification processes.

These vitamins, minerals, and antioxidants found in burdock root work synergistically to support overall health and well-being. Incorporating burdock into your diet or using it as a supplement may provide a wide range of nutritional benefits and promote optimal health.

Health Benefits of Burdock

Burdock root has been revered for centuries in traditional herbal medicine systems, including Traditional Chinese Medicine (TCM) and Ayurveda, for its numerous health benefits. Here are some of the key advantages of incorporating burdock into your wellness routine:

Digestive Support: Burdock root contains prebiotic fibers that promote the growth of beneficial gut bacteria, supporting digestive health and regularity. It is often used to alleviate symptoms of indigestion, bloating, and constipation.

Detoxification: Burdock root is prized for its diuretic and detoxifying properties, which help eliminate toxins and waste products from the body through the kidneys and urinary tract. It is believed to purify the blood and lymphatic system, supporting overall detoxification and cleansing.

Anti-inflammatory and Antioxidant Effects: Burdock root contains potent antioxidants, including phenolic acids and flavonoids, which help reduce inflammation and oxidative stress in the body. These properties may benefit conditions such as arthritis, eczema, and other inflammatory disorders.

Skin Health: Burdock root is often used topically to promote skin health and alleviate skin conditions such as acne, eczema, psoriasis, and dermatitis. Its anti-inflammatory and antibacterial properties help soothe irritation, reduce redness, and support healing.

Blood Sugar Regulation: Some studies suggest that burdock root may help regulate blood sugar levels and improve insulin sensitivity, making it potentially beneficial for individuals with diabetes or metabolic syndrome.

Versatile Uses of Burdock

Burdock root can be enjoyed in various forms, including fresh, dried, powdered, or as a supplement. Here are some common ways to incorporate burdock into your diet and skincare routine:

Nutritional Content

In 1 cup (about 155 grams) of cooked burdock root, the approximate nutritional content is as follows:

- Carbohydrates: Approximately 27 grams
- Protein: Approximately 2 grams
- Fiber: Approximately 6 grams
- Fat: Approximately 0.2 grams

Please note that these values are approximate and can vary slightly based on factors such as the cooking method and the specific variety of burdock.

Culinary Delights:

Burdock root is a versatile ingredient in culinary traditions around the world. It can be cooked and eaten as a vegetable, added to soups, stews, stir-fries, and salads, or pickled for a tangy and crunchy snack.

Herbal Teas and Infusions: Burdock root tea is a popular herbal remedy known for its detoxifying and diuretic properties. Simply steep dried burdock root slices or tea bags in hot water for a soothing and cleansing beverage.

Here are two delicious recipes featuring burdock:

1. **Burdock Root Stir-Fry:**
    - **Ingredients:**
        - 2 medium-sized burdock roots

- 2 tablespoons vegetable oil
- 2 cloves garlic, minced
- 1-inch piece of ginger, minced
- 2 carrots, julienned
- 1 bell pepper, thinly sliced
- 2 tablespoons soy sauce (or tamari for gluten-free option)
- 1 tablespoon rice vinegar
- 1 tablespoon maple syrup or honey
- Sesame seeds and chopped green onions for garnish (optional)

- **Instructions:**
  1. Peel the burdock roots and julienne them into thin strips.
  2. Heat vegetable oil in a large skillet or wok over medium heat. Add minced garlic and ginger and sauté for 1-2 minutes until fragrant.
  3. Add the julienned burdock roots to the skillet and stir-fry for 3-4 minutes until they begin to soften.
  4. Add julienned carrots and sliced bell pepper to the skillet and continue stir-frying for another 3-4 minutes until the vegetables are tender-crisp.
  5. In a small bowl, whisk together soy sauce, rice vinegar, and maple syrup or honey. Pour the sauce over the stir-fried vegetables and toss to coat evenly.
  6. Cook for an additional 1-2 minutes until the sauce thickens slightly and coats the vegetables.
  7. Remove from heat and garnish with sesame seeds and chopped green onions if desired. Serve hot as a side dish or over cooked rice or noodles.

2. **Burdock Root Tea:**
   - **Ingredients:**
     - 1 burdock root (about 6 inches long), washed and thinly sliced
     - 4 cups water
     - Honey or maple syrup (optional)
     - Lemon slices (optional)
   - **Instructions:**
     1. In a medium saucepan, combine the sliced burdock root and water. Bring to a boil over medium-high heat.
     2. Reduce the heat to low and simmer, covered, for 20-30 minutes, or until the burdock root has softened and the water has infused with its flavor.
     3. Remove the saucepan from heat and let the tea cool slightly.
     4. Strain the tea to remove the burdock root slices, then pour it into mugs.

5. Sweeten with honey or maple syrup if desired and garnish with lemon slices.
6. Serve hot and enjoy the earthy and aromatic flavor of burdock root tea.

These recipes showcase the versatility of burdock root and its ability to add unique flavor and nutritional value to dishes. Whether enjoyed in a savory stir-fry or brewed into a soothing tea, burdock root offers a delicious way to incorporate this nutritious ingredient into your diet.

Topical Treatments: Burdock root extract or oil can be applied topically to the skin to soothe irritation, reduce inflammation, and promote healing. It can be found in skincare products such as creams, lotions, and ointments.

Supplements: Burdock root supplements, available in various forms such as capsules, tablets, and tinctures, offer a convenient way to reap the health benefits of this botanical powerhouse.

Precautions and Considerations

While burdock root is generally safe for most people when consumed in moderate amounts, individuals with certain medical conditions, allergies, or sensitivities should exercise caution. It is advisable to consult with a healthcare professional before using burdock root, especially if you are pregnant, breastfeeding, taking medications, or have underlying health concerns.

In conclusion, burdock is a botanical treasure with a rich history of medicinal and culinary use. Whether enjoyed as a nourishing vegetable, brewed into a healing tea, or applied topically for skincare, burdock offers a multitude of benefits for health and well-being. Embrace the bounty of burdock and harness its potential to enhance your vitality and vitality.

Back to Table of Contents

Butternut Squash

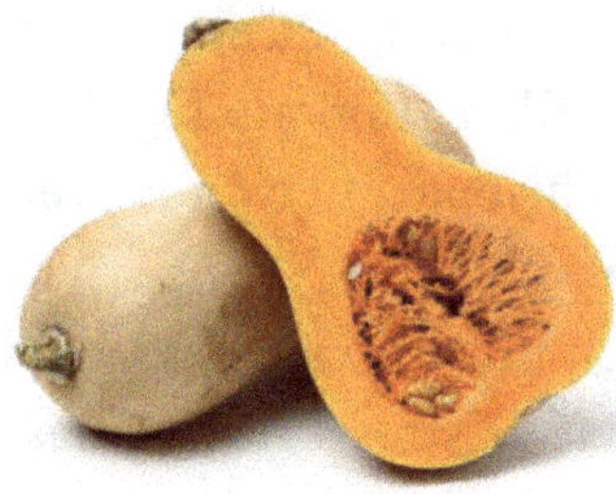

A Nutrient-Packed Gourd with Culinary Versatility

Butternut squash, with its distinct bell-like shape and vibrant orange flesh, is a versatile and nutritious vegetable that graces tables in various culinary creations. Beyond its rich, sweet flavor, butternut squash boasts an array of health benefits and can be incorporated into a multitude of dishes. In this article, we explore the numerous advantages of butternut squash and showcase its culinary versatility.

Nutritional Benefits:

Rich in Vitamin A:

- Butternut squash is a powerhouse of beta-carotene, a precursor to vitamin A. This nutrient is essential for maintaining healthy vision, supporting immune function, and promoting skin health.

Vitamin C:

Benefits:

- Boosts the immune system by supporting the production of white blood cells.
- Promotes collagen synthesis, contributing to healthy skin, gums, and blood vessels.
- Acts as an antioxidant, protecting cells from damage caused by free radicals.
- Enhances the absorption of non-heme iron from plant-based foods.

Vitamin E:

Benefits:

- Acts as an antioxidant, protecting cells from oxidative stress.
- Supports immune function and helps in maintaining healthy skin.
- Contributes to the protection of cell membranes.

Vitamin B6 (Pyridoxine):

Benefits:

- Plays a crucial role in brain development and function.
- Supports the metabolism of amino acids and neurotransmitters.
- Contributes to the formation of red blood cells.

- Helps regulate mood and sleep patterns.

High in Fiber:

- Fiber is crucial for digestive health, and butternut squash provides a significant amount. A diet rich in fiber supports regular bowel movements, helps maintain a healthy weight, and contributes to overall well-being.

Loaded with Antioxidants:

- Butternut squash is rich in antioxidants, including vitamin C and other compounds that help combat oxidative stress. Antioxidants play a key role in protecting cells from damage caused by free radicals.

Abundance of Minerals:

Butternut squash contains essential minerals such as potassium, manganese, and magnesium. These minerals contribute to heart health, bone health, and various physiological functions in the body.

Here are some minerals found in butternut squash and their benefits:

Potassium:

- **Benefits:**
    - Regulates blood pressure by balancing sodium levels in the body.
    - Supports proper fluid balance, which is crucial for kidney function.
    - Aids in muscle contraction and nerve transmission.

Manganese:

- **Benefits:**
    - Essential for bone formation and maintenance.
    - Plays a role in collagen production, contributing to skin health.
    - Acts as a cofactor for various enzymes involved in metabolism.

Magnesium:

- **Benefits:**
    - Supports muscle and nerve function.
    - Contributes to bone health by aiding in calcium absorption.
    - Plays a role in energy metabolism and protein synthesis.

Copper:

- **Benefits:**
    - Essential for the formation of red blood cells and hemoglobin.
    - Supports the development and maintenance of connective tissues.
    - Acts as a cofactor for enzymes involved in iron metabolism.

Health Benefits:

Supports Immune Function:

- The high vitamin A and C content in butternut squash plays a vital role in supporting the immune system, helping the body defend against infections and illnesses.

Aids in Weight Management:

- The fiber content in butternut squash promotes a feeling of fullness, which can be beneficial for those looking to manage their weight by reducing overall calorie intake.

Promotes Heart Health:

- Potassium in butternut squash helps regulate blood pressure and supports cardiovascular health, reducing the risk of heart-related issues.

Assists in Blood Sugar Control:

- The fiber content and low glycemic index of butternut squash make it a favorable choice for individuals looking to manage blood sugar levels.

Culinary Versatility:

Roasted Butternut Squash:

- Toss cubed butternut squash with olive oil, salt, and pepper, then roast until caramelized for a delicious side dish.

Butternut Squash Soup:

- Blend roasted or sautéed butternut squash with broth, seasonings, and cream for a creamy and comforting soup.

Butternut Squash Risotto:

- Incorporate cubed butternut squash into a creamy risotto for a hearty and flavorful dish.

Butternut Squash Salad:

- Roast slices of butternut squash and add them to salads for a burst of color, flavor, and nutrition.

Butternut squash is a versatile ingredient that can be used in both savory and sweet dishes. Here are two delicious recipes featuring butternut squash:

Roasted Butternut Squash Soup:

Ingredients:

- 1 medium-sized butternut squash, peeled, seeded, and cubed
- 1 large onion, chopped
- 2 carrots, peeled and chopped
- 2 cloves garlic, minced
- 2 tablespoons olive oil
- 4 cups vegetable broth
- 1 teaspoon ground cumin

- 1/2 teaspoon ground coriander
- 1/2 teaspoon smoked paprika
- Salt and pepper to taste
- 1/2 cup coconut milk (optional, for added creaminess)
- Fresh parsley or chives for garnish

Instructions:

1. Preheat the oven to 400°F (200°C).
2. Toss the cubed butternut squash, chopped onion, carrots, and minced garlic with olive oil, cumin, coriander, smoked paprika, salt, and pepper.
3. Spread the mixture on a baking sheet and roast in the preheated oven for about 30-40 minutes or until the vegetables are tender and slightly caramelized.
4. Transfer the roasted vegetables to a blender or food processor. Add vegetable broth and blend until smooth.
5. Pour the blended mixture into a pot and heat over medium heat. Stir in coconut milk if using.
6. Adjust seasoning to taste and simmer for an additional 10 minutes.
7. Serve hot, garnished with fresh parsley or chives.

Maple Glazed Butternut Squash with Pecans:

Ingredients:

- 1 medium-sized butternut squash, peeled, seeded, and cut into cubes
- 2 tablespoons maple syrup
- 2 tablespoons olive oil
- 1/2 teaspoon ground cinnamon
- 1/4 teaspoon ground nutmeg
- Salt and pepper to taste
- 1/2 cup pecans, chopped
- Fresh rosemary for garnish (optional)

Instructions:

1. Preheat the oven to 400°F (200°C).
2. In a bowl, toss the butternut squash cubes with maple syrup, olive oil, cinnamon, nutmeg, salt, and pepper until well coated.
3. Spread the coated squash on a baking sheet in a single layer.
4. Roast in the preheated oven for 25-30 minutes or until the squash is tender and caramelized.
5. In the last 5 minutes of roasting, sprinkle the chopped pecans over the squash and allow them to toast.
6. Remove from the oven and transfer to a serving dish.
7. Garnish with fresh rosemary if desired and serve as a delightful side dish.

These recipes showcase the versatility of butternut squash, whether used in a comforting soup or as a sweet and savory side dish. Enjoy!

Nutritional Content

In 1 cup (approximately 205 grams) of cooked butternut squash, the approximate nutritional content is as follows:

- Carbohydrates: Approximately 21 grams
- Protein: Approximately 2 grams
- Fiber: Approximately 6.6 grams
- Fat: Approximately 0.2 grams

Please note that these values are approximate and can vary slightly based on factors such as the cooking method and the specific variety of butternut squash.

Conclusion:

Butternut squash is not just a fall favorite; it's a year-round nutritional powerhouse that can elevate the taste and health benefits of your meals. Whether roasted, blended into soups, or featured in salads, the culinary versatility of butternut squash makes it a delightful addition to any kitchen. If you have specific health concerns or conditions, it's advisable to consult with a healthcare professional or a registered dietitian for personalized advice. Embrace this nutrient-packed gourd to savor its sweet, earthy flavor and reap the health benefits it brings to the table.

Back to Table of Contents

Cabbage

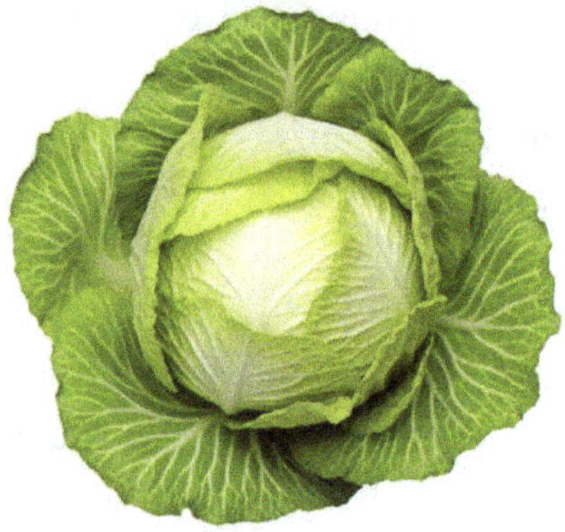

A Crunchy Cruciferous Wonder with Numerous Benefits and Culinary Versatility

Cabbage, a humble cruciferous vegetable, often finds its place in kitchens around the world, offering both culinary versatility and an impressive array of health benefits. Whether enjoyed raw in salads, fermented into sauerkraut, or cooked in various dishes, cabbage stands out as a nutrient-rich and budget-friendly addition to a well-balanced diet. In this article, we will explore the numerous advantages and creative uses that make cabbage a nutritional powerhouse.

Nutrient-Rich Composition:

Cabbage is renowned for its nutritional density, providing an assortment of vitamins, minerals, and antioxidants. Here's a closer look at the key components that make cabbage a healthy choice:

Vitamins:

Cabbage is a nutrient-rich vegetable that provides various vitamins essential for health. Here's a list of vitamins found in cabbage:

Vitamin C:

- Cabbage is an excellent source of vitamin C, a powerful antioxidant that supports the immune system, aids in collagen synthesis, and promotes skin health.

Vitamin K:

- Cabbage is rich in vitamin K, which is crucial for blood clotting and bone health. Adequate vitamin K intake contributes to proper bone metabolism.

Vitamin B6 (Pyridoxine):

- Cabbage contains vitamin B6, which is important for the metabolism of amino acids and the synthesis of neurotransmitters.

Folate (Vitamin B9):

- Folate is present in cabbage and is essential for DNA synthesis and cell division.

Vitamin B1 (Thiamine):

- Cabbage provides thiamine, a B-vitamin that plays a role in energy metabolism and nerve cell function.

Vitamin B2 (Riboflavin):

- Riboflavin is found in cabbage and is involved in energy production and **the metabolism of fats.**

Vitamin B3 (Niacin):

- Cabbage contains niacin, a B-vitamin important for energy metabolism and the health of the nervous system.

Vitamin B5 (Pantothenic Acid):

- Pantothenic acid is present in cabbage and is involved in the synthesis of essential molecules in the body.

Including cabbage in your diet can contribute to meeting your daily vitamin needs, supporting various physiological functions and promoting overall health. As with any food, it's important to consume a variety of nutrient-rich foods to ensure a balanced intake of vitamins and other essential nutrients.

Minerals:

Cabbage is a good source of several minerals that contribute to its nutritional value. Here's a list of minerals found in cabbage:

Calcium:

- Cabbage provides calcium, which is crucial for bone health, nerve function, and muscle contraction.

Potassium:

- Cabbage is a good source of potassium, an essential mineral that helps regulate fluid balance, nerve signals, and muscle contractions.

Phosphorus:

- Phosphorus is present in cabbage and is important for bone and teeth formation, DNA synthesis, and energy metabolism.

Magnesium:

- Magnesium in cabbage supports muscle and nerve function, regulates blood pressure, and contributes to bone health.

Sodium:

- While cabbage is not high in sodium, it naturally contains some sodium, contributing to electrolyte balance.

Iron:

- Iron is present in cabbage and is important for the formation of hemoglobin, the protein responsible for carrying oxygen in the blood.

Manganese:

- Manganese is a trace mineral found in cabbage, contributing to bone formation, blood clotting, and reducing inflammation.

Copper:

- Cabbage contains copper, which is essential for the formation of red blood cells, maintenance of healthy bones and nerves, and immune system function.

Including cabbage in your diet can help ensure a diverse intake of minerals, supporting various physiological functions and promoting overall health. As with any food, it's important to consume a variety of nutrient-rich foods to ensure a broad spectrum of minerals and other essential nutrients.

Dietary Fiber:

- Cabbage is rich in dietary fiber, promoting digestive health, regulating blood sugar levels, and contributing to a feeling of fullness.

Antioxidants:

- Cabbage is packed with antioxidants, including flavonoids and polyphenols, which help combat oxidative stress and reduce inflammation.

Health Benefits:

Digestive Health:

- The high fiber content in cabbage supports digestive health, preventing constipation and promoting a healthy gut microbiome.

Heart Health:

- Potassium, found in cabbage, contributes to heart health by helping regulate blood pressure and promoting cardiovascular function.

Anti-Inflammatory Properties:

- The antioxidants in cabbage, such as anthocyanins, help reduce inflammation and may lower the risk of chronic diseases.

Weight Management:

- Cabbage is low in calories and high in fiber, making it a satisfying and nutritious addition to weight management and healthy eating plans.

Nutritional Content

In 1 cup (approximately 89 grams) of raw cabbage, the approximate nutritional content is as follows:

- Carbohydrates: Approximately 5 grams
- Protein: Approximately 1 gram
- Fiber: Approximately 2 grams
- Fat: Approximately 0.1 grams

Please note that these values are approximate and can vary slightly based on factors such as the specific type of cabbage and its size. Additionally, the nutritional content may change if the cabbage is cooked or prepared in different ways.

Culinary Uses:

Coleslaw:

- Cabbage is a key ingredient in coleslaw, a classic side dish made with shredded cabbage, carrots, and a creamy dressing.

Stir-Fries and Soups:

- Add shredded cabbage to stir-fries and soups for a crunchy texture and a nutritional boost.

Fermented Foods:

- Cabbage is the main ingredient in sauerkraut, a fermented dish that not only enhances flavor but also provides gut-friendly probiotics.

Stuffed Cabbage Rolls:

- Create delicious stuffed cabbage rolls by wrapping cabbage leaves around a flavorful filling, often with ground meat or grains.

Cabbage is a versatile vegetable that can be used in a variety of dishes. Here are three delicious recipes featuring cabbage:

Jamaican Cabbage and Saltfish is a classic dish that combines the rich, savory flavor of salted codfish with the sweetness of cabbage and other aromatic ingredients. Here's a simple recipe for you to try:

Jamaican Cabbage and Saltfish

Ingredients:

- 1 lb salted codfish (saltfish), soaked and flaked
- 1 small head of green cabbage, shredded
- 1 large carrot, julienned
- 1 large onion, thinly sliced
- 2 tomatoes, diced
- 2 bell peppers (ideally one green and one red), thinly sliced
- 2 cloves garlic, minced
- 2 sprigs thyme
- 2 scallions, chopped
- 1 Scotch bonnet pepper, finely chopped (adjust to taste for spice)
- 2 tablespoons vegetable oil
- Black pepper to taste

- 2 tablespoons soy sauce (optional)
- 2 tablespoons fresh lime or lemon juice
- Steamed white rice, for serving

Instructions:

Prepare the Saltfish:

- Rinse the saltfish under cold water to remove excess salt. Place it in a bowl and cover with water. Allow it to soak for at least 4-6 hours, changing the water a few times. After soaking, boil the saltfish for about 15-20 minutes to further reduce saltiness. Drain and flake the fish, removing any bones or skin.

Sauté Aromatics:

- In a large skillet or wok, heat the vegetable oil over medium heat. Add the minced garlic, sliced onions, thyme, and Scotch bonnet pepper. Sauté until the onions are translucent and the garlic is fragrant.

Add Vegetables:

- Add the shredded cabbage, julienned carrots, sliced bell peppers, and diced tomatoes to the skillet. Toss the vegetables together and let them cook for about 5-7 minutes until they start to soften.

Incorporate Saltfish:

- Add the flaked saltfish to the vegetables. Mix everything well, ensuring that the saltfish is evenly distributed among the vegetables.

Seasoning:

- Season the mixture with black pepper and soy sauce (if using). Continue to stir and cook for an additional 5-7 minutes until the vegetables are tender but still have a slight crunch.

Finish and Serve:

- Add chopped scallions and fresh lime or lemon juice to the dish. Taste and adjust seasoning if needed. Continue to cook for an additional 2-3 minutes.

Serve:

- Serve the Jamaican Cabbage and Saltfish over steamed white rice. Garnish with additional scallions or fresh herbs if desired.

Enjoy this flavorful and satisfying Jamaican dish that brings together the vibrant taste of salted codfish with the goodness of cabbage and other aromatic vegetables. It's a perfect blend of savory and sweet, with a hint of spice to tantalize your taste buds.

Classic Cabbage Rolls:

Ingredients:

- 1 head of green cabbage
- 1 cup cooked rice
- 1 lb ground beef or plant-based alternative
- 1 onion, finely chopped

- 2 cloves garlic, minced
- 1 can (15 oz) tomato sauce
- 1 can (14.5 oz) diced tomatoes
- 1 teaspoon dried oregano
- 1 teaspoon dried thyme
- Salt and pepper to taste
- Olive oil for cooking

Instructions:

Prepare the Cabbage Leaves:

- Bring a large pot of water to a boil. Carefully remove the outer leaves of the cabbage and blanch them in the boiling water for about 2-3 minutes until they are pliable. Remove and set aside.

Prepare the Filling:

- In a skillet, heat olive oil over medium heat. Add chopped onions and garlic, sauté until softened. Add ground beef (or plant-based alternative) and cook until browned. Season with salt, pepper, dried oregano, and thyme. Stir in cooked rice.

Assemble the Cabbage Rolls:

- Place a spoonful of the filling onto each cabbage leaf. Roll them up, tucking in the sides to create neat rolls.

Cook the Cabbage Rolls:

- In a large baking dish, mix tomato sauce and diced tomatoes. Place the cabbage rolls in the dish, seam side down. Cover with the sauce. Bake in a preheated oven at 350°F (175°C) for about 45 minutes to 1 hour, until the cabbage is tender.

Serve:

- Serve the cabbage rolls hot, optionally garnished with fresh herbs.

Asian-inspired Cabbage Salad:

Ingredients:

- 1/2 head of green cabbage, thinly sliced
- 1 carrot, julienned
- 1 bell pepper, thinly sliced
- 1 cup edamame, cooked
- 1/4 cup soy sauce
- 2 tablespoons rice vinegar
- 1 tablespoon sesame oil
- 1 tablespoon honey or maple syrup
- 1 teaspoon grated ginger
- Sesame seeds and chopped green onions for garnish

Instructions:

Prepare the Vegetables:

- In a large bowl, combine sliced cabbage, julienned carrot, sliced bell pepper, and cooked edamame.

Prepare the Dressing:

- In a small bowl, whisk together soy sauce, rice vinegar, sesame oil, honey (or maple syrup), and grated ginger.

Assemble the Salad:

- Pour the dressing over the vegetables and toss until well coated.

Chill and Garnish:

- Refrigerate the salad for at least 30 minutes to allow the flavors to meld. Before serving, sprinkle sesame seeds and chopped green onions on top.

Serve:

- Enjoy the refreshing and crunchy Asian-inspired cabbage salad as a side or a light meal.

These recipes showcase the versatility of cabbage, whether used in hearty stuffed cabbage rolls or a vibrant Asian-inspired salad. Enjoy experimenting with this nutritious and budget-friendly vegetable in your kitchen!

Conclusion:

Cabbage, with its rich nutrient profile and versatility in the kitchen, deserves its status as a dietary staple. Whether raw, cooked, or fermented, incorporating cabbage into your meals can contribute to overall health and well-being. If you have specific health concerns, allergies, or conditions, it's advisable to consult with a healthcare professional or a registered dietitian before making significant changes to your diet.

Embrace the crunch and goodness of cabbage, and let this unassuming vegetable take center stage in your culinary adventures and on your journey to a balanced and nutritious diet.

Back to Table of Contents

Calendula

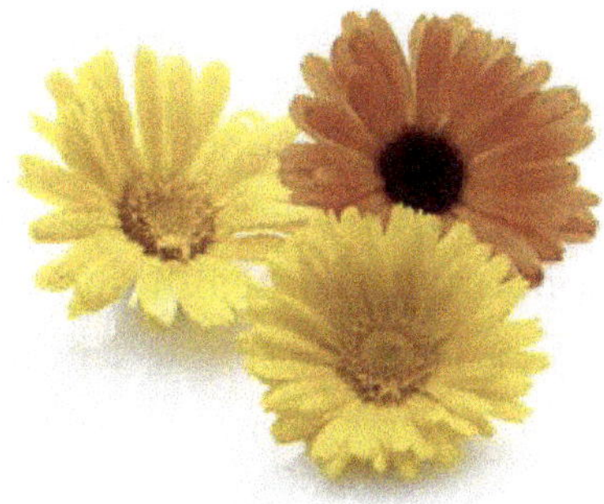

The Power of Calendula: A Comprehensive Guide to Benefits and Uses

Calendula, a vibrant and sun-loving herb, has been cherished for its medicinal properties and ornamental beauty for centuries. Also known as marigold, Calendula officinalis is a versatile plant that offers a wide array of benefits for both health and skincare. In this article, we will delve into the rich history, nutritional components, and diverse uses of calendula, exploring why it has become a beloved herb in traditional medicine and modern skincare.

History and Origin:

Calendula has a long history of cultivation, with its origins traced back to ancient Mediterranean civilizations. Egyptians and Greeks revered calendula for its symbolic significance, associating it with the sun and its golden petals. Throughout history, calendula has been utilized in various cultures for its healing properties, making it a staple in herbal medicine.

Nutritional Profile:

Calendula is not only admired for its aesthetic appeal but is also packed with valuable nutrients. Rich in flavonoids, carotenoids, and essential oils, calendula offers a spectrum of health-promoting compounds. These components contribute to its anti-inflammatory, antimicrobial, and antioxidant properties, making it a valuable addition to holistic wellness practices.

Calendula (Calendula officinalis) is a nutrient-rich herb that offers various health benefits due to its diverse array of compounds. Here are some key nutrients found in calendula and their associated benefits:

Flavonoids:

Benefits:

- *Antioxidant Activity:* Flavonoids in calendula, such as quercetin and rutin, exhibit strong antioxidant properties. Antioxidants help neutralize free radicals in the body, reducing oxidative stress and protecting cells from damage.

Carotenoids:

Benefits:

- ***Skin Health:*** Calendula contains carotenoids like beta-carotene, which contribute to its vibrant color. Beta-carotene is converted into vitamin A in the body, supporting skin health and promoting a healthy complexion. It also plays a role in maintaining eye health.

Essential Oils:

Benefits:

- ***Anti-Inflammatory Properties:*** The essential oils in calendula, including terpenoids and sesquiterpenes, contribute to its anti-inflammatory effects. These properties make calendula beneficial for soothing skin irritations, reducing inflammation, and promoting wound healing.

Triterpenoids:

Benefits:

- ***Wound Healing:*** Triterpenoids found in calendula, such as faradiol esters, are associated with accelerated wound healing. Calendula extracts are often used topically in creams and ointments to promote the healing of cuts, burns, and other skin injuries.

These nutrients work synergistically to provide a range of health benefits, making calendula a valuable herb for both internal and external use.

Health Benefits:

Skin Healing and Repair:

- Calendula's anti-inflammatory and antibacterial properties make it effective in promoting wound healing and preventing infections. It is commonly used in salves, creams, and ointments to soothe skin irritations, cuts, and burns.

Anti-Inflammatory Action:

- Calendula's anti-inflammatory compounds help alleviate inflammatory conditions, such as dermatitis and eczema. Its soothing effects can bring relief to irritated and sensitive skin.

Immune Support:

- The immune-boosting properties of calendula, attributed to its antioxidants, contribute to overall immune system health. Consuming calendula in various forms, such as teas or tinctures, may provide immune support.

Skincare Uses:

Calendula-infused Oil:

- Infuse carrier oils like olive or jojoba with dried calendula petals to create a soothing and nourishing oil. This infusion can be applied topically to moisturize and calm the skin.

Calendula Tea Compress:

- Brew calendula tea and let it cool. Soak a clean cloth in the tea and apply it as a compress to areas with skin irritations, rashes, or sunburn. The anti-inflammatory properties can help reduce redness and discomfort.

Calendula Creams and Balms:

- Calendula creams and balms are widely available for topical application. These products are crafted to harness the herb's healing properties and are used for conditions like dry skin, chapped lips, and minor skin irritations.

Culinary Uses:

Calendula Petal Salad:

- Harvest fresh calendula petals and add them to your salads for a burst of color and subtle floral notes. Calendula petals can be sprinkled over mixed greens or incorporated into a salad with other edible flowers and herbs. The petals not only enhance the visual appeal of the dish but also contribute a mild, earthy flavor.

Calendula Infused Honey:

- Create a delicately flavored calendula-infused honey by combining fresh or dried calendula petals with honey. Place the petals in a clean, dry jar and pour honey over them, ensuring the petals are fully submerged. Allow the mixture to infuse for a week or longer, depending on your desired intensity of flavor. Strain out the petals, and you'll have a sweet and floral-infused honey. Use it as a natural sweetener in teas, drizzled over desserts, or as a unique addition to marinades.

Calendula Tea or Herbal Infusion:

- Brew a soothing and aromatic tea by using fresh or dried calendula flowers. Infuse hot water with calendula petals, allowing them to steep for about 5 to 10 minutes. You can enjoy calendula tea on its own or mix it with other herbal teas for a unique blend. Additionally, calendula petals can be incorporated into herbal infusions with ingredients like chamomile or mint for a flavorful and calming beverage.

These culinary applications showcase the versatility of calendula in enhancing both the visual appeal and flavor profile of various dishes. Whether incorporated into salads, infused in honey, or brewed into a delightful tea, calendula adds a touch of uniqueness to your culinary creations.

Conclusion:

Calendula, with its sunny disposition and multifaceted benefits, has earned its place as a revered herb in both traditional and contemporary practices. Whether applied topically or consumed as a tea, calendula stands as a testament to the enduring relationship between nature and well-being. Embrace the golden powers of calendula to nurture your skin and promote a holistic approach to health and vitality.

Back to Table of Contents

Callaloo

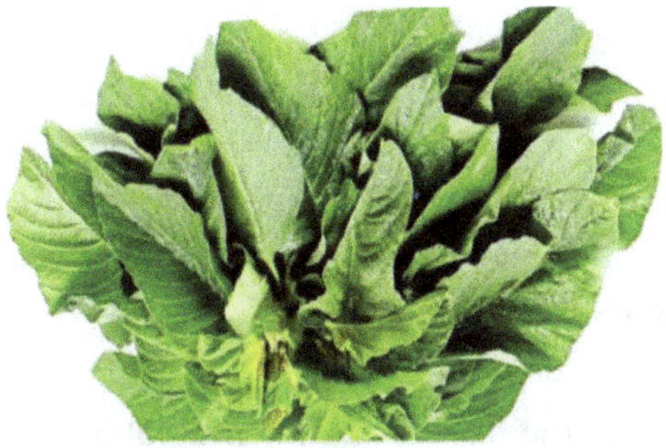

A Nutrient-Rich Green Powerhouse with Culinary Versatility

Callaloo, a leafy green vegetable native to the Caribbean and popular in many tropical regions, is not just a flavorful addition to dishes but also a nutritional powerhouse. Known for its vibrant green leaves and distinct flavor, callaloo offers a range of health benefits and versatile culinary uses. Let's explore the myriad advantages of including callaloo in your diet and discover creative ways to enjoy this nutritious leafy green.

Nutritional Bounty:

Callaloo is a rich source of essential nutrients, making it a valuable addition to a well-balanced diet. Packed with vitamins A, C, and K, callaloo contributes to eye health, immune support, and blood clotting. It also contains a variety of minerals, including iron, calcium, and potassium, vital for maintaining strong bones, healthy blood pressure, and overall electrolyte balance.

Vitamin A:

- **Benefits:** Callaloo is a rich source of vitamin A, essential for maintaining healthy vision, skin, and the immune system. Vitamin A also plays a crucial role in cell growth and differentiation, contributing to overall well-being.

Vitamin C:

- **Benefits:** Callaloo contains a significant amount of vitamin C, an antioxidant that supports the immune system and helps the body absorb iron. Vitamin C also promotes the health of skin, blood vessels, and connective tissues.

Iron:

- **Benefits:** Iron is essential for the formation of hemoglobin, the oxygen-carrying component of red blood cells. Adequate iron intake from foods like callaloo helps prevent iron deficiency anemia and ensures proper oxygen transport throughout the body.

Potassium:

- **Benefits:** Callaloo is a good source of potassium, a mineral that plays a crucial role in maintaining healthy blood pressure, fluid balance, and proper muscle and nerve function. Adequate potassium intake is associated with a lower risk of cardiovascular diseases.

Minerals

Calcium:

- **Benefits:** Callaloo is a good source of calcium, a mineral essential for building and maintaining strong bones and teeth. Adequate calcium intake also plays a role in muscle function, nerve transmission, and blood clotting.

Iron:

- **Benefits:** Iron is crucial for the formation of hemoglobin, the protein in red blood cells responsible for transporting oxygen throughout the body. Adequate iron intake from callaloo and other sources helps prevent iron deficiency anemia and supports overall energy levels.

Potassium:

- **Benefits:** Callaloo contains potassium, a mineral that plays a key role in maintaining proper fluid balance, supporting healthy blood pressure, and ensuring optimal nerve and muscle function. Adequate potassium intake is associated with a reduced risk of cardiovascular diseases.

Magnesium:

- **Benefits:** Magnesium is involved in more than 300 biochemical reactions in the body, including energy production, muscle function, and the maintenance of strong bones. Consuming callaloo as a source of magnesium contributes to overall health and well-being.

Heart-Healthy Properties:

The high fiber content in callaloo is beneficial for heart health. Dietary fiber helps lower cholesterol levels, reducing the risk of cardiovascular diseases. Potassium, present in significant amounts in callaloo, further supports heart health by regulating blood pressure and promoting proper heart function.

Antioxidant Boost:

Callaloo is a rich source of antioxidants, including beta-carotene and flavonoids. These compounds help neutralize harmful free radicals in the body, protecting cells from oxidative stress and reducing inflammation. Regular consumption of callaloo may contribute to a lower risk of chronic diseases associated with oxidative damage.

Historical Uses

Traditional Medicine in the Caribbean:

- **Historical Use:** In the Caribbean, callaloo has a history of use in traditional medicine. The leaves were often brewed into teas or infusions and used to alleviate various ailments, including digestive issues. The high fiber content in callaloo likely contributed to its use in promoting healthy digestion and preventing constipation.

African Culinary Traditions:

- **Historical Use:** Callaloo has its roots in African culinary traditions, particularly among communities brought to the Caribbean through the transatlantic slave trade. The leaves were commonly used in stews and soups, providing a nutritious and flavorful addition to meals. The consumption of callaloo was not only a culinary practice but also a way to maintain cultural connections and dietary traditions.

Nutrient-Rich Staple in Indigenous Cultures:

- **Historical Use:** Indigenous cultures in tropical regions historically relied on callaloo as a nutrient-rich staple in their diets. The leaves provided essential vitamins, minerals, and antioxidants, contributing to overall health and well-being. Incorporating callaloo into regular meals helped ensure a diverse and nutritionally balanced diet.

Symbol of Resilience and Survival:

- **Historical Use:** Callaloo became a symbol of resilience and survival in the face of adversity. During challenging times, the cultivation and consumption of callaloo played a crucial role in providing sustenance and nutrition. The plant's ability to thrive in various conditions made it a valuable resource, emphasizing its historical significance in sustaining communities.

Nutritional Content

The nutritional content of callaloo can vary depending on the specific preparation method and any additional ingredients used. However, here's a general approximation based on cooked callaloo greens:

In 1 cup (approximately 160 grams) of cooked callaloo:

- Carbohydrates: Approximately 7 grams
- Protein: Approximately 2 grams
- Fiber: Approximately 4 grams
- Fat: Approximately 0.5 grams

Please note that these values are approximate and can vary based on factors such as the specific ingredients used in the preparation and the cooking method. Additionally, if you're referring to callaloo as a dish, the nutritional content can vary greatly depending on the recipe.

Culinary Versatility:

Beyond its nutritional benefits, callaloo's versatility in the kitchen makes it a favorite ingredient in various culinary traditions. Here are some creative ways to incorporate callaloo into your meals:

Callaloo Soup: A popular Caribbean dish, callaloo soup often features a combination of callaloo leaves, coconut milk, and a medley of spices, creating a flavorful and comforting bowl.

Stir-Fries and Sautes: Add chopped callaloo leaves to stir-fries or sauté them with garlic and olive oil for a quick and nutritious side dish.

Smoothies: Blend callaloo leaves into your favorite smoothie for a nutrient-packed green boost. The mild flavor pairs well with fruits and other vegetables.

Callaloo Salad: Use callaloo leaves in salads for a fresh and vibrant addition. Combine them with other greens, vegetables, and a zesty dressing for a nutritious and delicious dish.

Tips on Growing Callaloo

The time it takes for callaloo to grow depends on various factors including the specific variety of callaloo, growing conditions, and desired size at harvest. However, callaloo typically matures relatively quickly compared to other leafy greens.

Here's a general timeline for growing callaloo:

1. **Germination**: Callaloo seeds usually germinate within 7 to 14 days after planting, provided they are kept in optimal conditions such as adequate moisture and warmth.
2. **Growth Stage**: Callaloo plants grow rapidly once they have germinated. They typically reach harvestable size within 4 to 6 weeks after germination. However, you can start harvesting leaves earlier if you prefer young and tender greens.
3. **Harvesting**: You can harvest callaloo leaves as soon as they reach the desired size, typically when they are 6 to 12 inches tall. Harvesting can be done by cutting the outer leaves, allowing the inner leaves to continue growing for future harvests.

It's important to note that callaloo is often grown as a cut-and-come-again crop, meaning you can harvest the outer leaves multiple times throughout the growing season as long as the plant continues to produce new growth.

Overall, callaloo is known for its relatively fast growth compared to other leafy greens, making it a popular choice for home gardeners and small-scale farmers.

Conclusion:

Callaloo stands out not only for its delightful taste but also for its impressive nutritional profile. Packed with vitamins, minerals, and antioxidants, callaloo offers a multitude of health benefits, from supporting heart health to boosting the immune system. Whether enjoyed in soups, salads, or smoothies, callaloo adds a touch of tropical goodness to your meals while contributing to your overall well-being. Embrace the culinary versatility and health advantages of callaloo, and elevate your dining experience with this green powerhouse.

Back to Table of Contents

Cantaloupe

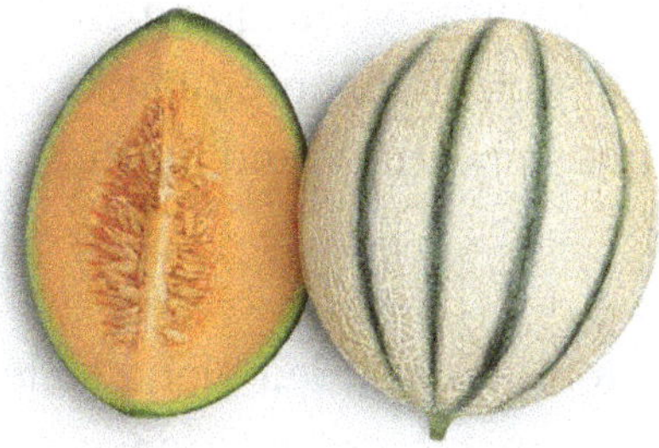

A Sweet and Nutrient-Rich Melon with Health Benefits

Cantaloupe, also known as muskmelon, is a delicious and refreshing fruit that belongs to the melon family. With its sweet, juicy flesh and distinctive aroma, cantaloupe is not only a favorite summer treat but also a nutritious addition to a well-balanced diet. In this article, we'll explore the many benefits of cantaloupe and highlight its versatile uses.

Nutritional Benefits:

Rich in Vitamin C:

Cantaloupe is a great source of vitamin C, an antioxidant that supports the immune system, promotes healthy skin, and aids in collagen synthesis.

Vitamins in Cantaloupe:

Vitamin C:

- **Benefits:**
    - Supports the immune system by enhancing the production and function of white blood cells.
    - Acts as an antioxidant, protecting cells from oxidative damage.
    - Promotes healthy skin by aiding in collagen synthesis.

Vitamin A (Beta-Carotene):

- **Benefits:**
    - Essential for maintaining healthy vision and preventing night blindness.
    - Supports immune function and helps maintain healthy skin and mucous membranes.
    - Acts as an antioxidant, contributing to overall cellular health.

Vitamin K:

- **Benefits:**
    - Plays a crucial role in blood clotting, preventing excessive bleeding.
    - Contributes to bone health by aiding in the regulation of calcium.
    - Supports cardiovascular health by preventing arterial calcification.

Minerals in Cantaloupe:

Potassium:

- **Benefits:**
    - Regulates blood pressure by balancing sodium levels in the body.
    - Supports proper muscle and nerve function.
    - Aids in maintaining a healthy fluid balance.

Copper:

- **Benefits:**
    - Essential for the formation of red blood cells and hemoglobin.
    - Supports the development and maintenance of connective tissues.
    - Contributes to the function of various enzymes involved in iron metabolism.

Magnesium:

- **Benefits:**
    - Important for muscle and nerve function.
    - Contributes to bone health by working with calcium and vitamin D.
    - Supports energy metabolism and protein synthesis.

High Water Content:

- With its high-water content, cantaloupe helps keep the body hydrated, especially important on hot days or after physical activity.

Beta-Carotene Content:

- The orange hue of cantaloupe is indicative of its beta-carotene content, which the body converts into vitamin A. Vitamin A is essential for vision, immune function, and skin health.

Low in Calories:

- Cantaloupe is a low-calorie fruit, making it a healthy option for those watching their calorie intake. It provides natural sweetness without added sugars.

Health Benefits:

Hydration and Electrolyte Balance:

- The water content in cantaloupe helps with hydration, while its natural electrolytes, such as potassium, assist in maintaining a proper fluid balance in the body.

Digestive Health:

- Cantaloupe is a good source of dietary fiber, supporting digestive health by promoting regular bowel movements and preventing constipation.

Antioxidant Protection:

- The presence of antioxidants, including vitamin C and beta-carotene, helps protect cells from oxidative stress, reducing the risk of chronic diseases.

Eye Health:

- The beta-carotene in cantaloupe is converted into vitamin A, which is crucial for maintaining healthy vision and preventing age-related macular degeneration.

Nutritional Content

In 1 cup (approximately 160 grams) of raw cantaloupe (also known as muskmelon or rockmelon), the approximate nutritional content is as follows:

- Carbohydrates: Approximately 13 grams
- Protein: Approximately 1.3 grams
- Fiber: Approximately 1.6 grams
- Fat: Approximately 0.3 grams

Please note that these values are approximate and can vary slightly based on factors such as the specific variety of cantaloupe and its ripeness.

Culinary Uses:

Cantaloupe Salad:

- Combine diced cantaloupe with fresh mint, feta cheese, and a drizzle of balsamic glaze for a refreshing summer salad.

Cantaloupe Smoothie:

- Blend cantaloupe chunks with yogurt, a splash of orange juice, and ice for a cool and hydrating smoothie.

Cantaloupe Salsa:

- Mix diced cantaloupe with red onion, jalapeño, cilantro, and lime juice for a sweet and spicy salsa, perfect for topping grilled chicken or fish.

Cantaloupe Sorbet:

- Freeze pureed cantaloupe with a touch of honey for a delightful and guilt-free sorbet.

Here are two delightful recipes featuring cantaloupe:

Cantaloupe and Prosciutto Skewers:

Ingredients:

- 1 cantaloupe, peeled, seeded, and cut into bite-sized cubes
- 10 slices of prosciutto, cut into strips
- Fresh mint leaves
- Balsamic glaze for drizzling (optional)

Instructions:

1. Thread a cube of cantaloupe, a strip of prosciutto, and a mint leaf onto small skewers or toothpicks.
2. Arrange the skewers on a serving platter.
3. Drizzle with balsamic glaze if desired.

4. Serve as a refreshing and elegant appetizer for gatherings.

Cantaloupe Gazpacho:

Ingredients:

- 1 cantaloupe, peeled, seeded, and diced
- 1 cucumber, peeled and diced
- 1 red bell pepper, diced
- 1 small red onion, finely chopped
- 2 cloves garlic, minced
- 3 cups tomato juice
- 1/4 cup red wine vinegar
- 1/4 cup extra-virgin olive oil
- Salt and pepper to taste
- Fresh basil or mint for garnish

Instructions:

1. In a blender, combine cantaloupe, cucumber, red bell pepper, red onion, garlic, and tomato juice.
2. Blend until smooth.
3. Add red wine vinegar and olive oil, and blend again until well combined.
4. Season with salt and pepper to taste.
5. Chill the gazpacho in the refrigerator for at least 2 hours before serving.
6. Garnish with fresh basil or mint before serving.
7. Serve the cantaloupe gazpacho as a refreshing chilled soup on a warm day.

These recipes showcase the versatility of cantaloupe, whether paired with prosciutto for a tasty appetizer or blended into a refreshing gazpacho. Enjoy the sweet and juicy flavors of cantaloupe in these creative dishes!

Conclusion:

Cantaloupe is not only a delicious and hydrating fruit but also a nutrient-packed addition to a healthy lifestyle. If you have specific health concerns or conditions, it's advisable to consult with a healthcare professional or a registered dietitian for personalized advice. Whether enjoyed on its own or incorporated into various dishes, the benefits of cantaloupe extend beyond its sweet taste. Embrace the goodness of this melon and savor the health benefits it brings to your plate.

Back to Table of Contents

Carrot

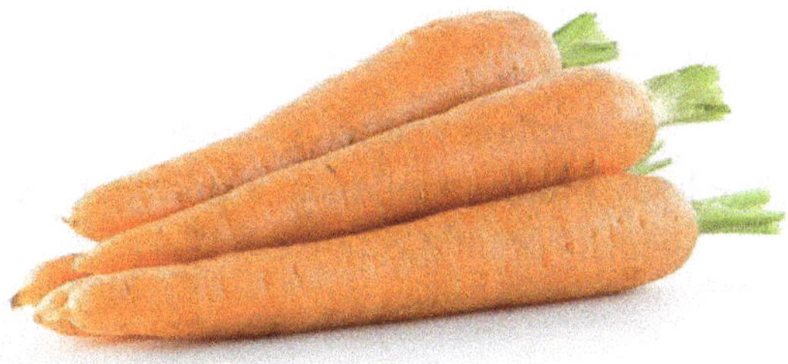

Health Benefits and Culinary Versatility of Carrots

Carrots, with their vibrant orange hue and sweet, crisp texture, have earned their place as a nutritional powerhouse in the world of fruits and vegetables. Beyond being a favorite snack, carrots boast an impressive array of health benefits and lend themselves to a wide range of culinary creations. In this article, we will explore the rich nutritional profile, health benefits, and diverse uses of carrots that make them a must-have in any well-balanced diet.

Nutritional Profile:

Carrots (Daucus carota) are rich in essential nutrients that contribute to overall health and well-being. Here are some key components of their nutritional profile:

Beta-Carotene:

- Carrots are famously known for their high beta-carotene content, a precursor to vitamin A. Beta-carotene is a potent antioxidant that promotes healthy vision, supports immune function, and contributes to skin health.

Fiber:

- Carrots are an excellent source of dietary fiber, which aids in digestion and promotes a feeling of fullness. The fiber content in carrots also supports a healthy gut, helping to prevent constipation and maintain bowel regularity.

Vitamins and Minerals:

Carrots provide essential vitamins such as vitamin K, vitamin C, and various B-vitamins. They also contain minerals like potassium, which plays a crucial role in maintaining proper fluid balance and supporting heart health.

Vitamin A:

Benefits:

- ***Eye Health:*** Carrots are renowned for their high content of beta-carotene, a precursor to vitamin A. Vitamin A is essential for maintaining healthy vision, particularly in low-light conditions. It contributes to the proper functioning of the retina and helps prevent conditions like night blindness.

Vitamin C:

Benefits:

- ***Immune Support:*** Carrots contain vitamin C, an antioxidant that supports the immune system. Vitamin C helps the body produce collagen, a protein crucial for skin health, wound healing, and maintaining the integrity of connective tissues.

Vitamin K:

Benefits:

- ***Blood Clotting and Bone Health:*** Vitamin K plays a vital role in blood clotting, helping prevent excessive bleeding. Additionally, vitamin K contributes to bone health by assisting in the regulation of calcium within bones and tissues.

Potassium:

Benefits:

- ***Heart Health:*** Potassium is crucial for maintaining proper fluid balance in the body and helps regulate blood pressure. Consuming potassium-rich foods like carrots may contribute to cardiovascular health by supporting blood pressure control.

Manganese:

Benefits:

- ***Antioxidant Defense:*** Manganese is an essential mineral that plays a role in the body's antioxidant defense system. It helps neutralize free radicals, reducing oxidative stress and supporting overall health.

Phosphorus:

Benefits:

- ***Bone Health:*** Phosphorus is a key mineral for bone health, working in conjunction with calcium to maintain strong and healthy bones. It also plays a role in various cellular processes and energy metabolism.

Magnesium:

Benefits:

- ***Nerve and Muscle Function:*** Magnesium is essential for nerve function and muscle contraction. It also contributes to maintaining a healthy heartbeat and supporting energy production within the body. Consuming magnesium-rich foods like carrots is important for overall neuromuscular health.

Incorporating carrots into your diet provides not only the vitamins that contribute to skin and eye health but also these essential minerals that play crucial roles in various physiological functions.

Health Benefits:

Eye Health:

- The beta-carotene in carrots is essential for maintaining healthy eyesight. It is converted into vitamin A, which is crucial for the proper functioning of the retina and can help prevent conditions such as night blindness.

Heart Health:

- The high fiber and potassium content in carrots contribute to heart health. Fiber helps regulate cholesterol levels, while potassium supports blood pressure control, reducing the risk of cardiovascular diseases.

Skin Health:

- Antioxidants in carrots, including beta-carotene and vitamin C, promote skin health by combating free radicals that can contribute to premature aging. Regular consumption of carrots may contribute to a radiant and healthy complexion.

Nutritional Content

In 1 cup (approximately 128 grams) of raw carrots, the approximate nutritional content is as follows:

- Carbohydrates: Approximately 12 grams
- Protein: Approximately 1 gram
- Fiber: Approximately 3.6 grams
- Sugar: Approximately 6 grams
- Fat: Approximately 0.2 grams

Please note that these values are approximate and can vary slightly based on factors such as the size and specific variety of carrots.

Culinary Uses:

Raw Snacking:

- Carrots make a convenient and nutritious snack when enjoyed raw. Slice them into sticks or rounds for a crunchy and satisfying treat. Pair them with hummus or yogurt-based dips for added flavor.

Cooked Dishes:

- Incorporate carrots into a variety of cooked dishes, including soups, stews, and stir-fries. Their natural sweetness adds depth to savory dishes, while their vibrant color enhances the visual appeal of the meal.

Juices and Smoothies:

- Carrots are a popular ingredient in juices and smoothies, providing a naturally sweet and nutrient-rich base. Combine them with fruits like oranges or apples for a refreshing and vitamin-packed beverage.

Historical Uses:

Medicinal Uses in Ancient Greece:

- **Benefit:** In ancient Greece, carrots were not only valued as a food but also for their medicinal properties. Historical records indicate that ancient Greek physicians, including Hippocrates, used carrots to treat various ailments. Carrots were believed to have diuretic properties and were used to promote urinary health.

Middle Ages: Carrot as a Medicinal Herb:

- **Benefit:** During the Middle Ages, carrots were cultivated not only as a culinary vegetable but also for their perceived medicinal benefits. Carrots were used as a herbal remedy to address digestive issues, and their seeds were believed to have properties that could expel worms. Additionally, carrot poultices were applied externally to soothe skin conditions.

World War II: Carrot as a Substitute for Scarcity:

- **Benefit:** In World War II, scarcity led to creative uses of available resources. Due to a shortage of traditional sweeteners, carrots were utilized as a substitute for sugar in some recipes. Carrot-based desserts and preserves became popular as a way to address the challenges posed by wartime rationing.

Traditional Chinese Medicine:

- **Benefit:** Carrots have been a part of traditional Chinese medicine for centuries. According to Chinese herbal medicine, carrots are believed to have cooling properties that can help balance the body's energy. Carrots were traditionally used to nourish the spleen, enhance digestion, and promote overall vitality.

These historical uses of carrots highlight their versatility beyond being a common culinary vegetable. Throughout different periods and cultures, carrots were recognized for their potential medicinal benefits, ranging from promoting urinary health to addressing digestive issues and even serving as a creative solution during times of scarcity. While some historical uses may not align with modern scientific understanding, they showcase the cultural significance and adaptability of carrots throughout history.

Tips on Growing Carrots

The time it takes for carrots to grow from seed to harvest depends on various factors including the variety of carrots, growing conditions, and desired size at harvest. However, here's a general timeline for growing carrots:

1. **Seed Germination**: Carrot seeds typically germinate within 1 to 3 weeks after planting, depending on factors such as soil temperature and moisture levels. Carrots prefer cooler soil temperatures for germination, ideally around 55°F to 75°F (13°C to 24°C).
2. **Growth Stage**: Once germinated, carrot plants grow relatively slowly during the early stages. Carrots require consistent moisture and loose, well-draining soil to develop properly. It usually takes about 2 to 4 months for carrot roots to reach maturity, depending on the variety and growing conditions.

3. **Harvesting**: Carrots are typically ready to harvest when they reach their mature size and color. Baby carrots can be harvested earlier, usually around 50 to 60 days after planting, while larger varieties may take up to 70 to 80 days or longer. The exact time to harvest depends on the variety and your preference for the size of the carrots.

It's important to note that carrots can be left in the ground even after reaching maturity, as they can withstand cooler temperatures and improve in flavor with time. However, it's best to harvest them before the ground freezes in colder climates to prevent damage to the roots.

Overall, with proper care and growing conditions, carrots can be grown successfully in most regions and climates.

Conclusion:

From supporting vision to promoting heart health, carrots are a versatile and nutritious addition to your daily diet. Whether enjoyed raw as a snack, cooked in savory dishes, or blended into beverages, the benefits of carrots extend far beyond their delicious flavor. Embrace the orange powerhouse and savor the goodness of carrots for a healthier and more vibrant lifestyle.

Back to Table of Contents

Cashews

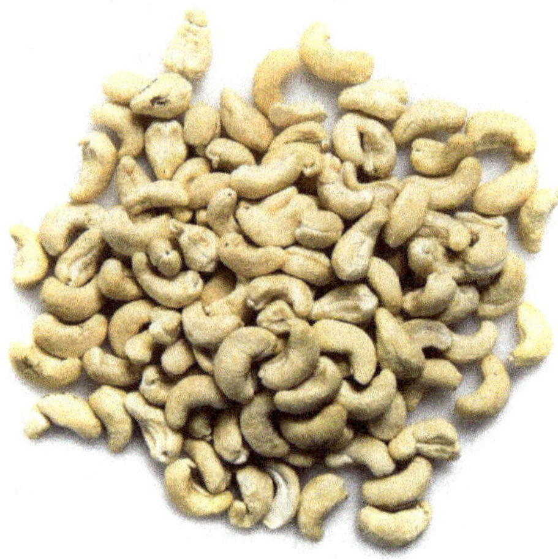

Nutrient-Rich Delights with Health Benefits and Culinary Versatility

Cashews, the kidney-shaped nuts native to Brazil, are not just a delicious snack but also pack a punch in terms of nutritional benefits. Known for their rich, buttery flavor and versatility, cashews have found their way into a variety of cuisines and dishes around the world. In this article, we will explore the myriad benefits and uses of cashews, shedding light on why these nuts are celebrated both for their taste and nutritional profile.

Nutritional Profile:

Cashews are nutritional powerhouses, offering a mix of essential nutrients that contribute to overall well-being. Here's a glimpse of the key nutrients found in cashews:

Healthy Fats:

- Cashews are rich in heart-healthy monounsaturated and polyunsaturated fats, including oleic acid, which is also found in olive oil.

Protein:

- As a plant-based protein source, cashews provide essential amino acids necessary for muscle repair, immune function, and overall growth.

Dietary Fiber:

- Cashews contain dietary fiber, promoting digestive health, regulating blood sugar levels, and supporting weight management.

Vitamins:

Cashews are a good source of vitamins, including vitamin E (an antioxidant), vitamin K, vitamin B6, and folate.

Vitamin K:

- Essential for blood clotting and bone health.

Vitamin E:

- A powerful antioxidant that protects cells from oxidative damage.

Vitamin B1 (Thiamine):

- Important for energy metabolism and the proper functioning of the nervous system.

Vitamin B2 (Riboflavin):

- Plays a key role in energy production and the maintenance of healthy skin.

Vitamin B3 (Niacin):

- Essential for DNA repair, energy metabolism, and the proper functioning of the nervous system.

Vitamin B6 (Pyridoxine):

- Important for brain development, the production of neurotransmitters, and the metabolism of amino acids.

Folate (Vitamin B9):

- Crucial for DNA synthesis and cell division. Adequate folate intake is particularly important during pregnancy for fetal development.

Pantothenic Acid (Vitamin B5):

- Involved in the synthesis of fatty acids, amino acids, and other important molecules.

It's important to note that while cashews provide a variety of vitamins, the specific nutrient content can vary based on factors such as the variety of cashews, growing conditions, and processing methods. Including cashews in a balanced and varied diet can contribute to meeting your daily vitamin requirements and supporting overall health.

Minerals:

Rich in essential minerals such as copper, magnesium, phosphorus, iron, and zinc, cashews contribute to bone health, immune function, and energy metabolism.

Copper:

- Critical for the formation of red blood cells, maintenance of bones and nerves, and the function of the immune system.

Magnesium:

- Important for muscle and nerve function, energy metabolism, and bone health.

Phosphorus:

- Vital for bone and teeth health, energy production, and the synthesis of DNA and RNA.

Zinc:

- Essential for immune function, wound healing, and DNA synthesis.

Iron:

- Important for the formation of hemoglobin, which carries oxygen in the blood.

Manganese:

- Plays a role in bone formation, blood clotting, and reducing inflammation.

Potassium:

- Important for maintaining proper heart and muscle function, regulating fluid balance, and supporting overall cardiovascular health.

Selenium:

- An antioxidant that supports thyroid function and immune system health.

Calcium:

- Essential for bone and teeth health, blood clotting, and muscle function.

Phytosterols:

- Plant compounds with potential health benefits, including cholesterol-lowering properties.

Sodium:

- While sodium is generally present in smaller amounts, it plays a role in maintaining fluid balance and nerve function.

The mineral content of cashews can vary depending on factors such as the variety of cashews, growing conditions, and processing methods. Including cashews in your diet can contribute to meeting your daily mineral requirements and supporting various physiological functions in the body.

Health Benefits:

Heart Health:

- The monounsaturated fats in cashews, along with magnesium and antioxidants, contribute to heart health by lowering bad cholesterol levels and supporting overall cardiovascular function.

Weight Management:

- The combination of healthy fats, protein, and fiber in cashews can help promote satiety, making them a satisfying and nutritious snack that may aid in weight management.

Blood Sugar Regulation:

- The fiber content in cashews helps regulate blood sugar levels, making them a suitable choice for individuals with diabetes or those aiming to manage their blood sugar.

Bone Health:

- Cashews are a good source of minerals like magnesium, phosphorus, and copper, which play a crucial role in maintaining strong and healthy bones.

Antioxidant Defense:

- The presence of antioxidants, including vitamin E and other compounds, helps protect cells from oxidative stress and inflammation.

Nutritional Content

In 1 cup (about 137 grams) of raw cashew nuts, the approximate nutritional content is as follows:

- Carbohydrates: Approximately 27 grams
- Protein: Approximately 18 grams
- Fiber: Approximately 3 grams
- Sugar: Approximately 6 grams
- Fat: Approximately 55 grams

Please note that these values are approximate and can vary slightly based on factors such as the specific variety and preparation of the cashews. Additionally, these values are for raw cashew nuts and may differ for roasted or salted varieties.

Culinary Uses:

Cashews are not just enjoyed as a snack; their creamy texture and mild flavor make them a versatile ingredient in various culinary creations. Here are some popular uses:

Dairy-Free Creaminess:

- Cashews can be blended into a smooth and creamy texture, making them an excellent base for dairy-free alternatives like cashew milk, cashew cream, or even vegan cheese.

Nut Butter:

- Cashew butter is a delicious and nutritious spread that can be used on toast, in sandwiches, or as a dip for fruits and vegetables.

Curries and Stir-Fries:

- Crushed or ground cashews are often used in Indian and Asian cuisines to add richness and a nutty flavor to curries, stir-fries, and sauces.

Baked Goods:

- Chopped or ground cashews can be incorporated into cookies, cakes, and other baked goods for added texture and flavor.

Salads and Snacks:

- Whole or roasted cashews are a popular addition to salads, providing a satisfying crunch. They also make a convenient and nutritious snack on their own or in trail mixes.

Cashews are incredibly versatile and can be used in both savory and sweet dishes. **Here are two delicious recipes featuring cashews:**

Vegan Cashew Alfredo Pasta:

Ingredients:

- 1 cup raw cashews, soaked in water for at least 4 hours or overnight
- 1 lb fettuccine or your favorite pasta
- 2 tablespoons olive oil
- 4 cloves garlic, minced

- 1 cup unsweetened almond milk (or any plant-based milk)
- 1/2 cup nutritional yeast
- Juice of 1 lemon
- Salt and pepper to taste
- Fresh parsley for garnish

Instructions:

1. **Prepare the Cashew Cream:**
    - Drain the soaked cashews and blend them with almond milk, nutritional yeast, and lemon juice until smooth. Set aside.
2. **Cook the Pasta:**
    - Cook the pasta according to package instructions. Drain and set aside.
3. **Make the Alfredo Sauce:**
    - In a large skillet, heat olive oil over medium heat. Add minced garlic and sauté until fragrant.
4. **Combine Pasta and Sauce:**
    - Pour the cashew cream into the skillet with the sautéed garlic. Stir until the sauce thickens slightly. Add salt and pepper to taste.
5. **Toss with Pasta:**
    - Add the cooked pasta to the skillet, tossing to coat evenly with the cashew Alfredo sauce.
6. **Serve:**
    - Garnish with fresh parsley and additional nutritional yeast if desired. Serve the Vegan Cashew Alfredo Pasta immediately.

Maple Cinnamon Cashew Energy Bites:

Ingredients:

- 1 cup raw cashews
- 1 cup pitted dates
- 1/4 cup rolled oats
- 2 tablespoons maple syrup
- 1 teaspoon ground cinnamon
- 1/2 teaspoon vanilla extract
- Pinch of salt
- Desiccated coconut for rolling (optional)

Instructions:

1. **Prepare Cashew Mixture:**
    - In a food processor, combine cashews, dates, rolled oats, maple syrup, cinnamon, vanilla extract, and a pinch of salt. Process until the mixture forms a sticky dough.
2. **Form Energy Bites:**

- With your hands, roll the mixture into bite-sized balls. If the mixture is too sticky, you can wet your hands slightly.

3. **Optional Coating:**
    - Roll the energy bites in desiccated coconut for an extra layer of flavor.
4. **Chill:**
    - Place the energy bites in the refrigerator for at least 30 minutes to firm up.
5. **Serve and Enjoy:**
    - Once chilled, these Maple Cinnamon Cashew Energy Bites are ready to be enjoyed as a wholesome snack or a sweet treat.

These recipes showcase the versatility of cashews, from creating a creamy vegan Alfredo sauce to crafting nutritious energy bites. Whether you're in the mood for a savory pasta dish or a sweet and satisfying snack, cashews can be a delicious and nutritious addition to your culinary repertoire.

Conclusion:

Cashews, with their delightful taste and nutritional richness, have rightfully earned their place as a beloved nut in the world of culinary arts and health-conscious eating. Whether enjoyed as a wholesome snack, blended into creamy sauces, or sprinkled on salads and desserts, cashews offer a delightful fusion of flavor and nutrition. If you have specific health concerns, allergies, or conditions, it's advisable to consult with a healthcare professional or a registered dietitian before making significant changes to your diet.

As you savor the buttery goodness of cashews, you're not just indulging in a tasty treat but also nourishing your body with a wealth of essential nutrients that contribute to overall vitality and well-being.

Back to Table of Contents

Cauliflower

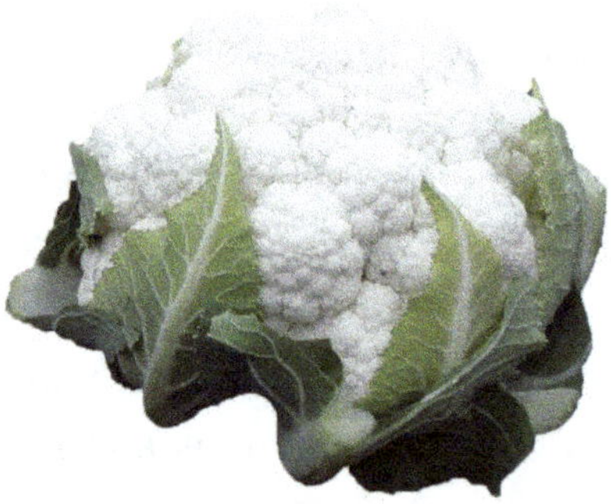

A Cruciferous Wonder with Health Benefits and Culinary Versatility

Cauliflower, a member of the Brassicaceae family, is a cruciferous vegetable celebrated for its versatility in the kitchen and a myriad of health benefits. While its mild flavor might make it seem unassuming, cauliflower's nutritional profile and adaptability in various culinary applications make it a powerhouse in both taste and wellness.

Nutritional Highlights:

Cauliflower is a low-calorie, nutrient-dense vegetable that provides a range of essential vitamins, minerals, and antioxidants. A single serving of cauliflower (about one cup, chopped) offers:

Vitamin C:

- Crucial for immune health, collagen synthesis, and antioxidant defense.

Vitamin K:

- Important for blood clotting and bone metabolism.

Vitamin B6:

- Involved in various metabolic processes, including amino acid metabolism.

Folate:

- Essential for DNA synthesis and cell division, particularly important during pregnancy.

Fiber:

- Supports digestive health, helps maintain a healthy weight, and contributes to a feeling of fullness.

Choline:

- Plays a role in brain development and supports various metabolic functions.

Potassium:

- Important for maintaining proper fluid balance, nerve transmission, and muscle contraction.

Antioxidants:

Cauliflower contains antioxidants like glucosinolates and carotenoids, which may help protect cells from oxidative stress.

Glucosinolates:

- **Benefits:** Glucosinolates are sulfur-containing compounds that are known for their potential anti-cancer properties. They can activate detoxification enzymes in the body and may help inhibit the growth of cancer cells.

Vitamin C:

- **Benefits:** Vitamin C is a powerful antioxidant that supports the immune system, helps in the synthesis of collagen for skin health, and contributes to the protection of cells from oxidative stress.

Carotenoids (Beta-Carotene):

- **Benefits:** Beta-carotene, a precursor to vitamin A, acts as an antioxidant that supports vision, skin health, and immune function. It may also help protect against certain cancers and cardiovascular diseases.

Quercetin:

- **Benefits:** Quercetin is a flavonoid with anti-inflammatory and antioxidant properties. It may help reduce inflammation, support heart health, and contribute to overall antioxidant defense.

Kaempferol:

- **Benefits:** Kaempferol is a flavonoid with antioxidant and anti-inflammatory effects. It may have protective effects on the cardiovascular system and potential anti-cancer properties.

Beta-Cryptoxanthin:

- **Benefits:** Beta-cryptoxanthin is a carotenoid with antioxidant properties. It may contribute to joint health and has anti-inflammatory effects.

Caffeic Acid:

- **Benefits:** Caffeic acid is a polyphenol with antioxidant and anti-inflammatory properties. It may help protect against oxidative stress and inflammation.

Quinones:

- **Benefits:** Quinones are compounds with antioxidant properties that may contribute to the overall protection of cells from damage caused by free radicals.

Health Benefits:

Cancer Prevention:

- The presence of glucosinolates in cauliflower has been linked to a reduced risk of certain cancers, including lung, colorectal, and breast cancers.

Anti-Inflammatory Properties:

- Cauliflower's rich supply of antioxidants contributes to its anti-inflammatory effects, potentially reducing the risk of chronic diseases.

Heart Health:

- The fiber, potassium, and antioxidants in cauliflower support cardiovascular health by promoting healthy blood pressure levels and reducing oxidative stress.

Digestive Health:

- The fiber content aids in digestion and promotes a healthy gut by supporting the growth of beneficial gut bacteria.

Weight Management:

- With its low-calorie content and high fiber content, cauliflower can be a valuable ally in weight management by promoting satiety.

Nutritional Content

In 1 cup (about 107 grams) of raw cauliflower florets, the approximate nutritional content is as follows:

- Carbohydrates: Approximately 5 grams
- Protein: Approximately 2 grams
- Fiber: Approximately 2 grams
- Fat: Approximately 0.3 grams

Please note that these values are approximate and can vary slightly based on factors such as the size of the cauliflower florets and the specific variety of cauliflower.

Culinary Versatility:

One of cauliflower's most intriguing aspects is its ability to transform into various textures and flavors based on cooking techniques. Here are some popular culinary uses:

Cauliflower Rice:

- Finely grated cauliflower can substitute for rice, providing a low-carb and nutrient-packed alternative.

Cauliflower Mash:

- Mashed cauliflower, seasoned and blended, makes a delicious, low-carb alternative to mashed potatoes.

Cauliflower Steaks:

- Thick slices of cauliflower roasted or grilled can serve as a hearty and satisfying main course.

Cauliflower Pizza Crust:

- A gluten-free and lower-carb pizza crust option that allows for creative and healthy pizza toppings.

Cauliflower Soup:

- Creamy cauliflower soup is a comforting and nutritious option, often flavored with herbs and spices.

Cauliflower Wings:

- Baked or fried cauliflower florets coated in flavorful sauces provide a healthier take on traditional buffalo wings.

Here are two delicious and versatile recipes using cauliflower:

Roasted Cauliflower with Garlic and Parmesan:

Ingredients:

- 1 head of cauliflower, cut into florets
- 3 tablespoons olive oil
- 4 cloves garlic, minced
- 1/2 cup grated Parmesan cheese
- 1 teaspoon dried thyme
- Salt and black pepper to taste
- Fresh parsley for garnish (optional)

Instructions:

1. Preheat the oven to 425°F (220°C).
2. In a large bowl, toss cauliflower florets with olive oil, minced garlic, Parmesan cheese, dried thyme, salt, and black pepper until evenly coated.
3. Spread the cauliflower mixture on a baking sheet in a single layer.
4. Roast in the preheated oven for 25-30 minutes or until the cauliflower is golden brown and crispy at the edges, stirring halfway through for even cooking.
5. Garnish with fresh parsley if desired and serve as a flavorful side dish.

Cauliflower and Chickpea Curry:

Ingredients:

- 1 head of cauliflower, cut into florets
- 1 can (15 oz) chickpeas, drained and rinsed
- 1 onion, finely chopped
- 3 cloves garlic, minced
- 1 can (14 oz) diced tomatoes
- 1 can (14 oz) coconut milk
- 2 tablespoons curry powder
- 1 teaspoon ground cumin
- 1 teaspoon ground coriander
- 1/2 teaspoon turmeric
- Salt and black pepper to taste
- Fresh cilantro for garnish

- Cooked rice for serving

Instructions:

1. In a large pot or skillet, sauté the chopped onion and minced garlic in a bit of oil until softened.
2. Add the cauliflower florets, chickpeas, diced tomatoes, and coconut milk to the pot.
3. Stir in the curry powder, ground cumin, ground coriander, turmeric, salt, and black pepper.
4. Bring the mixture to a simmer, cover, and let it cook for 20-25 minutes or until the cauliflower is tender.
5. Adjust seasoning if necessary and serve the cauliflower and chickpea curry over cooked rice.
6. Garnish with fresh cilantro and enjoy this flavorful and satisfying vegetarian curry.

These recipes showcase the versatility of cauliflower, whether roasted for a simple side dish or used as a star ingredient in a delicious curry. Feel free to customize the recipes based on your preferences and dietary needs.

Tips on Growing Cauliflower

Cauliflower typically takes about 55 to 100 days to grow from seed to harvest, depending on the variety and growing conditions. Here's a general timeline for growing cauliflower:

1. **Seedling Stage**: Cauliflower seeds are usually started indoors about 4 to 6 weeks before the last spring frost date. They are then transplanted outdoors when they have grown to about 4 to 6 inches tall, which typically takes about 3 to 4 weeks.
2. **Growth Stage**: Once transplanted, cauliflower plants continue to grow and develop. They require consistent watering, adequate sunlight, and proper nutrition during this stage. Cauliflower heads begin to form when the plants reach a certain size and maturity.
3. **Head Formation**: Cauliflower heads develop within the center of the plant, surrounded by the large outer leaves. The heads are typically ready to harvest when they reach a desirable size and density. This process may take anywhere from 55 to 100 days after transplanting, depending on the variety and growing conditions.
4. **Blanching**: Some growers choose to "blanch" cauliflower heads by tying the outer leaves over the developing heads to protect them from sunlight. This helps keep the heads white and prevents them from turning green or developing a bitter taste.
5. **Harvesting**: Cauliflower heads are typically ready to harvest when they are firm, compact, and the curds (the edible parts) are tightly closed. Harvesting usually occurs when the heads reach 6 to 8 inches in diameter, but this can vary depending on the variety.

It's important to monitor cauliflower plants closely during the growth stage and provide proper care to ensure healthy development. Additionally, factors such as temperature, soil quality, and pest management can also affect the growth rate of cauliflower plants.

Conclusion:

Cauliflower's rise to stardom in the culinary world is not only due to its adaptability but also its impressive nutritional profile and health benefits. Whether enjoyed raw, roasted, mashed, or transformed into creative alternatives for traditional dishes, cauliflower stands out as a versatile vegetable that adds both flavor and wellness to the plate. If you have specific health concerns, allergies, or conditions, it's advisable to consult with a healthcare professional or a registered dietitian before making significant changes to your diet.

Embrace the cruciferous wonder that is cauliflower and discover the countless ways it can contribute to a delicious and health-conscious diet.

Back to Table of Contents

Cayenne Pepper

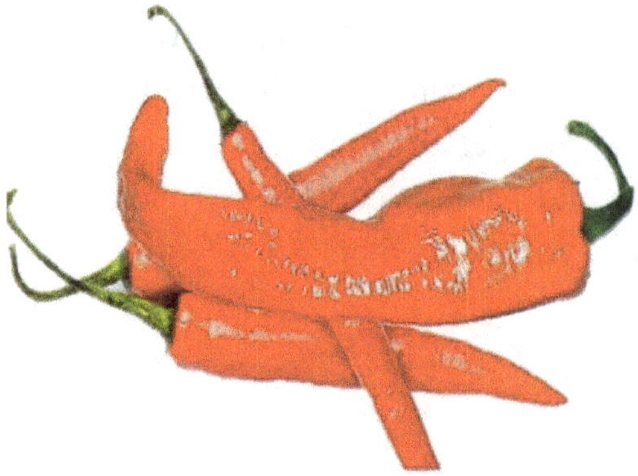

Unveiling the Fiery Wonder

Cayenne pepper, a staple in kitchens worldwide, is not just an ordinary spice that adds heat to dishes; it's a powerhouse of flavor and health benefits. Derived from dried and ground chili peppers, particularly Capsicum annuum, cayenne pepper has been revered for centuries for its culinary and medicinal properties. Let's delve into the fiery wonder of cayenne pepper, exploring its myriad benefits and versatile uses.

Cayenne pepper is a potent source of various vitamins, minerals, and antioxidants, each offering unique benefits to health and well-being. Here's a list of some of the key nutrients found in cayenne pepper and their associated benefits:

Vitamins:

Vitamin A:

- Benefits: Essential for maintaining healthy vision, supporting immune function, promoting skin health, and aiding in cell growth and development.

Vitamin C:

- Benefits: Boosts immune system function, acts as an antioxidant to protect cells from damage caused by free radicals, supports collagen production for healthy skin, and enhances iron absorption.

Minerals:

Potassium:

- Benefits: Regulates fluid balance, supports proper muscle function, helps maintain healthy blood pressure levels, and plays a role in nerve transmission.

Manganese:

- Benefits: Necessary for bone formation, wound healing, metabolism of carbohydrates and cholesterol, and antioxidant defense.

Magnesium:

- Benefits: Supports muscle and nerve function, regulates blood sugar levels, aids in energy production, promotes bone health, and contributes to heart health.

Iron:

- Benefits: Essential for the production of hemoglobin, which carries oxygen in the blood, supports energy metabolism, and helps prevent iron deficiency anemia.

Antioxidants:

Capsaicin:

- Benefits: Acts as a potent antioxidant, reducing inflammation and oxidative stress, promoting heart health, supporting weight loss by increasing metabolism, and potentially reducing the risk of certain cancers.

Carotenoids (including beta-carotene):

- Benefits: Function as antioxidants to protect cells from damage, support eye health, boost immune function, and may reduce the risk of chronic diseases such as heart disease and cancer.

Flavonoids:

- Benefits: Possess antioxidant and anti-inflammatory properties, support cardiovascular health by improving blood flow and reducing the risk of blood clots, and may help lower blood pressure and cholesterol levels.

Vitamin E:

- Benefits: Acts as an antioxidant, protecting cells from damage caused by free radicals, supports immune function, promotes skin health, and may help prevent age-related cognitive decline.

Caffeic Acid:

- Benefits: Exhibits antioxidant and anti-inflammatory properties, potentially reducing the risk of chronic diseases such as heart disease and cancer and supporting overall health and well-being.

These vitamins, minerals, and antioxidants found in cayenne pepper contribute to its numerous health benefits, including immune support, improved cardiovascular health, enhanced skin health, and reduced inflammation. Incorporating cayenne pepper into your diet in moderation can be a flavorful way to reap these nutritional benefits and support overall health and wellness.

Health Benefits:

Weight Management:

- Cayenne pepper is celebrated for its ability to boost metabolism and promote weight loss. It contains capsaicin, a compound that can increase calorie burning and reduce appetite, making it a valuable tool for individuals looking to shed pounds.

Digestive Health:

- Incorporating cayenne pepper into your diet can aid digestion and alleviate digestive issues. It stimulates the production of gastric juices, which helps in the breakdown of food and facilitates smooth digestion. Additionally, it can relieve gas and bloating.

Cardiovascular Health:

- Studies suggest that cayenne pepper may have cardiovascular benefits, including the ability to improve circulation and lower blood pressure. Capsaicin helps to relax blood vessels, promoting better blood flow and reducing the risk of heart disease.

Pain Relief:

- Topical applications of cayenne pepper have been used for centuries to alleviate pain. Capsaicin can inhibit the transmission of pain signals, offering relief from conditions such as arthritis, muscle soreness, and nerve pain.

Immune Support:

- Rich in vitamins A and C, cayenne pepper provides immune-boosting properties that help the body fend off infections and illnesses. Its anti-inflammatory effects further support immune function by reducing inflammation in the body.

Versatile Uses:

Culinary Delights:

- Sprinkle cayenne pepper onto grilled meats, vegetables, soups, and stews for a fiery kick.
- Add it to marinades, dressings, and sauces to elevate the flavor profile of your dishes.
- Incorporate it into homemade spice blends for a unique and vibrant seasoning.

Herbal Remedies:

- Create a soothing tea by steeping cayenne pepper with honey and lemon to relieve cold and flu symptoms.
- Make a topical pain relief salve by combining cayenne pepper with coconut oil or beeswax.

Natural Cleaning Agent:

- Cayenne pepper's antibacterial properties make it an effective ingredient in homemade cleaning solutions. Mix it with vinegar or baking soda to create a powerful cleaner for kitchen and bathroom surfaces.

Garden Aid:

- Sprinkle cayenne pepper around plants to deter pests such as slugs, snails, and squirrels without resorting to harmful chemicals.

Culinary Marvel:

Cayenne pepper boasts a distinct, fiery flavor profile that adds depth and intensity to a variety of dishes. From spicy curries to savory sauces and marinades, its versatile nature makes it a favorite among chefs and home cooks alike. Its culinary uses extend beyond just flavor enhancement; it can also serve as a natural preservative, aiding in food preservation.

Here are two delicious recipes featuring Cayenne Pepper:

Spicy Cajun Shrimp Pasta:

Ingredients:

- 1 pound shrimp, peeled and deveined
- 8 ounces fettuccine or your preferred pasta
- 2 tablespoons olive oil
- 4 cloves garlic, minced
- 1 bell pepper, sliced
- 1 onion, diced
- 1 teaspoon paprika
- 1/2 teaspoon **cayenne pepper** (adjust to taste)
- 1 teaspoon dried thyme
- 1 cup heavy cream
- Salt and pepper to taste
- Fresh parsley, chopped (for garnish)
- Grated Parmesan cheese (optional)

Instructions:

1. Cook the pasta according to package instructions until al dente. Drain and set aside.
2. In a large skillet, heat olive oil over medium heat. Add minced garlic, sliced bell pepper, and diced onion. Cook until softened, about 5 minutes.
3. Add shrimp to the skillet and season with paprika, cayenne pepper, dried thyme, salt, and pepper. Cook until the shrimp are pink and cooked through, about 3-4 minutes.
4. Pour in the heavy cream and stir well to combine. Allow the sauce to simmer for a few minutes until slightly thickened.
5. Add the cooked pasta to the skillet and toss until well coated in the sauce.
6. Serve the spicy Cajun shrimp pasta hot, garnished with chopped parsley and grated Parmesan cheese if desired.

Honey Glazed Cayenne Roasted Carrots:

Ingredients:

- 1 pound carrots, peeled and sliced into sticks
- 2 tablespoons olive oil
- 2 tablespoons honey

- 1/2 teaspoon **cayenne pepper** (adjust to taste)
- Salt and pepper to taste
- Fresh parsley, chopped (for garnish)

Instructions:

1. Preheat the oven to 400°F (200°C). Line a baking sheet with parchment paper.
2. In a large bowl, toss the carrot sticks with olive oil, honey, cayenne pepper, salt, and pepper until evenly coated.
3. Spread the carrots in a single layer on the prepared baking sheet.
4. Roast in the preheated oven for 20-25 minutes, or until the carrots are tender and caramelized, stirring halfway through.
5. Once roasted, remove the carrots from the oven and transfer to a serving dish.
6. Garnish the honey glazed cayenne roasted carrots with chopped parsley before serving.

These recipes showcase the versatility of cayenne pepper, adding a flavorful kick to both savory and sweet dishes. Enjoy the spicy goodness in every bite!

Historical Uses

Historically, cayenne pepper has been used for various medicinal purposes. Here are few examples:

Pain Relief:

- Cayenne pepper contains capsaicin, a compound that has been used for centuries as a natural pain reliever. When applied topically, capsaicin creams or ointments derived from cayenne peppers can help alleviate pain associated with conditions such as arthritis, neuropathy, and muscle soreness. Capsaicin works by desensitizing nerve endings and reducing the transmission of pain signals.

Digestive Aid:

- Cayenne pepper has traditionally been used to improve digestive health. It stimulates the production of saliva, which aids in the breakdown of food, and promotes the secretion of gastric juices, which can enhance digestion. Additionally, cayenne pepper is believed to help alleviate symptoms of indigestion, bloating, and gas.

Circulatory Support:

- Cayenne pepper has a long history of use in traditional medicine to support cardiovascular health. It is believed to help improve circulation by dilating blood vessels and promoting better blood flow. This improved circulation can have beneficial effects on heart health and may help reduce the risk of blood clots and related cardiovascular issues.

Respiratory Support:

- Cayenne pepper has been used historically as a remedy for respiratory conditions such as coughs, colds, and sinus congestion. Its spicy properties can help stimulate mucus flow and clear congestion in the respiratory passages, making it easier to breathe. Additionally, the heat from cayenne pepper may have mild antibacterial properties that can help fight respiratory infections.

While cayenne pepper has been valued for its medicinal properties throughout history, it's essential to use it judiciously and in appropriate forms.

Tips on Growing Cayenne Pepper

Growing cayenne peppers is a rewarding experience, but it requires patience and attention to detail. Here's a detailed breakdown of the typical timeline for growing cayenne peppers from seed to harvest:

1. Seed Germination (7-14 days):

- Start by planting cayenne pepper seeds indoors in small pots or trays filled with seed starting mix.
- Keep the soil consistently moist but not waterlogged and maintain a warm temperature between 70-80°F (21-27°C) to encourage germination.
- Cayenne pepper seeds typically germinate within 7 to 14 days, although some may sprout earlier or later.

2. Seedling Stage (4-6 weeks):

- Once the seeds have germinated, they will develop into seedlings with two sets of true leaves.
- Continue to keep the soil moist and provide adequate light. You can use grow lights or place seedlings near a sunny window.
- As the seedlings grow, you may need to transplant them into larger pots to provide more space for root development.

3. Transplanting (6-8 weeks):

- After 6 to 8 weeks, when the seedlings have grown to about 6 inches tall and have several sets of true leaves, they are ready to be transplanted outdoors (if growing in a garden) or into larger containers (if growing in pots).
- Choose a sunny location with well-drained soil for planting. Space the plants about 18-24 inches apart to allow for adequate air circulation.

4. Vegetative Growth (2-3 months):

- Once transplanted, cayenne pepper plants will enter a period of vegetative growth, during which they will continue to develop foliage and establish a strong root system.
- Water the plants regularly, ensuring that the soil remains evenly moist but not waterlogged. Mulching around the base of the plants can help retain moisture and suppress weeds.

5. Flowering and Fruit Set (2-3 months):

- Around 2 to 3 months after transplanting, cayenne pepper plants will begin to flower. The flowers are small and white, and they will eventually give way to small green fruits.
- Bees and other pollinators will help facilitate the pollination process, which is necessary for fruit development.

6. Fruit Ripening (2-3 months):

- After the flowers have been pollinated, the small green fruits will gradually begin to mature and ripen.
- Cayenne peppers typically take 2 to 3 months to reach full maturity, depending on growing conditions and the specific variety being grown.
- As the peppers ripen, they will change color from green to yellow, orange, or red, depending on the variety.

7. Harvesting:

- Harvest ripe cayenne peppers as needed by snipping them from the plant using scissors or pruners.
- The peppers can be harvested individually as they ripen, or you can wait until the entire plant has produced a full crop before harvesting all at once.
- Avoid pulling or twisting the peppers, as this can damage the plant.

By following these guidelines and providing proper care and attention, you can expect to harvest a bountiful crop of flavorful cayenne peppers to enjoy in your culinary creations.

Precautions:

While cayenne pepper offers numerous benefits, it's essential to use it in moderation, especially for individuals with sensitive stomachs or gastrointestinal issues. Additionally, topical application may cause skin irritation, so it's advisable to perform a patch test before using it extensively. If you have specific health concerns, allergies, or conditions, it's advisable to consult with a healthcare professional or a registered dietitian before making significant changes to your diet.

In conclusion, cayenne pepper is not just a spice; it's a treasure trove of culinary delights and health-promoting properties. Whether you're adding a pinch to your favorite recipe or harnessing its healing potential in herbal remedies, cayenne pepper stands as a testament to nature's bounty and its ability to nourish and heal the body and soul.

Back to Table of Contents

Celery

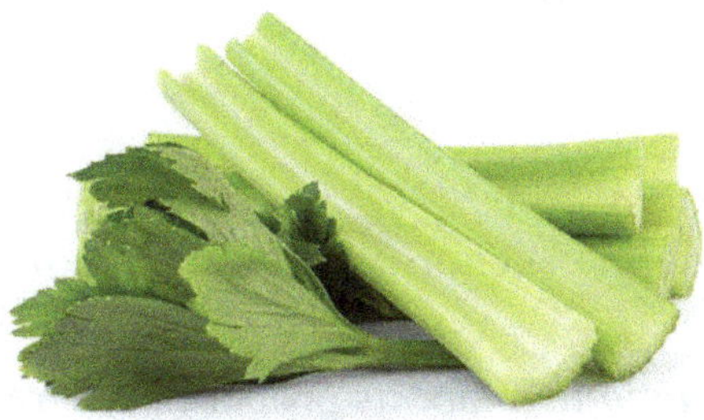

The Crisp Wonder: Exploring the Benefits and Versatile Uses of Celery

Celery, with its crunchy texture and refreshing flavor, is more than just a popular addition to salads and snacks. This humble vegetable boasts an array of health benefits and is a versatile ingredient in the kitchen. In this article, we'll delve into the nutritional advantages of celery and explore the creative ways it can be used in various culinary applications.

Nutritional Benefits:

Celery is low in calories but high in essential nutrients, making it a healthy addition to any diet. Here are some key nutritional components found in celery:

Dietary Fiber:

- **Benefits:**
  - ***Digestive Health:*** The high fiber content aids in digestion and helps prevent constipation.
  - ***Weight Management:*** Fiber contributes to a feeling of fullness, supporting weight management by reducing overeating.

Vitamin K:

- **Benefits:**
  - ***Bone Health:*** Vitamin K is essential for bone health, playing a role in bone mineralization and density.
  - ***Blood Clotting:*** Supports proper blood clotting and wound healing.

Vitamin C:

- **Benefits:**
  - ***Immune System Support:*** Acts as an antioxidant, helping protect cells from damage and boosting the immune system.
  - ***Collagen Synthesis:*** Contributes to the synthesis of collagen, promoting healthy skin and connective tissues.

Potassium:

- **Benefits:**
  - ***Heart Health:*** Potassium helps regulate blood pressure, promoting cardiovascular health.
  - ***Muscle Function:*** Essential for proper muscle contraction and nerve signaling.

Calcium:

- **Benefits:**

  Bone Health: Calcium is a crucial mineral for maintaining strong and healthy bones.

  Nerve Function: Supports proper nerve transmission and muscle function.

Phosphorus:

- ***Benefits:***

  Bone and Teeth Health: Phosphorus, in conjunction with calcium, contributes to bone and teeth formation.

  Energy Metabolism: Plays a role in energy metabolism and the synthesis of ATP, the body's primary energy currency.

Nutritional Content

In 1 cup (about 101 grams) of raw celery, the approximate nutritional content is as follows:

- Carbohydrates: Approximately 3 grams
- Protein: Approximately 0.7 grams
- Fiber: Approximately 1.6 grams
- Fat: Approximately 0.2 grams

Please note that these values are approximate and can vary slightly based on factors such as the specific size and variety of celery.

Versatile Culinary Uses:

Celery's mild flavor and crisp texture make it a versatile ingredient in the kitchen. Here are some creative ways to incorporate celery into your meals:

Snack on Celery Sticks:

- Enjoy celery sticks with your favorite dip, such as hummus or peanut butter, for a healthy and satisfying snack.

Add to Salads:

- Include chopped celery in salads to add crunch and freshness. It pairs well with a variety of greens and other vegetables.

Use in Soups and Stews:

- Dice celery and add it to soups, stews, and casseroles for added flavor and nutrition.

Juicing:

- Incorporate celery into your fresh juice blends for a nutritious and hydrating beverage.

Classic Celery and Peanut Butter Snack Recipe:

Ingredients:

- Fresh celery stalks, washed and trimmed
- Peanut butter (or any nut or seed butter of your choice)

Instructions:

1. Cut celery stalks into manageable lengths, typically 4 to 6 inches.
2. Spread peanut butter generously on one side of each celery stalk.

Enjoy this classic and nutritious snack that combines the crispness of celery with the creamy goodness of peanut butter.

Chicken and Celery Stir-Fry:

Ingredients:

- 1 lb boneless, skinless chicken breasts, thinly sliced
- 2 cups celery, sliced diagonally
- 1 bell pepper, thinly sliced
- 1 onion, thinly sliced
- 2 cloves garlic, minced
- 1 tablespoon soy sauce
- 1 tablespoon oyster sauce
- 1 teaspoon sesame oil
- 2 tablespoons vegetable oil
- Cooked rice for serving
- Sesame seeds and chopped green onions for garnish (optional)

Instructions:

1. Heat vegetable oil in a wok or large skillet over medium-high heat.
2. Add sliced chicken and stir-fry until browned and cooked through. Remove from the wok and set aside.
3. In the same wok, add a bit more oil if needed and stir-fry sliced celery, bell pepper, onion, and minced garlic until vegetables are crisp-tender.
4. Return the cooked chicken to the wok with the vegetables.
5. In a small bowl, mix soy sauce, oyster sauce, and sesame oil. Pour the sauce over the chicken and vegetables, tossing to coat evenly.
6. Continue to stir-fry for an additional 2-3 minutes until everything is well combined and heated through.
7. Serve the chicken and celery stir-fry over cooked rice.
8. Garnish with sesame seeds and chopped green onions if desired.

These recipes showcase the versatility of celery, whether enjoyed as a simple and healthy snack or incorporated into a flavorful stir-fry for a satisfying meal.

Benefits of Celery Consumption:

Hydration and Detoxification:

- Celery has a high water content, aiding in hydration, and contains compounds that may support the body's natural detoxification processes.

Anti-Inflammatory Properties:

- Certain antioxidants in celery, including flavonoids and polyphenols, have anti-inflammatory effects that may contribute to overall health.

Heart Health:

- The potassium content in celery helps regulate blood pressure, reducing the risk of cardiovascular diseases.

Weight Management:

- Celery's low-calorie content and high fiber contribute to a feeling of fullness, making it a valuable snack for those aiming to manage their weight.

Digestive Health:

- The fiber in celery promotes regular bowel movements and supports a healthy digestive system.

Historical uses:

Ancient Medicinal Uses:

- **Historical Use:**
    - Celery has a long history of medicinal use, dating back to ancient civilizations such as Egypt, Greece, and Rome.
    - Ancient Egyptians used celery for medicinal purposes, including treating ailments like arthritis and promoting relaxation.
- **Benefits:**
    - The anti-inflammatory properties of celery may have contributed to its use in addressing conditions like arthritis.
    - Celery's calming effects might have been utilized to alleviate stress and promote relaxation in ancient medicinal practices.

Ancient Culinary Use in Greece and Rome:

- **Historical Use:**
    - Celery was cultivated in ancient Greece and Rome, where it was used not only for medicinal purposes but also as a culinary ingredient.
    - Ancient Greeks and Romans appreciated the aromatic and flavorful qualities of celery, incorporating it into various dishes.
- **Benefits:**
    - Culinary use of celery in ancient times provided a source of essential nutrients, including vitamins and minerals, contributing to overall well-being.

- The unique flavor and texture of celery enhanced the taste of ancient dishes, making them more palatable and enjoyable.

These historical uses of celery highlight its dual role as both a medicinal plant and a culinary ingredient in different cultures throughout the ages. Celery's versatility has allowed it to play a significant role not only in promoting health but also in enhancing the flavors of various traditional dishes.

Tips on Growing Celery

Celery is a biennial plant, but it's typically grown as an annual for its edible stalks. Here's a general timeline for growing celery:

1. **Seed Starting**: Celery seeds are usually started indoors 10 to 12 weeks before the last spring frost date. Celery seeds can be slow to germinate, often taking up to 2 to 3 weeks to sprout. Starting seeds indoors gives them a head start before transplanting them outdoors.
2. **Transplanting**: Once the seedlings have developed several true leaves and are strong enough, usually when they are about 8 to 10 weeks old, they can be transplanted outdoors. This is typically done when the soil has warmed up and there is no longer a risk of frost.
3. **Growing Stage**: Celery plants require consistent moisture and regular feeding with a balanced fertilizer to support healthy growth. They also prefer cool temperatures and may benefit from shade during hot summer months. Celery grows slowly, taking about 3 to 4 months from transplanting to reach maturity.
4. **Harvesting**: Celery stalks can be harvested as soon as they reach the desired size, usually when they are 12 to 18 inches tall. Harvesting typically begins around 90 to 120 days after transplanting, but this can vary depending on the specific variety and growing conditions.

It's important to keep celery well-watered and free from weeds throughout the growing season. Additionally, blanching celery by covering the stalks with paper or cardboard tubes can help reduce bitterness and improve the flavor.

Conclusion: Celery's crispness, mild flavor, and nutritional profile make it a standout vegetable in both the realm of health benefits and culinary creativity. Whether enjoyed as a refreshing snack, added to salads, or incorporated into various recipes, celery proves to be a versatile and nutritious addition to your diet. Embrace the many uses of celery to not only tantalize your taste buds but also to promote overall well-being with its array of health benefits.

Back to Table of Contents

Chamomile

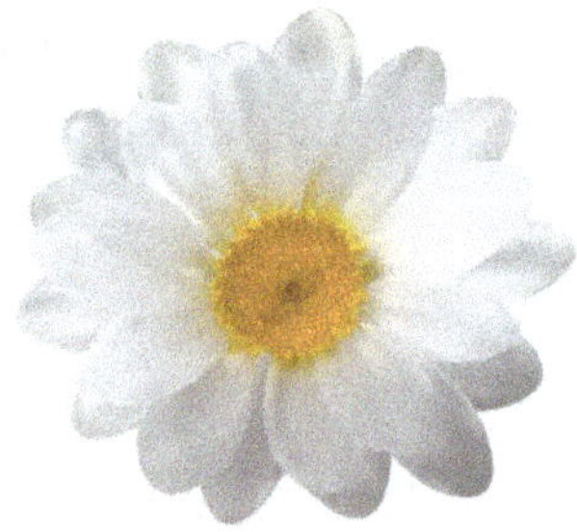

A Comprehensive Exploration of Its Benefits

Chamomile, derived from the Asteraceae family of plants, has been utilized for centuries for its myriad health benefits and soothing properties. This document delves into the origins, types, and the extensive range of advantages associated with chamomile.

Origins and Types of Chamomiles:

Chamomile comes in two primary varieties: German chamomile (Matricaria chamomilla) and Roman chamomile (Chamaemelum nobile). Both types have distinct characteristics and are used for various purposes. German chamomile is often preferred for its high content of chamazulene, a compound with anti-inflammatory properties. Roman chamomile, on the other hand, is known for its sweet fragrance and is frequently used in aromatherapy.

Historical Significance:

The use of chamomile dates to ancient civilizations. Egyptians revered chamomile for its healing properties, using it in medicinal concoctions. Greeks and Romans also recognized its therapeutic value, often employing chamomile in teas to promote relaxation and alleviate digestive issues. This historical significance highlights the enduring reputation of chamomile as a medicinal herb.

Health Benefits of Chamomile:

Promotes Better Sleep:

Chamomile is renowned for its calming effects, making it a popular remedy for insomnia and sleep disorders. The herb contains apigenin, an antioxidant that binds to specific receptors in the brain, inducing a sense of tranquility and aiding in sleep.

Alleviates Digestive Issues:

Chamomile has been traditionally used to soothe digestive problems such as indigestion, bloating, and gas. Its anti-inflammatory properties may help reduce inflammation in the gastrointestinal tract, providing relief from discomfort.

Anxiety and Stress Reduction:

Consuming chamomile tea has been linked to a reduction in anxiety and stress levels. The compounds in chamomile interact with the brain receptors, promoting relaxation and potentially mitigating symptoms of anxiety disorders.

Skin Health Improvement:

Chamomile's anti-inflammatory and antioxidant properties extend to skincare. It is often used topically to soothe skin irritations, reduce redness, and promote healing. Chamomile extracts are prevalent in skincare products due to their gentle and calming effects.

Menstrual Pain Relief:

Women experiencing menstrual cramps may find relief in chamomile. Its muscle-relaxant properties can help alleviate the discomfort associated with menstrual pain when consumed as a tea or in supplement form.

Preparation and Consumption:

Chamomile can be consumed in various forms, including tea, essential oil, capsules, and topical applications. Chamomile tea remains one of the most popular methods of ingestion. To prepare chamomile tea, dried chamomile flowers are steeped in hot water. The essential oil is extracted from the flowers and can be used in aromatherapy or diluted for topical application.

Ways Chamomile can be Used:

Chamomile Tea:

Ingredients: Dried chamomile flowers, hot water.

Method: Place a tablespoon of dried chamomile flowers in a teapot or tea infuser. Pour hot water over the flowers and steep for 5-10 minutes. Strain the tea and sweeten with honey or lemon if desired.

Chamomile Essential Oil Blend:

Ingredients: Chamomile essential oil, carrier oil (such as jojoba or sweet almond).

Method: Mix a few drops of chamomile essential oil with a carrier oil to create a soothing massage oil or an aromatherapy blend. This can be applied to the skin or used in a diffuser for a calming atmosphere.

Chamomile Infused Honey:

Ingredients: Dried chamomile flowers, honey.

Method: Place dried chamomile flowers in a clean, dry jar. Pour honey over the flowers and let it infuse for a week, shaking the jar occasionally. The chamomile-infused honey can be used as a sweetener in tea or drizzled over desserts.

Chamomile Bath Soak:

Ingredients: Chamomile tea bags, Epsom salts.

Method: Brew a strong chamomile tea using multiple tea bags. Allow the tea to cool. Mix the chamomile tea with Epsom salt and add it to a warm bath. Soak for a relaxing experience that can help soothe muscles and promote calmness.

Chamomile Lemonade:

Ingredients: Chamomile tea (cooled), freshly squeezed lemon juice, honey, ice.

Method: Prepare chamomile tea and let it cool. Mix the chamomile tea with freshly squeezed lemon juice and sweeten with honey to taste. Serve over ice for a refreshing chamomile-infused lemonade.

These diverse preparations showcase the versatility of chamomile, allowing individuals to incorporate it into their daily routines in ways that suit their preferences and wellness goals. Whether enjoyed as a warm tea, in a relaxing bath, or as an essential oil blend, chamomile offers a range of options for harnessing its soothing properties.

Considerations and Precautions:

While chamomile is generally considered safe, individuals with allergies to plants in the Asteraceae family should exercise caution. Pregnant women and those on blood-thinning medications should consult a healthcare professional before incorporating chamomile into their routine. Additionally, excessive consumption of chamomile tea may lead to drowsiness, so it is advisable to avoid driving or operating heavy machinery after consumption.

In conclusion, chamomile's rich history and diverse range of benefits make it a versatile and valuable herb. From promoting better sleep to alleviating digestive issues and reducing anxiety, chamomile has rightfully earned its status as a revered natural remedy. As with any herbal supplement, it is essential to approach chamomile with a balanced understanding of its potential benefits and any associated precautions. Incorporating chamomile into a wellness routine may offer a holistic approach to health and well-being.

Back to Table of Contents

Cherry

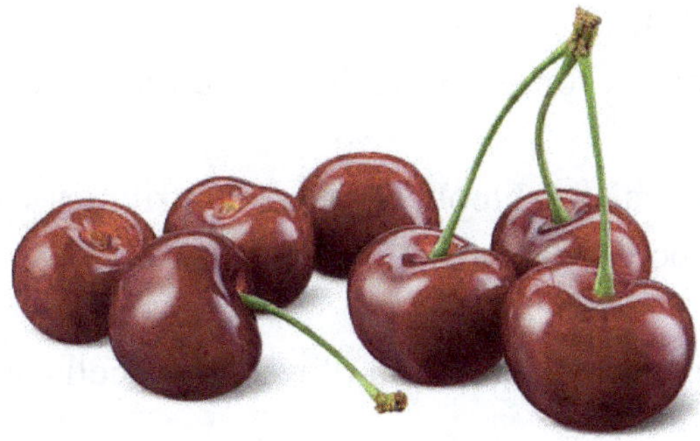

The Vibrant Elegance of Cherries: Health Benefits and Culinary Delights

Cherries, with their bold and juicy presence, are not only a delight for the taste buds but also a nutritional powerhouse. Whether enjoyed fresh, dried, or incorporated into various culinary creations, cherries bring a burst of color and flavor to the table. In this article, we will explore the numerous benefits of cherries, from their rich nutritional profile to their versatile uses in the kitchen.

Nutritional Richness:

Cherries boast an impressive array of nutrients that contribute to overall health and well-being. Here are some key nutritional components found in cherries:

Antioxidants:

- **Benefits:** Cherries are rich in antioxidants, including anthocyanins and quercetin, which help combat oxidative stress and inflammation in the body.

Vitamin C:

- **Benefits:** Boosts the immune system, supports skin health, aids in collagen production.

Dietary Fiber:

- **Benefits:** Promotes digestive health, helps regulate blood sugar levels, contributes to a feeling of fullness.

Potassium:

- **Benefits:** Helps regulate blood pressure, supports heart and muscle function, aids in fluid balance.

Vitamin A:

- **Benefits:** Essential for vision health, supports immune function, maintains healthy skin.

Melatonin:

- **Benefits:** Cherries contain melatonin, a hormone that regulates sleep-wake cycles, making them a natural option for promoting better sleep.

B Vitamins (B1, B2, B3, B5, B6):

- **Benefits:** Essential for energy metabolism, support nerve function, and contribute to overall well-being.

Folate (Vitamin B9):

- **Benefits:** Important for DNA synthesis and repair, aids in red blood cell formation.

Vitamin K:

- **Benefits:** Essential for blood clotting, contributes to bone health, helps regulate calcium in the body.

Copper:

- **Benefits:** Supports the formation of red blood cells, aids in iron absorption.

Manganese:

- **Benefits:** Contributes to bone formation, supports metabolism, acts as an antioxidant.

Iron:

- **Benefits:** Important for oxygen transport in the blood, supports energy metabolism.

Magnesium:

- **Benefits:** Important for muscle and nerve function, supports bone health.

2. **Phosphorus:**
   - **Benefits:** Essential for bone and teeth health, involved in energy metabolism.

Zinc:

- **Benefits:** Supports immune function, involved in wound healing, essential for DNA synthesis.

Calcium:

- **Benefits:** Important for bone and teeth health, supports muscle and nerve function.

Sodium:

- **Benefits:** Plays a role in fluid balance, nerve function, and muscle contractions.

Cherries' nutritional profile makes them a wholesome and delicious addition to a balanced diet, offering a variety of vitamins and minerals that contribute to overall health and well-being.

Health Benefits:

Anti-Inflammatory Properties:

- The antioxidants in cherries, particularly anthocyanins, have been linked to reduced inflammation, potentially alleviating symptoms of conditions like arthritis.

Heart Health:

- Potassium in cherries contributes to heart health by helping regulate blood pressure and supporting overall cardiovascular function.

Improved Sleep:

- The melatonin content in cherries may aid in improving sleep quality and duration, making them a natural and delicious sleep-promoting option.

Exercise Recovery:

- Cherries have been studied for their potential to reduce muscle soreness and inflammation, making them a popular choice for post-exercise recovery.

Cancer Prevention:

- The antioxidants in cherries, especially anthocyanins, have been studied for their potential anti-cancer properties. While more research is needed, cherries show promise in supporting cancer prevention.

Nutritional Content

In 1 cup (approximately 154 grams) of raw cherries (sweet cherries), the approximate nutritional content is as follows:

- Carbohydrates: Approximately 22 grams
- Protein: Approximately 1 gram
- Fiber: Approximately 3 grams
- Fat: Approximately 0.3 grams

Please note that these values are approximate and can vary slightly based on factors such as the specific variety and ripeness of the cherries. Sour cherries may have slightly different nutritional content compared to sweet cherries.

Culinary Versatility:

Cherries lend themselves to a variety of culinary applications, making them a versatile and delicious addition to both sweet and savory dishes. Here are some popular uses:

Fresh Snacking:

- Enjoy cherries fresh as a simple and satisfying snack. Their natural sweetness makes them a delightful treat on their own.

Baking and Desserts:

- Incorporate cherries into pies, tarts, muffins, and cakes for a burst of fruity flavor. Cherry compotes and sauces also make excellent toppings for desserts.

Salads:

- Add fresh or dried cherries to salads for a pop of color, sweetness, and a unique flavor dimension. They pair well with greens, nuts, and cheese.

Smoothies and Juices:

- Blend cherries into smoothies or juices for a refreshing and nutritious beverage. Combine them with other fruits, yogurt, or greens for a flavorful mix.

Here are two delightful recipes that showcase the deliciousness of cherries:

Fresh Cherry and Almond Clafoutis:

Ingredients:

- 2 cups fresh cherries, pitted
- 1 cup whole milk
- 3 large eggs
- 1/2 cup granulated sugar
- 1 teaspoon vanilla extract
- 1/2 cup all-purpose flour
- 1/4 teaspoon almond extract
- Pinch of salt
- Powdered sugar for dusting (optional)

Instructions:

1. Preheat the oven to 350°F (175°C). Grease a baking dish or tart pan.
2. Arrange the pitted cherries evenly in the greased dish.
3. In a blender, combine milk, eggs, granulated sugar, vanilla extract, almond extract, flour, and a pinch of salt. Blend until smooth.
4. Pour the batter over the cherries in the dish.
5. Bake in the preheated oven for 40-45 minutes or until the clafoutis is set and golden brown.
6. Allow it to cool slightly before slicing. Dust with powdered sugar if desired.
7. Serve this cherry and almond clafoutis as a delightful dessert, either warm or at room temperature.

Grilled Chicken and Cherry Salad with Balsamic Vinaigrette:

Ingredients:

- 2 boneless, skinless chicken breasts
- Salt and pepper to taste
- 1 tablespoon olive oil
- 4 cups mixed salad greens
- 1 cup fresh cherries, pitted and halved
- 1/2 cup feta cheese, crumbled
- 1/4 cup sliced almonds, toasted
- Balsamic vinaigrette dressing

Instructions:

1. Season the chicken breasts with salt and pepper. Grill or pan-sear them until fully cooked. Slice into thin strips.
2. In a large salad bowl, combine the mixed greens, cherry halves, sliced grilled chicken, crumbled feta cheese, and toasted sliced almonds.

3. Drizzle the salad with balsamic vinaigrette dressing and toss gently to combine.
4. Serve this grilled chicken and cherry salad as a flavorful and satisfying meal.

These recipes showcase the versatility of cherries, whether baked into a classic French dessert or featured in a vibrant and savory salad. Enjoy the sweet and tart flavors of cherries in these creative and delicious dishes!

Ancient Medicinal Remedies:

Cherries have a rich history of use, both for culinary purposes and traditional medicinal applications. Here are three historical uses of cherries and their associated benefits:

Ancient remedies:

- **Benefit:**
  - Cherries were utilized in ancient times for their perceived medicinal properties. The compounds found in cherries, including anthocyanins and antioxidants, were believed to have anti-inflammatory and pain-relieving effects.
  - Traditional medicine often employed cherries to address conditions such as arthritis and gout. The natural anti-inflammatory properties of cherries made them a popular remedy for managing joint pain.

Culinary Delights in Ancient Rome:

- **Benefit:**
  - Cherries were prized in ancient Rome for their delicious flavor and versatility in culinary creations. Romans incorporated cherries into various dishes, and they were particularly fond of using cherries in desserts and alcoholic beverages.
  - The appreciation for cherries as a culinary delight highlighted their appeal beyond medicinal uses, emphasizing their role as a delectable fruit enjoyed for taste and pleasure.

Cherry Orchards in Persia (Modern-day Iran):

- **Benefit:**
  - Historical records indicate that cherry orchards were established in Persia, showcasing the cultivation and appreciation of cherries in ancient times.
  - The benefits of cherries extended beyond their consumption, as the cultivation of cherry orchards contributed to the economic and agricultural prosperity of the regions where they were grown. Cherries became not only a dietary staple but also an essential part of local economies.

These historical uses of cherries reflect their significance in various cultures throughout the ages. Whether valued for their medicinal properties, culinary appeal, or economic contributions, cherries have played a diverse and enduring role in human history.

In **conclusion**, cherries stand as not only a delectable and vibrant fruit but also a nutritional powerhouse offering an array of health benefits. From their antioxidant-rich nature to their culinary versatility, cherries are a welcome addition to a well-balanced diet. If you have specific health concerns, allergies, or conditions, it's advisable to consult with a healthcare professional or a registered dietitian before making significant changes to your diet.

Embrace the sweet elegance of cherries as you explore the delicious ways they can enhance your meals while contributing to your overall health and vitality.

Back to Table of Contents

Chia Seeds

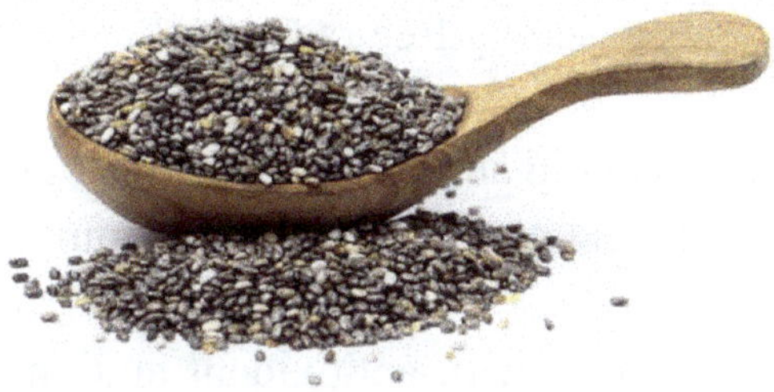

Tiny Powerhouses of Nutrition and Versatility

Chia seeds, the tiny black or white seeds derived from the Salvia hispanica plant, have gained immense popularity in the health and wellness community due to their impressive nutritional profile and versatile applications. These tiny seeds pack a powerful punch of nutrients, making them a valuable addition to a balanced and nutrient-rich diet.

Nutritional Powerhouse:

Rich in Omega-3 Fatty Acids:

- Chia seeds are one of the best plant-based sources of alpha-linolenic acid (ALA), a type of omega-3 fatty acid. Omega-3s are known for their anti-inflammatory properties and their role in supporting heart and brain health.

High in Fiber:

- Chia seeds are an excellent source of dietary fiber, both soluble and insoluble. This high fiber content aids in digestion, promotes a feeling of fullness, and helps regulate blood sugar levels.

Protein Packed:

- Despite their small size, chia seeds are surprisingly high in protein, making them a valuable addition for individuals following vegetarian or vegan diets. Protein is essential for muscle repair, immune function, and overall body maintenance.

Loaded with Antioxidants:

Chia seeds contain antioxidants that help protect the body's cells from oxidative damage. These antioxidants contribute to overall health and may play a role in reducing the risk of chronic diseases.

Quercetin:

- Quercetin is a flavonoid antioxidant with anti-inflammatory properties. It may help combat oxidative stress and contribute to overall health.

Chlorogenic Acid:

- Chlorogenic acid is a polyphenol antioxidant known for its potential anti-inflammatory and anti-diabetic effects. It is also found in coffee beans.

Caffeic Acid:

- Caffeic acid is another polyphenol with antioxidant properties. It may help protect cells from damage caused by free radicals.

Kaempferol:

- Kaempferol is a flavonoid antioxidant found in various fruits and vegetables. It has been studied for its potential anti-cancer and anti-inflammatory effects.

Myricetin:

- Myricetin is a flavonoid with antioxidant and anti-inflammatory properties. It is found in various plant-based foods, including chia seeds.

Quercetin Glycosides:

- Quercetin glycosides are a form of quercetin bound to sugar molecules. They contribute to the antioxidant capacity of chia seeds.

Alpha-Linolenic Acid (ALA):

- While not a traditional antioxidant, ALA is an essential omega-3 fatty acid found in chia seeds. It has anti-inflammatory properties and contributes to overall health.

Tocopherols (Vitamin E):

- Chia seeds contain various tocopherols, including alpha-tocopherol, which is a form of vitamin E. Vitamin E is a fat-soluble antioxidant that protects cells from oxidative damage.

Beta-Carotene:

- Beta-carotene is a precursor to vitamin A and serves as a provitamin antioxidant. It contributes to the overall antioxidant capacity of chia seeds.

Ascorbic Acid (Vitamin C):

- While present in smaller amounts, chia seeds contain vitamin C, which acts as an antioxidant. Vitamin C is essential for immune function and collagen synthesis.

It's important to note that the antioxidant content of chia seeds may vary depending on factors such as the growing conditions and storage. Incorporating a variety of antioxidant-rich foods into your diet can contribute to overall health and well-being.

Abundant in Essential Nutrients:

Chia seeds are a good source of various essential nutrients, including calcium, phosphorus, magnesium, and manganese. These minerals are crucial for bone health, energy metabolism, and enzyme function.

Vitamins in Chia Seeds:

Vitamin A:

- Chia seeds contain beta-carotene, a precursor to vitamin A, which is important for vision, immune function, and skin health.

Vitamin B1 (Thiamine):

- Thiamine plays a crucial role in energy metabolism and is necessary for the proper functioning of the nervous system.

Vitamin B2 (Riboflavin):

- Riboflavin is involved in energy production, cell growth, and maintenance of healthy skin.

Vitamin B3 (Niacin):

- Niacin is important for energy metabolism and supports the health of the skin, nerves, and digestive system.

Vitamin B5 (Pantothenic Acid):

- Pantothenic acid is essential for the synthesis of coenzyme A, which plays a role in various metabolic processes.

Vitamin B6 (Pyridoxine):

- Pyridoxine is involved in amino acid metabolism, neurotransmitter synthesis, and the formation of red blood cells.

Vitamin B9 (Folate):

- Folate is crucial for DNA synthesis and cell division, especially important during periods of rapid growth and development.

Vitamin E:

- Chia seeds contain tocopherols, including alpha-tocopherol, a form of vitamin E. Vitamin E is a fat-soluble antioxidant that protects cells from oxidative damage.

Minerals in Chia Seeds:

Calcium:

- Calcium is essential for bone and teeth health, muscle function, and blood clotting.

Phosphorus:

- Phosphorus is crucial for bone and teeth formation, energy metabolism, and acid-base balance.

Magnesium:

- Magnesium is involved in muscle and nerve function, blood glucose control, and bone health.

Potassium:

- Potassium is necessary for maintaining fluid balance, nerve transmission, and muscle contraction.

Zinc:

- Zinc supports immune function, wound healing, and DNA synthesis.

Manganese:

- Manganese is important for bone formation, blood clotting, and reducing inflammation.

Copper:

- Copper is essential for iron metabolism, connective tissue formation, and antioxidant function.

Iron:

- Iron is crucial for the formation of hemoglobin and oxygen transport in the blood.

Selenium:

- Selenium functions as an antioxidant and plays a role in thyroid hormone metabolism.

Trace Amounts of Other Minerals:

- Chia seeds also contain trace amounts of other minerals, including sodium and potassium.

Incorporating chia seeds into your diet can contribute to meeting your daily requirements for these essential vitamins and minerals, supporting overall health and well-being.

Health Benefits:

Heart Health:

- The omega-3 fatty acids in chia seeds have been associated with improved cardiovascular health. They may help reduce inflammation, lower blood pressure, and decrease the risk of heart disease.

Weight Management:

- The combination of fiber, protein, and healthy fats in chia seeds can contribute to feelings of fullness, potentially aiding in weight management by curbing overeating.

Blood Sugar Regulation:

- The soluble fiber in chia seeds can help regulate blood sugar levels by slowing down the digestion and absorption of carbohydrates. This can be particularly beneficial for individuals with diabetes or those looking to manage blood sugar levels.

Nutritional Content

In 1 cup (approximately 172 grams) of chia seeds, the approximate nutritional content is as follows:

- Carbohydrates: Approximately 12 grams
- Protein: Approximately 17 grams
- Fiber: Approximately 34 grams
- Fat: Approximately 31 grams

Chia seeds are nutrient-dense and known for their high content of omega-3 fatty acids, fiber, and protein. Please note that these values are approximate and can vary slightly based on factors such as the specific brand or variety of chia seeds.

Culinary Versatility:

Chia Pudding:

- Chia seeds absorb liquid and develop a gel-like consistency, making them ideal for creating chia pudding. Mix them with your favorite milk, add sweeteners or flavors, and refrigerate for a nutritious and delicious dessert or breakfast.

Smoothie Booster:

- Sprinkle chia seeds into your smoothies for an added nutritional boost. They not only provide texture but also contribute essential nutrients.

Baking Ingredient:

- Chia seeds can be incorporated into baking recipes such as muffins, pancakes, or bread, enhancing the nutritional content of these treats.

Salad Topping:

- Sprinkle chia seeds over salads to add a crunchy texture and a nutrient boost.

Egg Replacement:

- Chia seeds can be used as an egg substitute in baking. Combine chia seeds with water, and let the mixture sit until it forms a gel-like consistency, mimicking the binding properties of eggs.

Chia seeds are incredibly versatile and can be used in a variety of recipes. **Here are two delicious and nutritious recipes featuring chia seeds:**

Chia Seed Pudding:

Ingredients:

- 1/4 cup chia seeds
- 1 cup almond milk (or any milk of your choice)
- 1-2 tablespoons maple syrup or honey (adjust to taste)
- 1/2 teaspoon vanilla extract
- Fresh berries or sliced fruits for topping

Instructions:

1. In a bowl, mix chia seeds, almond milk, maple syrup (or honey), and vanilla extract.
2. Stir well and let the mixture sit for about 5 minutes.
3. Stir the mixture again to break up any clumps of chia seeds.
4. Cover the bowl and refrigerate for at least 2 hours or overnight.
5. Before serving, stir the pudding and adjust sweetness if needed.
6. Top with fresh berries or sliced fruits before serving.

This chia seed pudding is not only delicious but also packed with fiber, omega-3 fatty acids, and various nutrients. It makes for a delightful breakfast or a healthy dessert.

Chia Seed Smoothie:

Ingredients:

- 1 cup frozen mixed berries (strawberries, blueberries, raspberries)
- 1 ripe banana
- 1 cup spinach leaves
- 1 tablespoon chia seeds
- 1 cup almond milk (or any milk of your choice)
- Ice cubes (optional)
- Honey or agave syrup for sweetness (optional)

Instructions:

1. In a blender, combine frozen berries, banana, spinach, chia seeds, and almond milk.
2. Blend until smooth. If the smoothie is too thick, you can add more almond milk or water to achieve your desired consistency.
3. Taste the smoothie and add honey or agave syrup if additional sweetness is desired.
4. Optionally, add ice cubes and blend again until smooth.
5. Pour the smoothie into a glass and sprinkle a few chia seeds on top for texture.

This chia seed smoothie is a nutrient-packed, refreshing beverage that combines the goodness of fruits, vegetables, and chia seeds. It's an excellent way to start your day or enjoy as a midday snack.

Feel free to customize these recipes based on your preferences and dietary needs!

Conclusion:

Incorporating chia seeds into your diet offers a simple and delicious way to enhance your nutritional intake. Whether you enjoy them in puddings, smoothies, or as a topping for various dishes, these tiny seeds provide a wealth of health benefits. Embracing the versatility of chia seeds allows you to tap into their nutritional prowess and elevate both the flavor and nutrient content of your meals. As with any food, moderation is key, and it's advisable to consult with a healthcare professional or nutritionist for personalized dietary advice.

Back to Table of Contents

Chickpeas

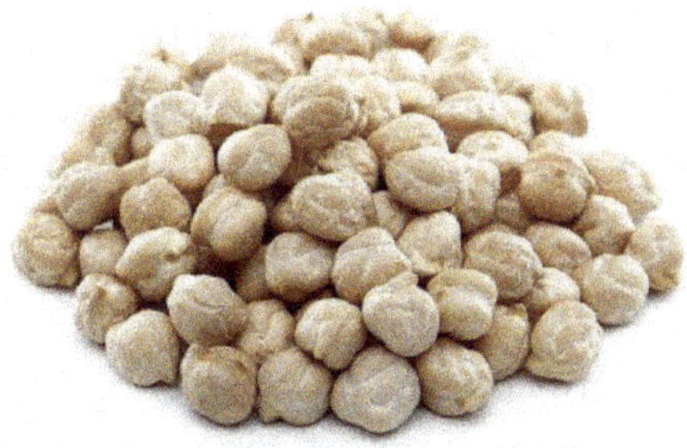

A Nutrient-Rich Superfood with Versatility and Health Benefits

Chickpeas, also known as garbanzo beans, are a versatile legume that has been a dietary staple in various cultures for centuries. These small, round legumes are not only delicious but also offer a wealth of nutritional benefits. Whether enjoyed in salads, soups, or as the star ingredient in hummus, chickpeas have earned their reputation as a superfood. In this article, we will explore the numerous health benefits and culinary uses that make chickpeas a valuable addition to a balanced and wholesome diet.

Nutritional Powerhouse:

Chickpeas are a nutritional powerhouse, providing a well-rounded array of essential nutrients that contribute to overall health and well-being. Key nutritional components of chickpeas include:

Protein:

- Chickpeas are an excellent source of plant-based protein, making them an essential component for vegetarians and vegans. Protein is crucial for muscle repair, immune function, and overall growth and maintenance.

Dietary Fiber:

- Rich in both soluble and insoluble fiber, chickpeas support digestive health by promoting regular bowel movements, preventing constipation, and fostering a healthy gut microbiota. Fiber also plays a role in heart health and blood sugar regulation.

Complex Carbohydrates:

- Chickpeas provide complex carbohydrates, offering a gradual release of energy. They have a low glycemic index, making them suitable for individuals aiming to manage blood sugar levels.

Vitamins and Minerals:

Chickpeas contain essential vitamins such as folate, vitamin B6, thiamine, and minerals including iron, magnesium, phosphorus, and potassium. These nutrients play vital roles in various bodily functions, including blood formation, energy metabolism, and bone health.

Essential Vitamins in Chickpeas:

Folate (Vitamin B9):

- **Benefits:** Folate is essential for DNA synthesis and repair. Adequate folate intake is crucial during periods of rapid cell division, such as pregnancy, and it helps prevent neural tube defects in developing fetuses.

Vitamin B6:

- **Benefits:** Vitamin B6 is involved in over 100 enzymatic reactions in the body, including the metabolism of amino acids and the production of neurotransmitters. It plays a role in immune function, cognitive development, and the regulation of mood.

Thiamine (Vitamin B1):

- **Benefits:** Thiamine is vital for energy metabolism, playing a key role in converting carbohydrates into energy. It also supports proper nerve function and is essential for the synthesis of neurotransmitters.

Vitamin C:

- **Benefits:** Vitamin C is an antioxidant that supports the immune system, helps the body absorb iron, and contributes to collagen formation, which is important for skin health.

Essential Minerals in Chickpeas:

Iron:

- **Benefits:** Iron is essential for the formation of hemoglobin, the oxygen-carrying component of red blood cells. Adequate iron intake is crucial for preventing iron-deficiency anemia and supporting overall energy levels.

Magnesium:

- **Benefits:** Magnesium is involved in various physiological processes, including muscle and nerve function, bone health, and energy metabolism. It contributes to the regulation of blood pressure and supports the immune system.

Phosphorus:

- **Benefits:** Phosphorus is a structural component of DNA, RNA, and ATP (adenosine triphosphate), the primary energy carrier in cells. It is essential for bone health, kidney function, and the metabolism of macronutrients.

Zinc:

- **Benefits:** Zinc is crucial for immune function, wound healing, and DNA synthesis. It also plays a role in the sense of taste and smell and supports normal growth and development.

Health Benefits:

Heart Health:

- The combination of fiber, potassium, and magnesium in chickpeas contributes to heart health. Fiber helps lower cholesterol levels, potassium regulates blood pressure, and magnesium supports overall cardiovascular function.

Blood Sugar Regulation:

- Chickpeas have a low glycemic index, providing a slow and steady release of glucose. This property makes them a suitable choice for individuals aiming to manage blood sugar levels and prevent insulin spikes.

Weight Management:

- The protein and fiber content in chickpeas promotes a feeling of fullness, aiding in weight management. Including chickpeas in meals can help control appetite and reduce overall calorie intake.

Digestive Health:

- The fiber in chickpeas supports digestive health by promoting regular bowel movements and contributing to a healthy gut microbiome. This can help prevent constipation and support overall gastrointestinal well-being.

Nutritional Content

In 1 cup (approximately 164 grams) of cooked chickpeas (garbanzo beans), the approximate nutritional content is as follows:

- Carbohydrates: Approximately 45 grams
- Protein: Approximately 15 grams
- Fiber: Approximately 13 grams
- Fat: Approximately 3 grams

Please note that these values are approximate and can vary slightly based on factors such as the cooking method and any added ingredients.

Culinary Versatility:

Chickpeas are incredibly versatile in the kitchen, adapting well to various cooking methods and flavor profiles. Some common culinary uses include:

Hummus:

- A popular Middle Eastern dip made from blended chickpeas, tahini, olive oil, lemon juice, and garlic. Hummus is not only delicious but also a nutritious snack or spread.

Chickpea Salad:

- A refreshing salad featuring chickpeas, fresh vegetables, herbs, and a zesty dressing. Chickpea salads are both satisfying and nutrient-packed.

Chickpea Curry:

- A flavorful and protein-rich curry featuring chickpeas, tomatoes, onions, and aromatic spices. Chickpea curry is a staple in many Indian and Middle Eastern cuisines.

Roasted Chickpea Snack:

- Chickpeas can be roasted with various spices for a crunchy and satisfying snack. Roasted chickpeas are a healthy alternative to traditional snacks.

Here are two delicious and nutritious recipes featuring chickpeas:

Chickpea and Spinach Curry:

Ingredients:

- 2 cans (15 ounces each) chickpeas, drained and rinsed
- 1 onion, finely chopped
- 3 cloves garlic, minced
- 1 tablespoon ginger, grated
- 1 can (14 ounces) diced tomatoes
- 1 can (14 ounces) coconut milk
- 1 bunch spinach, washed and chopped
- 2 tablespoons curry powder
- 1 teaspoon ground cumin
- 1 teaspoon ground coriander
- 1/2 teaspoon turmeric
- Salt and pepper to taste
- 2 tablespoons cooking oil
- Fresh cilantro, chopped (for garnish)
- Cooked rice or naan bread (for serving)

Instructions:

1. In a large pan, heat the cooking oil over medium heat. Add the chopped onion and cook until softened.
2. Add minced garlic and grated ginger to the pan, sautéing for an additional 1-2 minutes until fragrant.
3. Stir in the curry powder, ground cumin, ground coriander, and turmeric. Cook for another minute to toast the spices.
4. Add the diced tomatoes (with their juices) and coconut milk to the pan. Stir well to combine.
5. Add the drained and rinsed chickpeas to the curry sauce. Simmer for 15-20 minutes, allowing the flavors to meld.
6. Just before serving, add the chopped spinach to the curry. Cook until the spinach wilts.

7. Season the curry with salt and pepper to taste.
8. Serve the chickpea and spinach curry over cooked rice or with naan bread. Garnish with fresh chopped cilantro.

Roasted Chickpea Salad:

Ingredients:

- 2 cans (15 ounces each) chickpeas, drained and rinsed
- 2 tablespoons olive oil
- 1 teaspoon ground cumin
- 1 teaspoon smoked paprika
- 1/2 teaspoon garlic powder
- Salt and pepper to taste
- Mixed salad greens (lettuce, arugula, or spinach)
- Cherry tomatoes, halved
- Cucumber, sliced
- Red onion, thinly sliced
- Feta cheese, crumbled
- Balsamic vinaigrette dressing

Instructions:

1. Preheat the oven to 400°F (200°C).
2. In a bowl, toss the drained and rinsed chickpeas with olive oil, ground cumin, smoked paprika, garlic powder, salt, and pepper.
3. Spread the seasoned chickpeas in a single layer on a baking sheet.
4. Roast the chickpeas in the preheated oven for 25-30 minutes or until they become golden and crispy.
5. While the chickpeas are roasting, prepare the salad by arranging mixed greens, cherry tomatoes, cucumber slices, and thinly sliced red onion on a serving platter.
6. Once the chickpeas are done roasting, let them cool slightly before adding them to the salad.
7. Sprinkle crumbled feta cheese over the salad.
8. Drizzle the salad with balsamic vinaigrette dressing just before serving.
9. Toss the salad gently to combine, ensuring the roasted chickpeas are evenly distributed.
10. Serve the roasted chickpea salad as a hearty and flavorful main course or side dish.

These recipes showcase the versatility of chickpeas, whether in a rich and aromatic curry or as crispy roasted additions to a vibrant salad. Chickpeas not only add a satisfying texture but also provide a healthy dose of protein and fiber.

Conclusion:

Incorporating chickpeas into your diet is a delicious and health-conscious choice. Whether enjoyed in salads, curries, or as a dip, chickpeas offer a nutrient-dense addition to meals. While chickpeas are generally safe and healthy to consume as part of a balanced diet. As with any food, moderation is key. If you have specific health concerns, allergies, or conditions, it's advisable to consult with a healthcare professional or a registered dietitian before making significant changes to your diet.

With their robust nutritional profile, culinary versatility, and ability to contribute to various health benefits, chickpeas stand as a testament to the idea that wholesome foods can be both delightful and beneficial for overall health and well-being.

Back to Table of Contents

Chili Peppers

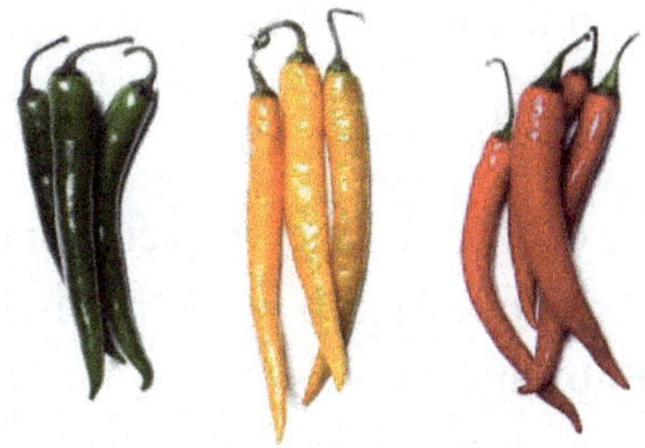

The Fiery Elixir: Unlocking the Benefits and Culinary Magic of Chili Peppers

Chili peppers, with their fiery kick and vibrant colors, have been an integral part of global cuisines for centuries. Scientifically classified under the genus Capsicum, these spicy gems not only add zest to dishes but also boast an array of health benefits. In this article, we'll explore the various advantages of consuming chili peppers and delve into their versatile uses in the kitchen.

Nutritional Profile:

Chili peppers are not just about heat; they are packed with essential nutrients that contribute to overall well-being. Here's a glimpse into the nutritional bounty offered by these fiery pods:

Capsaicin: The compound responsible for the heat in chili peppers, capsaicin is linked to various health benefits, including pain relief and metabolism boost.

Vitamin C: An antioxidant that supports the immune system, promotes skin health, and aids in the absorption of iron.

Vitamin A: Essential for vision, immune function, and skin health.

Potassium: Contributes to heart health and helps maintain proper blood pressure.

Fiber: Supports digestive health and helps maintain a feeling of fullness.

Some Vitamins in Chili Peppers:

Vitamin C:

- **Benefits:**
  - Boosts the immune system.
  - Supports collagen synthesis for healthy skin.
  - Acts as an antioxidant, protecting cells from oxidative stress.

Vitamin A:

- **Benefits:**
  - Essential for maintaining healthy vision.
  - Supports immune function.
  - Contributes to skin health and cell growth.

Vitamin B6 (Pyridoxine):

- **Benefits:**
  - Supports brain development and function.
  - Aids in the production of neurotransmitters.
  - Plays a role in the metabolism of proteins, carbohydrates, and fats.

Vitamin K:

- **Benefits:**
  - Essential for blood clotting, preventing excessive bleeding.
  - Contributes to bone health by aiding in calcium regulation.

Some Minerals in Chili Peppers:

Potassium:

- **Benefits:**
  - Helps regulate blood pressure.
  - Supports proper muscle and nerve function.
  - Contributes to fluid balance in the body.

Copper:

- **Benefits:**
  - Plays a role in the formation of collagen and connective tissues.
  - Supports the absorption and utilization of iron.
  - Contributes to the health of bones and nerves.

Iron:

- **Benefits:**
  - Essential for the formation of hemoglobin and red blood cells.
  - Supports oxygen transport in the blood.
  - Plays a role in energy metabolism.

Magnesium:

- **Benefits:**
  - Supports muscle and nerve function.
  - Contributes to bone health and calcium absorption.
  - Plays a role in energy metabolism.

Chili peppers provide a notable array of vitamins and minerals, offering various health benefits, from immune support to bone health and beyond. Consuming them in moderation can be a flavorful and nutritious way to enhance your diet.

Health Benefits:

Metabolism Boost: Capsaicin has been shown to increase metabolism, aiding in weight management and fat loss.

Pain Relief: Topical application of capsaicin has analgesic properties, providing relief from certain types of pain, such as arthritis and neuropathy.

Heart Health: The capsaicin in chili peppers may help lower blood pressure and reduce cholesterol levels, supporting cardiovascular health.

Anti-Inflammatory Properties: Chili peppers contain compounds with anti-inflammatory effects, which may help alleviate inflammation in the body.

Improved Digestion: Capsaicin stimulates the production of digestive enzymes, promoting better digestion and nutrient absorption.

Culinary Uses:

Spicy Sauces: Chili peppers are the backbone of numerous spicy sauces, from classic hot sauce to exotic salsas. They add depth and heat to dishes without overwhelming the palate.

Curries and Stews: In various global cuisines, chili peppers play a central role in creating flavorful and spicy curries, stews, and chili con carne.

Salsas and Dips: Diced or blended, chili peppers contribute heat and flavor to salsas, guacamole, and other dips, providing a perfect accompaniment to chips or as a topping for various dishes.

Pickles and Preserves: Pickling chili peppers preserves their heat and imparts a tangy flavor, making them a zesty addition to sandwiches, salads, and charcuterie boards.

Marinades and Rubs: Ground or minced chili peppers are essential components of marinades and rubs, adding spiciness to grilled meats and vegetables.

Here are two flavorful recipes that showcase the versatile use of chili peppers:

Spicy Chicken Fajitas

Ingredients:

- 1 pound boneless, skinless chicken breasts, thinly sliced
- 2 bell peppers (red and green), thinly sliced
- 1 onion, thinly sliced
- 2 cloves garlic, minced
- 2 tablespoons olive oil
- 1 teaspoon ground cumin
- 1 teaspoon chili powder
- 1/2 teaspoon smoked paprika
- Salt and pepper to taste
- Flour tortillas
- Toppings: Salsa, guacamole, sour cream, shredded cheese, lime wedges

Instructions:

1. In a large skillet, heat olive oil over medium-high heat.
2. Add sliced chicken and cook until browned and cooked through.
3. Add minced garlic, sliced bell peppers, and sliced onions to the skillet. Cook until vegetables are tender-crisp.
4. Sprinkle ground cumin, chili powder, smoked paprika, salt, and pepper over the chicken and vegetables. Toss to coat evenly.

5. Warm flour tortillas in a dry skillet or microwave.
6. Serve the spicy chicken fajita mixture in warm tortillas with your favorite toppings.

Thai Red Curry

Ingredients:

- 1 pound shrimp, chicken, or tofu, cut into bite-sized pieces
- 1 can (14 ounces) coconut milk
- 2 tablespoons red curry paste
- 1 red bell pepper, sliced
- 1 yellow bell pepper, sliced
- 1 zucchini, sliced
- 1 cup snap peas
- 2 tablespoons fish sauce (or soy sauce for a vegetarian version)
- 1 tablespoon brown sugar
- Fresh basil or cilantro for garnish
- Cooked rice or noodles

Instructions:

1. In a large pan or wok, heat coconut milk over medium heat. Add red curry paste and stir until well combined.
2. Add your choice of protein (shrimp, chicken, or tofu) and cook until almost done.
3. Add sliced bell peppers, zucchini, and snap peas to the pan. Stir and cook until the vegetables are tender.
4. Season the curry with fish sauce (or soy sauce) and brown sugar. Adjust the seasoning to taste.
5. Simmer for a few minutes until everything is heated through and well-cooked.
6. Serve the Thai red curry over cooked rice or noodles. Garnish with fresh basil or cilantro.

These recipes offer a delightful mix of flavors and showcase how chili peppers can add a spicy kick to different cuisines, from Mexican-inspired fajitas to the bold and aromatic Thai red curry. Adjust the level of spiciness according to your taste preferences for a satisfying and spicy culinary experience.

Conclusion:

Chili peppers are more than just a culinary indulgence; they offer a fiery elixir with an array of health benefits. Whether you savor the intense heat of a Carolina Reaper or appreciate the milder kick of a jalapeño, chili peppers bring a unique flavor profile to the table. Additionally, individuals with known allergies or sensitivities should exercise caution and seek guidance from a medical professional.

Embrace the zest and spice of chili peppers in your cooking, and let these vibrant pods elevate both the taste and health quotient of your meals.

Back to Table of Contents

Chinese Rhubarb / Rheum Officinale

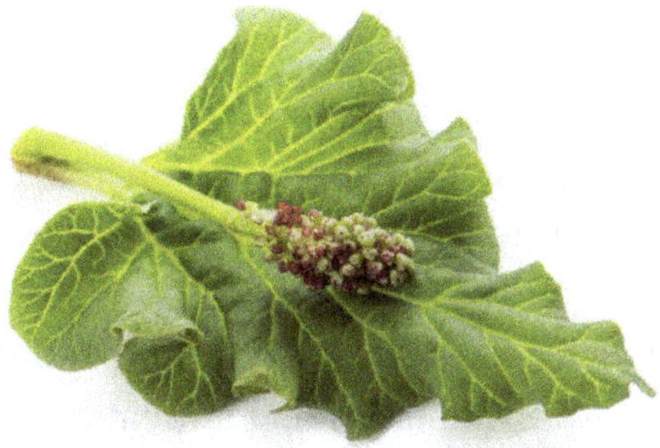

Exploring the Potent Benefits and Versatile Uses of Chinese Rhubarb

Chinese rhubarb, scientifically known as Rheum palmatum, is a perennial herb native to China and Tibet, where it has been cultivated and used for centuries for its medicinal properties. Renowned for its vibrant red stems and potent health benefits, Chinese rhubarb has earned a significant place in traditional Chinese medicine (TCM) and is increasingly recognized worldwide for its therapeutic potential.

Health Benefits:

Digestive Health: Chinese rhubarb is celebrated for its digestive properties. It contains compounds like anthraquinones and tannins, which have been shown to promote healthy digestion by stimulating the production of digestive juices, enhancing intestinal motility, and relieving constipation.

Liver Support: This herb is widely used to support liver health and detoxification. Studies suggest that Chinese rhubarb may help protect the liver from damage caused by toxins and oxidative stress, thus promoting overall liver function.

Anti-inflammatory Properties: Chinese rhubarb contains bioactive compounds that exhibit potent anti-inflammatory effects. These properties make it beneficial for alleviating symptoms associated with inflammatory conditions such as arthritis and inflammatory bowel disease.

Antimicrobial Action: Traditional uses of Chinese rhubarb include its application as an antimicrobial agent. Research indicates that certain constituents of rhubarb possess antimicrobial properties, which may help combat bacterial and fungal infections.

Cardiovascular Support: Chinese rhubarb has been investigated for its potential cardiovascular benefits. Studies suggest that it may help lower cholesterol levels, reduce blood pressure, and improve blood circulation, thus supporting heart health.

Chinese rhubarb (Rheum palmatum) contains a variety of vitamins, minerals, and antioxidants, each with its own set of potential health benefits. Here's a breakdown of some of these nutrients and their associated benefits:

Vitamin C:
- **Benefits:** Supports immune function, collagen synthesis, wound healing, and acts as an antioxidant to protect cells from damage caused by free radicals.

Vitamin K:
- **Benefits:** Essential for blood clotting, bone health, and may contribute to heart health by helping to prevent arterial calcification.

Vitamin A (beta-carotene):
- **Benefits:** Important for vision, skin health, immune function, and may have antioxidant properties to protect against oxidative stress.

Vitamin E (tocopherols and tocotrienols):
- **Benefits:** Acts as a potent antioxidant, protecting cells from oxidative damage, and may contribute to heart health by reducing inflammation and improving blood vessel function.

B Vitamins (thiamine, riboflavin, niacin, vitamin B6, folate):
- **Benefits:** Play crucial roles in energy metabolism, nervous system function, red blood cell formation, and support overall health and well-being.

Calcium:
- **Benefits:** Essential for bone and teeth health, muscle function, nerve transmission, and may also play a role in cardiovascular health.

Potassium:
- **Benefits:** Helps regulate fluid balance, muscle contractions, nerve signals, and blood pressure, supporting heart and kidney health.

Magnesium:
- **Benefits:** Important for muscle and nerve function, energy production, bone health, and may help regulate blood sugar levels and blood pressure.

Manganese:
- **Benefits:** Acts as a cofactor for various enzymes involved in metabolism, bone formation, and antioxidant defense.

Iron:
- **Benefits:** Essential for the production of hemoglobin and red blood cells, oxygen transport, energy metabolism, and overall vitality.

Zinc:
- **Benefits:** Supports immune function, wound healing, DNA synthesis, and may have antioxidant properties to protect against cellular damage.

Copper:

- **Benefits:** Necessary for the formation of red blood cells, collagen production, and may support immune function and antioxidant defenses.

Antioxidants and Other Phytonutrients:

Anthraquinones (such as emodin, rhein, and aloe-emodin):

- **Benefits**: Possess anti-inflammatory, antioxidant, and laxative properties, supporting digestive health and potentially offering protection against oxidative stress-related diseases.

Tannins:

- **Benefits**: Have antioxidant properties and may support digestive health by promoting the balance of gut microflora.

Flavonoids:

- **Benefits:** Act as antioxidants, may have anti-inflammatory effects, and contribute to cardiovascular health by supporting blood vessel function and reducing the risk of heart disease.

Polyphenols:

- **Benefits:** Possess antioxidant and anti-inflammatory properties, supporting overall health and potentially reducing the risk of chronic diseases such as cancer and cardiovascular disease.

Quercetin:

- **Benefits:** Exhibits antioxidant and anti-inflammatory effects, supports cardiovascular health, immune function, and may have anticancer properties.

Resveratrol:

- **Benefits:** Known for its antioxidant properties, potential anti-inflammatory effects, and may support cardiovascular health and longevity.

Catechins:

- **Benefits**: Found in green tea and certain other foods, catechins have antioxidant properties and may support cardiovascular health, brain function, and weight management.

These vitamins, minerals, and antioxidants found in Chinese rhubarb contribute to its overall health-promoting properties, including antioxidant, anti-inflammatory, digestive, and cardiovascular benefits. Incorporating Chinese rhubarb into a balanced diet or using it as a supplement may help support overall health and well-being. However, it's important to consume Chinese rhubarb in moderation and consult with a healthcare professional before using it for medicinal purposes, especially if you are allergic, have any underlying health conditions or are taking medications.

Uses:

Traditional Medicine: Chinese rhubarb has a long history of use in traditional medicine systems, including TCM. It is commonly prescribed in various formulations to address digestive disorders, liver ailments, and other health concerns.

Herbal Preparations: Chinese rhubarb is utilized in various herbal preparations, including decoctions, tinctures, and powders. These formulations are often tailored to specific health needs and may be combined with other herbs for synergistic effects.

Dietary Supplement: Due to its beneficial properties, Chinese rhubarb is also available in supplemental forms such as capsules and tablets. These supplements are commonly used to support digestive health, liver function, and overall well-being.

Nutritional Content

Chinese rhubarb, also known as medicinal rhubarb (Rheum palmatum), is primarily used for its medicinal properties rather than as a food. However, if you're referring to the edible stalks of Chinese rhubarb that are occasionally used in cooking, here's an approximate nutritional breakdown based on the USDA's data for rhubarb:

In 1 cup (about 122 grams) of diced raw rhubarb:

- Carbohydrates: Approximately 5.5 grams
- Protein: Approximately 0.6 grams
- Fiber: Approximately 2 grams
- Fat: Approximately 0.2 grams

Please note that the nutritional values provided here are approximate and can vary depending on factors such as the specific variety of Chinese rhubarb and its growing conditions. Additionally, Chinese rhubarb stalks are typically tart and fibrous, and they are often cooked and sweetened before consumption.

Culinary Use:

While Chinese rhubarb is primarily valued for its medicinal properties, its tart flavor and vibrant color also make it a popular ingredient in certain culinary dishes, particularly in Chinese cuisine. It is used in jams, sauces, desserts, and savory dishes to add flavor and visual appeal.

Chinese rhubarb, particularly the stalks, can be used in a variety of culinary dishes, especially in Chinese cuisine. Here are two recipes that incorporate Chinese rhubarb:

Chinese Rhubarb Stir-Fry:

Ingredients:

- 300g Chinese rhubarb stalks, washed and chopped into bite-sized pieces
- 200g lean pork, thinly sliced
- 2 cloves garlic, minced
- 1 tablespoon soy sauce
- 1 tablespoon oyster sauce
- 1 tablespoon vegetable oil

- Salt and pepper to taste
- Optional: sliced green onions for garnish

Instructions:

1. Heat vegetable oil in a wok or large skillet over medium-high heat.
2. Add minced garlic and sliced pork to the hot oil. Stir-fry until the pork is browned and cooked through.
3. Add chopped Chinese rhubarb to the skillet and stir-fry for about 3-4 minutes until tender but still crisp.
4. Season with soy sauce, oyster sauce, salt, and pepper. Stir to combine.
5. Cook for another 1-2 minutes, allowing the flavors to meld together.
6. Serve hot, garnished with sliced green onions if desired. Enjoy this savory and nutritious Chinese rhubarb stir-fry with steamed rice!

Chinese Rhubarb Compote:

Ingredients:

- 500g Chinese rhubarb stalks, washed and chopped into small pieces
- 1 cup water
- 1/2 cup granulated sugar (adjust to taste)
- Zest and juice of 1 orange
- 1 cinnamon stick
- Optional: vanilla extract or a vanilla bean pod

Instructions:

1. In a medium saucepan, combine chopped Chinese rhubarb, water, sugar, orange zest, orange juice, and cinnamon stick.
2. If using vanilla extract, add it to the mixture. If using a vanilla bean pod, split it open lengthwise and scrape the seeds into the saucepan, then add the pod itself.
3. Bring the mixture to a gentle boil over medium heat, then reduce the heat to low and let it simmer for about 15-20 minutes, stirring occasionally, until the rhubarb is soft and cooked down.
4. Taste the compote and adjust the sweetness if needed by adding more sugar or a squeeze of lemon juice.
5. Remove the cinnamon stick and vanilla bean pod if used.
6. Allow the compote to cool slightly before serving. Serve warm or chilled, either as a topping for yogurt, ice cream, or oatmeal, or as a standalone dessert. Enjoy the tangy-sweet flavor of this delightful Chinese rhubarb compote!

These recipes showcase the versatility of Chinese rhubarb in both savory and sweet dishes, allowing you to enjoy its unique flavor and reap its nutritional benefits. Adjust the seasonings and ingredients according to your taste preferences for a personalized culinary experience.

Conclusion: Chinese rhubarb stands out as a versatile herb with a rich history of medicinal use and a growing body of scientific research supporting its health benefits. Whether incorporated into traditional remedies, herbal formulations, or dietary supplements, this herb continues to offer promising potential for promoting digestive health, liver function, and overall well-being. As interest in natural remedies and herbal medicine continues to rise, Chinese rhubarb remains a valuable botanical with much to offer in the pursuit of optimal health.

Back to Table of Contents

Chives

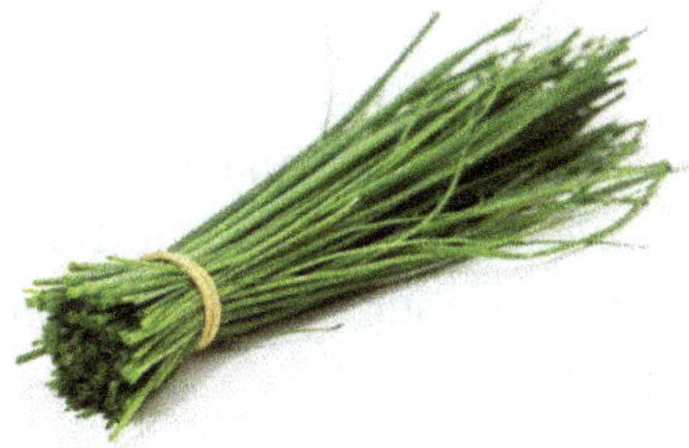

The Petite Herb with Big Flavor and Health Benefits

Chives, with their slender green stalks and mild onion flavor, have earned a special place in culinary traditions around the world. Often considered a garnish, these petite herbs pack more than just a punch of flavor. In this article, we'll explore the benefits and versatile uses of chives, shedding light on why this herb is cherished by chefs and health enthusiasts alike.

Rich in Nutrients:

Despite their small size, chives are surprisingly nutrient-dense. They are a good source of essential vitamins and minerals, including vitamin K, vitamin C, folate, and potassium. Incorporating chives into your diet can contribute to overall health by providing a boost of essential nutrients.

Vitamin K:

- *Benefits:* Vitamin K is crucial for blood clotting and bone health. It plays a vital role in the synthesis of proteins involved in bone mineralization and blood coagulation. Adequate vitamin K intake supports overall bone density and helps in maintaining a healthy cardiovascular system.

Vitamin C:

- *Benefits:* Vitamin C is a powerful antioxidant that helps protect cells from damage caused by free radicals. It is also essential for collagen synthesis, promoting healthy skin, blood vessels, and connective tissues. Vitamin C supports the immune system and aids in the absorption of non-heme iron from plant-based foods.

Folate (Vitamin B9):

- *Benefits:* Folate is important for DNA synthesis and cell division. It plays a crucial role in preventing neural tube defects during fetal development, making it particularly important for pregnant women. Folate also supports overall cell function and helps in the formation of red blood cells.

Potassium:

- *Benefits:* Potassium is an electrolyte that plays a crucial role in maintaining proper fluid balance, nerve signals, and muscle contractions. Adequate potassium intake supports cardiovascular health by helping regulate blood pressure and supporting proper heart function.

Calcium:

- *Benefits:* Calcium is essential for the formation and maintenance of strong bones and teeth. It also plays a role in muscle function, blood clotting, and nerve signaling. Including chives in your diet can contribute to your overall calcium intake, supporting bone health and various physiological processes.

Phosphorus:

- Benefits: Phosphorus is a key mineral involved in the formation and maintenance of bones and teeth. It is also essential for energy metabolism, kidney function, and the synthesis of DNA and RNA. Adequate phosphorus intake is crucial for overall health and well-being.

Magnesium:

- Benefits: Magnesium is involved in numerous biochemical processes in the body, including muscle and nerve function, energy production, and the synthesis of DNA and proteins. Adequate magnesium intake supports cardiovascular health, muscle function, and overall metabolic processes.

In addition to these minerals, chives also contain trace amounts of other essential minerals such as iron, zinc, copper, and manganese. The combination of these minerals contributes to chives' nutritional value and their potential role in supporting various aspects of health.

Antioxidant Properties:

Chives contain antioxidants, including quercetin and other flavonoids, which play a role in neutralizing free radicals in the body. Antioxidants are essential for protecting cells from oxidative stress, supporting overall health, and potentially reducing the risk of chronic diseases.

Quercetin:

- *Antioxidant Property:* Quercetin is a flavonoid antioxidant present in chives.

  Benefits:

  - **Anti-Inflammatory:** Quercetin has anti-inflammatory properties, helping to reduce inflammation in the body. Chronic inflammation is associated with various health conditions, and quercetin's anti-inflammatory effects may contribute to overall well-being.
  - **Immune Support:** Quercetin has been studied for its potential to support the immune system by enhancing the activity of certain immune cells. This may contribute to the body's defense against infections and illnesses.

Allicin:

- *Antioxidant Property:* Chives belong to the Allium family, which includes garlic and onions. Allicin is a sulfur-containing compound with antioxidant properties found in Allium vegetables, including chives.

  Benefits:
  - **Cardiovascular Health:** Allicin has been associated with cardiovascular benefits, including potential effects on lowering blood pressure and improving cholesterol levels. These benefits contribute to overall heart health.

Flavonoids:

- *Antioxidant Property:* Chives contain various flavonoids, which are plant compounds with antioxidant properties.

  Benefits:
  - **Cellular Protection:** Flavonoids help protect cells from oxidative stress by neutralizing free radicals. This antioxidant activity may play a role in preventing cellular damage and reducing the risk of chronic diseases.
  - **Cognitive Health:** Some flavonoids have been studied for their potential cognitive benefits. While more research is needed, the antioxidant properties of flavonoids may contribute to brain health.

Digestive Health:

Chives belong to the Allium family, which also includes onions and garlic. Like their aromatic relatives, chives contain sulfur compounds that may have beneficial effects on digestion. These compounds may help promote a healthy digestive system and reduce the risk of certain gastrointestinal issues.

Immune System Support:

The vitamin C content in chives contributes to immune system health. Vitamin C is known for its role in supporting the body's defenses against infections and illnesses. Including chives in your diet can be a flavorful way to boost your immune system and maintain overall well-being.

Nutritional Content

In 1 cup (about 65 grams) of chopped chives, the approximate nutritional content is as follows:

- Carbohydrates: Approximately 4 grams
- Protein: Approximately 1 gram
- Fiber: Approximately 2 grams
- Fat: Approximately 0.3 grams

Please note that these values are approximate and can vary slightly based on factors such as the specific variety and growing conditions of the chives. Additionally, chives are typically consumed in smaller quantities as a garnish or flavoring agent rather than as a main ingredient in dishes.

Culinary Delight:

Chives are celebrated for their delicate onion flavor, making them a delightful addition to a variety of dishes. From soups and salads to omelets and dips, chives bring a subtle and fresh taste that enhances the overall culinary experience. They are often used as a garnish to add a burst of color and flavor to finished dishes.

Versatile Uses:

- *Garnish:* Chopped chives make a vibrant and flavorful garnish for a wide range of dishes, from creamy soups to baked potatoes.
- *Salads:* Add chives to salads for a mild onion flavor and a pop of green color.
- *Omelets and Scrambles:* Sprinkle chopped chives over omelets or scrambled eggs to enhance the taste and visual appeal.
- *Herb Butter:* Mix finely chopped chives with butter to create a flavorful herb butter that can be used on bread, vegetables, or grilled meats.

Chives, with their mild onion flavor and vibrant green color, are a versatile herb that can be prepared in various ways for consumption. Here are four popular methods:

Fresh Chopped Chives:

Preparation: Harvest fresh chives by cutting them with scissors or a knife. Rinse them thoroughly to remove any dirt.

Usage: Chopped chives can be sprinkled as a garnish over a wide range of dishes, including soups, salads, omelets, baked potatoes, and more. Their mild onion flavor adds a burst of freshness to the finished dish.

Chive Pesto:

Preparation: Blend fresh chives with garlic, pine nuts or walnuts, Parmesan cheese, and olive oil in a food processor.

Usage: Chive pesto can be used as a flavorful spread on bread, a topping for pasta, or a sauce for grilled meats. It offers a unique twist to traditional pesto with its mild onion undertones.

Herb Butter with Chives:

Preparation: Mix finely chopped chives into softened butter along with a pinch of salt.

Usage: Chive-infused herb butter is a delightful addition to baked potatoes, steamed vegetables, or grilled meats. It can also be spread on bread for a flavorful accompaniment.

Chive Cream Cheese:

Preparation: Blend finely chopped chives into cream cheese.

Usage: Chive cream cheese makes for a delicious spread on bagels or crackers. It can also be used as a flavorful filling for sandwiches or as a dip for fresh vegetables.

These preparation methods highlight the versatility of chives and showcase how they can be incorporated into a wide range of dishes. Whether used as a garnish, blended into spreads, or infused into butter, chives contribute a subtle onion flavor that enhances the overall taste of various culinary creations.

Growing Your Own:

Chives are easy to grow at home, making them a convenient addition to your culinary repertoire. Whether in a garden or a pot on the windowsill, cultivating chives allows you to have a fresh supply at your fingertips for year-round enjoyment.

Growing chives at home is a simple and rewarding process. Here's one common way to grow chives indoors or in your garden:

Container Gardening:

1. **Select a Container:** Choose a pot or container with good drainage. Chives can be grown in small individual pots or in a larger container with other herbs.
2. **Use Well-Draining Soil:** Fill the container with well-draining potting soil. Chives prefer soil that is fertile and well-drained.
3. **Planting Chive Seeds or Transplants:**
    - *From Seeds:* If starting from seeds, sprinkle chive seeds evenly over the soil surface and cover them lightly with a thin layer of soil. Water gently.
    - *From Transplants:* If using chive transplants, plant them at a depth of about 1-2 inches, leaving enough space between each plant.
4. **Sunlight:** Place the container in a location that receives at least 4-6 hours of sunlight per day. Chives thrive in partial to full sunlight.
5. **Watering:** Keep the soil consistently moist but not waterlogged. Water when the top inch of soil feels dry.
6. **Fertilization:** Chives generally don't require heavy fertilization. You can use a balanced, water-soluble fertilizer once every 4-6 weeks during the growing season.
7. **Harvesting:** Once the chives have reached a height of at least 6 inches, you can start harvesting. Use scissors or shears to snip the leaves near the base, allowing the plant to continue growing.
8. **Pruning Flowers:** Chives produce edible flowers, but continuous harvesting of leaves is encouraged. If flowers appear and you prefer to focus on leaf production, consider pruning the flowers to redirect the plant's energy.

Growing chives in containers allows you to have a fresh and convenient supply of this flavorful herb right at your fingertips. Whether placed on a sunny windowsill or a balcony, container gardening makes it easy to cultivate chives in a space-saving and manageable way.

Tips on Growing Chives

Chives are relatively quick-growing herbs and can be harvested multiple times throughout the growing season. Here's a general timeline for growing chives:

1. **Germination**: Chive seeds typically germinate within 7 to 14 days after planting, provided they are kept in optimal conditions such as consistent moisture and moderate temperatures. Alternatively, you can propagate chives from existing plants by dividing the clumps.
2. **Establishment**: Chive plants establish quickly and begin producing leaves within a few weeks of germination or division. The leaves are typically ready for harvest when they reach about 6 to 8 inches in length, which can occur within 4 to 6 weeks after planting or dividing.
3. **Continuous Harvest**: Chives are a perennial herb, meaning they can regrow year after year. Once established, chive plants can be harvested multiple times throughout the growing season. As you harvest the leaves, new growth continues to emerge from the base of the plant.
4. **Maturity**: Chive plants reach full maturity within the first growing season. While they can be harvested at any stage of growth, they are typically considered fully mature when they are well-established and producing abundant foliage.
5. **Overwintering**: In regions with cold winters, chive plants may die back to the ground in the winter months but will regrow from the roots in the spring. Mulching around the base of the plants can help protect them during the winter.

Overall, chives are easy to grow and require minimal maintenance. With regular harvesting and proper care, you can enjoy a continuous supply of fresh chives throughout the growing season and beyond.

Conclusion:

Chives may be small in size, but their impact on both flavor and health is substantial. From their nutrient density to their culinary versatility, chives bring a lot to the table. It's advisable to consult with healthcare professionals before making significant changes to one's diet, allergies or lifestyle based on specific compounds in foods. Whether you're looking to enhance the taste of your dishes or add a nutritional boost, consider incorporating chives into your culinary creations for a delightful and health-conscious experience.

Back to Table of Contents

Chlorella

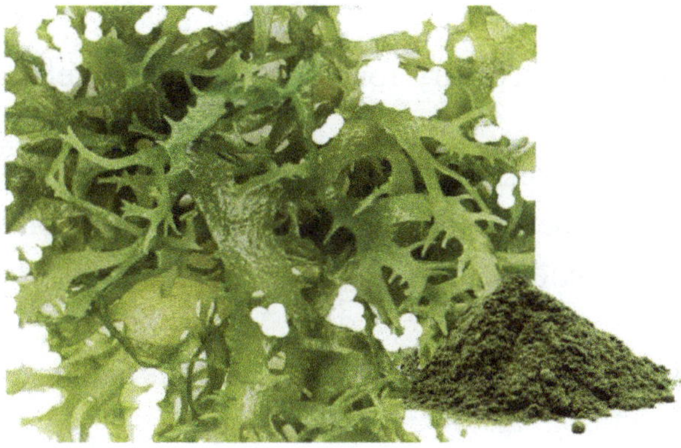

The Superfood Algae Powerhouse

Chlorella, a single-celled green freshwater algae, has gained popularity in recent years as a potent superfood with numerous health benefits. Packed with essential nutrients and unique compounds, chlorella offers a wide range of health-promoting properties and culinary uses. Let's dive into the world of chlorella and explore its benefits and uses.

Nutritional Profile:

Chlorella is a nutritional powerhouse, containing a wide array of vitamins, minerals, antioxidants, and other beneficial compounds. Here's a glimpse of what chlorella has to offer:

- **Protein:** Chlorella is a rich source of complete protein, containing all essential amino acids necessary for muscle repair, growth, and overall health.
- **Chlorophyll:** Chlorella owes its vibrant green color to chlorophyll, a plant pigment with powerful detoxifying and antioxidant properties.

Vitamins:

Chlorella is loaded with vitamins, including vitamin A, vitamin C, vitamin E, vitamin K, and various B vitamins, which support immune function, skin health, and energy metabolism.

Vitamin A: Chlorella contains beta-carotene, a precursor to vitamin A, which is important for vision health, immune function, and skin health.

Vitamin B1 (Thiamine): Necessary for energy metabolism and nerve function.

Vitamin B2 (Riboflavin): Essential for energy production, cell growth, and antioxidant activity.

Vitamin B3 (Niacin): Supports energy metabolism, nervous system function, and skin health.

Vitamin B5 (Pantothenic Acid): Involved in energy metabolism, hormone synthesis, and nutrient metabolism.

Vitamin B6 (Pyridoxine): Important for amino acid metabolism, neurotransmitter synthesis, and immune function.

Vitamin B9 (Folate): Necessary for DNA synthesis, cell division, and red blood cell formation.

Vitamin B12: Some forms of chlorella may contain small amounts of vitamin B12, which is essential for nerve function, DNA synthesis, and red blood cell production.

Vitamin C: An antioxidant that supports immune function, collagen synthesis, and wound healing.

Vitamin E: Provides antioxidant protection to cells and tissues and supports skin health and immune function.

Vitamin K: Important for blood clotting, bone health, and heart health.

These vitamins play crucial roles in various physiological processes in the body, including energy metabolism, immune function, and overall health and vitality. Incorporating chlorella into your diet can be a beneficial way to ensure you're getting a wide range of essential vitamins.

Minerals:

Chlorella provides essential minerals such as iron, magnesium, potassium, calcium, and zinc, which are important for bone health, muscle function, and overall well-being.

1. **Calcium:** Important for bone and teeth health, muscle function, and nerve transmission.
2. **Magnesium:** Crucial for nerve function, muscle contraction, and energy metabolism.
3. **Iron:** Necessary for oxygen transport in the blood and energy production.
4. **Phosphorus:** Essential for bone and teeth formation, DNA synthesis, and energy metabolism.
5. **Potassium:** Important for nerve function, muscle contraction, and maintaining fluid balance in the body.
6. **Sodium:** Necessary for maintaining fluid balance, nerve function, and muscle contraction.
7. **Zinc:** Essential for immune function, wound healing, and DNA synthesis.
8. **Copper:** Important for iron metabolism, antioxidant defense, and connective tissue formation.
9. **Manganese:** Necessary for bone formation, metabolism, and antioxidant activity.
10. **Selenium:** Acts as an antioxidant, supports thyroid function, and may have anti-inflammatory properties.
11. **Chromium:** Supports glucose metabolism and may help regulate blood sugar levels.
12. **Iodine:** Essential for thyroid hormone production and regulation of metabolic rate.
13. **Sulfur:** Found in various organic compounds, including amino acids like cysteine and methionine, and plays a role in protein synthesis and overall cellular function.

These minerals play critical roles in various bodily functions, including bone health, immune function, energy metabolism, and antioxidant defense. Incorporating chlorella into your diet can be a nutritious way to ensure you're getting these important minerals.

Antioxidants:

Chlorella contains a variety of antioxidants, including beta-carotene, lutein, and zeaxanthin, which help protect cells from damage caused by free radicals and oxidative stress.

Chlorophyll: Chlorella owes its green color to chlorophyll, a powerful antioxidant that helps neutralize free radicals and supports detoxification processes in the body.

Beta-carotene: A precursor to vitamin A, beta-carotene is a potent antioxidant that supports immune function, vision health, and skin health.

Lutein: Found in high amounts in chlorella, lutein is a carotenoid antioxidant that supports eye health and may reduce the risk of age-related macular degeneration.

Zeaxanthin: Another carotenoid antioxidant present in chlorella, zeaxanthin helps protect the eyes from oxidative damage and supports overall eye health.

Vitamin C: Chlorella contains vitamin C, a water-soluble antioxidant that supports immune function, collagen production, and wound healing.

Vitamin E: Chlorella provides vitamin E, a fat-soluble antioxidant that protects cell membranes from oxidative damage and supports skin health.

Superoxide dismutase (SOD): An enzyme found in chlorella, SOD helps convert superoxide radicals into less harmful molecules, reducing oxidative stress in the body.

Glutathione: Chlorella contains glutathione, a potent antioxidant that plays a key role in detoxification and helps protect cells from damage caused by free radicals.

These antioxidants work together to neutralize free radicals, reduce inflammation, and support overall health and well-being. Incorporating chlorella into your diet can be a valuable way to boost your antioxidant intake and promote optimal health.

Omega-3 Fatty Acids:

Chlorella contains omega-3 fatty acids, including alpha-linolenic acid (ALA), which have anti-inflammatory properties and support heart health.

Health Benefits:

Detoxification: Chlorella is renowned for its detoxifying properties, helping to remove heavy metals, toxins, and pollutants from the body. Its high chlorophyll content binds to toxins and facilitates their elimination through the digestive tract.

Immune Support: The vitamins, minerals, and antioxidants found in chlorella help support immune function, protect against infections, and enhance overall health and vitality.

Digestive Health: Chlorella contains dietary fiber and beneficial bacteria that support digestive health, promote regular bowel movements, and improve gut flora balance.

Anti-Inflammatory: Chlorella's omega-3 fatty acids and antioxidants have anti-inflammatory properties, which may help reduce inflammation, alleviate joint pain, and support cardiovascular health.

Energy Boost: Chlorella's nutrient-rich composition provides a natural energy boost, helping to combat fatigue, increase stamina, and improve physical performance.

Culinary Uses:

Chlorella can be incorporated into your diet in various ways, including:

- **Smoothies:** Add a scoop of chlorella powder to your favorite smoothie recipe for an extra nutritional boost.
- **Salads:** Sprinkle chlorella flakes or powder over salads or vegetable dishes for added flavor and nutrition.
- **Soups and Stews:** Stir chlorella powder into soups, stews, or broths to enhance their nutritional content and color.
- **Baked Goods:** Incorporate chlorella powder into baked goods such as bread, muffins, or energy bars for a nutritious twist.
- **Sauces and Dressings:** Mix chlorella powder into sauces, dressings, or dips for a vibrant green color and added nutrients.

Here are two delicious recipes featuring chlorella:

Chlorella Smoothie Bowl

Ingredients:

- 1 ripe banana, frozen
- 1 cup mixed berries (such as strawberries, blueberries, raspberries)
- 1/2 cup spinach leaves
- 1/2 cup almond milk (or any milk of your choice)
- 1 tablespoon chlorella powder
- Toppings: sliced banana, fresh berries, granola, chia seeds, shredded coconut, etc.

Instructions:

1. In a blender, combine the frozen banana, mixed berries, spinach leaves, almond milk, and chlorella powder.
2. Blend until smooth and creamy, adding more milk if needed to reach your desired consistency.
3. Pour the smoothie into a bowl.
4. Top with sliced banana, fresh berries, granola, chia seeds, shredded coconut, or any other toppings of your choice.
5. Serve immediately and enjoy this nutritious and refreshing chlorella smoothie bowl!

Chlorella Energy Bites

Ingredients:

- 1 cup pitted dates
- 1/2 cup almonds
- 1/4 cup rolled oats
- 2 tablespoons chlorella powder
- 2 tablespoons unsweetened shredded coconut
- 1 tablespoon almond butter (or any nut butter of your choice)
- 1 tablespoon honey or maple syrup (optional, for sweetness)
- Pinch of salt

Instructions:

1. In a food processor, combine the pitted dates, almonds, rolled oats, chlorella powder, shredded coconut, almond butter, honey or maple syrup (if using), and a pinch of salt.
2. Pulse the mixture until it comes together and forms a sticky dough.
3. Using your hands, roll the dough into small balls, about 1 inch in diameter.
4. Place the energy bites on a parchment-lined baking sheet and refrigerate for at least 30 minutes to firm up.
5. Once firm, store the chlorella energy bites in an airtight container in the refrigerator for up to one week.
6. Enjoy these nutritious and energizing chlorella energy bites as a healthy snack on the go!

These recipes showcase the versatility of chlorella and its ability to be incorporated into a variety of delicious and nutritious dishes. Feel free to customize the recipes with your favorite ingredients for a personalized touch!

Conclusion:

Chlorella is a nutrient-dense superfood that offers a wide range of health benefits and culinary uses. Whether you're looking to support detoxification, boost your immune system, or enhance your overall health and vitality, chlorella is a valuable addition to any diet. Incorporate chlorella into your daily routine and experience the transformative power of this green superfood algae.

If you have specific health concerns, allergies, or conditions, it's advisable to consult with a healthcare professional or a registered dietitian before making significant changes to your diet.

Back to Table of Contents

Cilantro

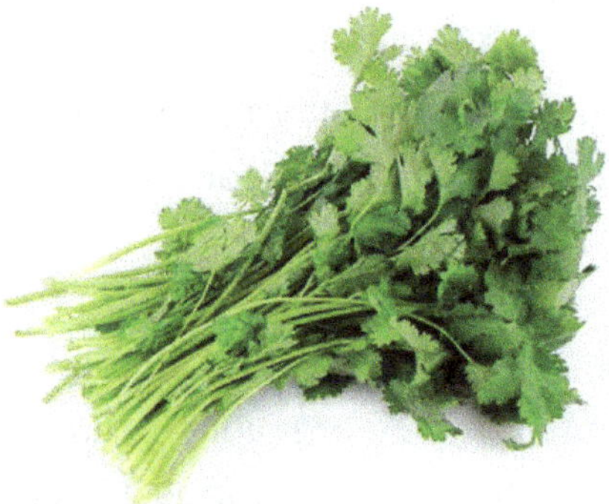

The Versatile Cilantro Plant: Unveiling Its Benefits and Culinary Wonders

Cilantro, also known as coriander leaves, is a popular herb that has been embraced across various culinary traditions for its unique flavor and numerous health benefits. This vibrant green herb, native to regions spanning from Southern Europe to Western Asia, plays a significant role in enhancing the taste of dishes and contributing to overall well-being. In this article, we will explore the diverse benefits and versatile uses of the cilantro plant.

Rich in Nutrients:

Cilantro is a nutritional powerhouse, packed with essential vitamins and minerals. It is a good source of vitamin K, vitamin A, and vitamin C. Additionally, cilantro contains folate, potassium, and small amounts of calcium and iron. Including cilantro in your diet can be a flavorful way to boost your nutrient intake.

Cilantro is a nutrient-rich herb that provides a variety of essential vitamins and minerals. Here are a few key nutrients found in cilantro and their associated benefits:

Vitamin K:

- *Benefits:* Vitamin K is crucial for blood clotting and bone health. It plays a vital role in the synthesis of proteins involved in bone mineralization and blood coagulation. Adequate vitamin K intake supports overall bone density and helps in maintaining a healthy cardiovascular system.

Vitamin A:

- *Benefits:* Vitamin A is essential for maintaining healthy vision, skin, and mucous membranes. It also plays a role in immune function and cell growth. Cilantro's contribution to vitamin A intake supports these vital bodily functions, promoting overall health and well-being.

Vitamin C:

- *Benefits:* Vitamin C is a powerful antioxidant that helps protect cells from damage caused by free radicals. It is also essential for collagen synthesis, promoting healthy skin, blood vessels, and connective tissues. Vitamin C supports the immune system and aids in the absorption of non-heme iron from plant-based foods.

Folate (Vitamin B9):

- *Benefits:* Folate is important for DNA synthesis and cell division. It plays a crucial role in preventing neural tube defects during fetal development, making it particularly important for pregnant women. Folate also supports overall cell function and helps in the formation of red blood cells.

Potassium:

- *Benefits:* Potassium is an electrolyte that plays a crucial role in maintaining proper fluid balance, nerve signals, and muscle contractions. Adequate potassium intake supports cardiovascular health by helping regulate blood pressure and supporting proper heart function.

Calcium:

- *Benefits:* Calcium is essential for the development and maintenance of strong bones and teeth. It also plays a role in muscle function, blood clotting, and nerve signaling. Including cilantro in your diet contributes to your overall calcium intake, promoting bone health and proper bodily functions.

Iron:

- *Benefits:* Iron is vital for the formation of hemoglobin, the protein in red blood cells that carries oxygen to tissues throughout the body. Adequate iron intake is essential for preventing iron-deficiency anemia, which can lead to fatigue and weakness.

Magnesium:

- *Benefits:* Magnesium is involved in numerous biochemical processes in the body, including muscle and nerve function, blood glucose control, and bone health. It also plays a role in energy production and supports the immune system. Cilantro's magnesium content contributes to these essential functions.

In addition to these minerals, cilantro also contains trace amounts of other minerals such as phosphorus, manganese, and zinc, which play roles in various physiological processes.

Digestive Aid:

One of the notable benefits of cilantro lies in its digestive properties. Cilantro contains compounds such as cineole and linoleic acid, which have been studied for their potential to aid digestion. The herb may help alleviate bloating, gas, and indigestion, making it a valuable addition to meals.

Antioxidant Powerhouse:

Cilantro is rich in antioxidants, including quercetin, beta-carotene, and flavonoids. These antioxidants help combat oxidative stress in the body, neutralizing free radicals and contributing to overall cellular health. Regular consumption of cilantro may play a role in supporting the body's defense against oxidative damage.

Detoxification Support:

Cilantro has been studied for its potential to aid in detoxification processes. It is believed to bind to heavy metals and facilitate their elimination from the body. Including cilantro in your diet may offer a natural and flavorful way to support the body's detoxification mechanisms.

Culinary Marvel:

Cilantro is a staple in kitchens around the world, and its fresh, citrusy flavor adds a zing to various dishes. From salsas and chutneys to soups, salads, and main courses, cilantro enhances the taste and aroma of a wide range of culinary creations. It is particularly prominent in Mexican, Indian, Middle Eastern, and Southeast Asian cuisines.

Versatile Uses:

- *Garnish:* Fresh cilantro leaves make a vibrant and aromatic garnish for a variety of dishes.
- *Sauces and Chutneys:* Cilantro is a key ingredient in sauces and chutneys, adding a refreshing and herbaceous flavor.
- *Soups and Stews:* Chopped cilantro is often used as a finishing touch in soups and stews, infusing them with a burst of freshness.
- *Marinades:* Cilantro is an excellent addition to marinades, contributing to the flavor profile of grilled meats and vegetables.

Here are four ways in which cilantro can be prepared for consumption:

Fresh Cilantro Leaves:

Preparation: Harvest fresh cilantro leaves by snipping them from the stems. Rinse the leaves thoroughly to remove any dirt or impurities.

Usage: Fresh cilantro leaves can be added as a garnish to salads, soups, tacos, curries, and many other dishes. Their bright flavor enhances the overall taste and adds a burst of freshness.

Cilantro Pesto:

Preparation: Blend fresh cilantro leaves with garlic, pine nuts, Parmesan cheese, olive oil, and a touch of salt in a food processor.

Usage: Cilantro pesto can be used as a flavorful spread on sandwiches, a topping for grilled meats or vegetables, or a sauce for pasta. It offers a unique twist to the traditional basil pesto.

Cilantro Chutney:

Preparation: Blend cilantro leaves with green chilies, garlic, ginger, lime juice, and salt to create a vibrant green chutney.

Usage: Cilantro chutney is a popular condiment in Indian cuisine and can be served with snacks, grilled meats, or used as a dipping sauce. It adds a zesty and spicy kick to the dish.

Cilantro Lime Rice:

Preparation: Chop fresh cilantro leaves and mix them into cooked rice along with lime juice and a pinch of salt.

Usage: Cilantro lime rice is a flavorful side dish that pairs well with Mexican and Asian cuisines. It can be served alongside main dishes, used as a base for burrito bowls, or enjoyed on its own.

Cilantro in Global Cuisine:

Cilantro's versatility has made it a beloved herb in global cuisine. In Mexican cuisine, it is a crucial component of salsa and guacamole. In Indian cuisine, it is a key ingredient in chutneys and curries. The herb's ability to complement a wide range of flavors has led to its inclusion in diverse culinary traditions.

Tips on Growing Cilantro

Cilantro, also known as coriander or Chinese parsley, is an annual herb that grows relatively quickly compared to some other herbs. Here's a general timeline for growing cilantro:

1. **Germination**: Cilantro seeds typically germinate within 7 to 10 days after planting, provided they are kept in optimal conditions such as consistent moisture and moderate temperatures.
2. **Establishment**: Cilantro plants establish quickly and begin producing leaves within a few weeks of germination. You can start harvesting cilantro leaves as soon as they are large enough to use, usually when they are about 3 to 4 inches tall. This stage can be reached within 3 to 4 weeks after planting.
3. **Bolting**: Cilantro has a tendency to bolt, or produce flowers and go to seed, especially in warmer temperatures. This process can occur relatively quickly, within 4 to 6 weeks after planting. Once cilantro bolts, the flavor of the leaves can become bitter.
4. **Continuous Harvest**: To prolong the harvest period, you can sow cilantro seeds successively every few weeks throughout the growing season. This ensures a continuous supply of fresh leaves and reduces the likelihood of the plants bolting all at once.

5. **Maturity**: Cilantro plants are typically fully mature when they bolt and produce seeds. At this point, you can allow the seeds to mature on the plant and collect them for culinary use or to replant cilantro in the future.

Overall, cilantro is a relatively fast-growing herb that can be grown successfully in a variety of climates. With proper care and attention to temperature and watering, you can enjoy a continuous supply of fresh cilantro leaves for use in cooking and garnishing dishes throughout the growing season.

Conclusion:

The cilantro plant stands out not only for its culinary versatility but also for its potential health benefits. Whether you're seeking to enhance the flavor of your dishes or harness the nutritional and digestive advantages, cilantro proves to be a delightful addition to a well-balanced diet. It's advisable to consult with healthcare professionals before making significant changes to one's diet, allergies or lifestyle based on specific compounds in foods. Embrace the vibrancy of cilantro in your cooking, and let this versatile herb elevate both the taste and health quotient of your meals.

Back to Table of Contents

Cinnamon

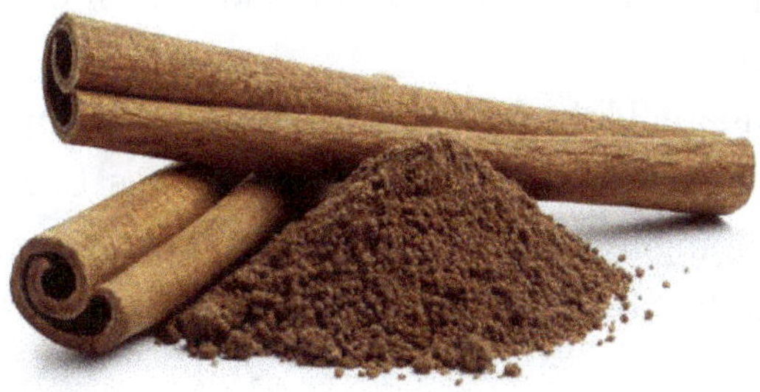

The Sweet and Spicy Wonder: The Benefits and Versatile Uses of Cinnamon

Cinnamon, with its warm and inviting aroma, has been cherished for centuries for its delightful flavor and medicinal properties. Derived from the bark of trees belonging to the Cinnamomum family, cinnamon is not only a culinary delight but also a spice with a rich history of traditional use. In this article, we will explore the various health benefits and versatile uses of cinnamon.

Nutritional Profile:

Cinnamon is not just a spice that adds depth to your favorite dishes; it also offers a range of essential nutrients and bioactive compounds. While the specific nutritional content can vary between types of cinnamon, the common varieties include Cassia and Ceylon cinnamon. Cinnamon is a good source of antioxidants, including polyphenols, and it contains trace amounts of essential minerals such as manganese and calcium.

Here are few essential nutrients and bioactive compounds found in cinnamon and their associated benefits:

Polyphenols:

- **Benefits:** Polyphenols are powerful antioxidants found in cinnamon. These compounds help neutralize free radicals in the body, protecting cells from oxidative stress. The antioxidant properties of polyphenols are associated with anti-aging effects and a reduced risk of chronic diseases.

Manganese:

- **Benefits:** Cinnamon is a good source of manganese, an essential trace mineral. Manganese plays a role in bone formation, blood clotting, and reducing inflammation. It also contributes to the proper functioning of enzymes involved in metabolism.

Fiber:

- **Benefits:** While cinnamon is not a significant source of dietary fiber, it does contain trace amounts. Fiber is essential for digestive health, supporting regular bowel movements, preventing constipation, and contributing to overall gut health.

Cinnamaldehyde:

- **Benefits:** Cinnamaldehyde is the main active compound in cinnamon responsible for its flavor and aroma. This compound has been studied for its antimicrobial properties, helping to inhibit the growth of bacteria and fungi. Cinnamaldehyde also contributes to the potential anti-inflammatory effects of cinnamon.

Cinnamic Acid:

- **Benefits:** Cinnamic acid, another bioactive compound in cinnamon, is known for its antioxidant and anti-inflammatory properties. It may play a role in reducing oxidative stress in the body and mitigating inflammation, contributing to overall health.

Essential Oils:

- **Benefits:** Cinnamon contains essential oils, including eugenol and linalool, which contribute to its aromatic and therapeutic qualities. These oils have been associated with potential antimicrobial, anti-inflammatory, and analgesic effects. Additionally, the scent of cinnamon essential oil is often used in aromatherapy for relaxation and mood enhancement.

Health Benefits:

Antioxidant Powerhouse:

- Cinnamon is rich in polyphenols, which are potent antioxidants. Antioxidants play a crucial role in neutralizing free radicals in the body, thereby protecting cells from oxidative stress. This property is linked to potential anti-aging effects and a reduced risk of chronic diseases.

Anti-Inflammatory Properties:

- The compounds found in cinnamon have been shown to have anti-inflammatory effects. Chronic inflammation is associated with various health issues, including heart disease and certain types of cancer. Cinnamon's anti-inflammatory properties may contribute to overall health and well-being.

Blood Sugar Regulation:

- Cinnamon has demonstrated the ability to improve insulin sensitivity and lower blood sugar levels. This makes it particularly valuable for individuals with insulin resistance or type 2 diabetes. Incorporating cinnamon into the diet may help regulate blood glucose and reduce the risk of complications related to diabetes.

Heart Health Support:

- Cinnamon has been associated with heart health benefits, including the potential to reduce risk factors for cardiovascular disease. It may help lower levels of bad cholesterol (LDL) while maintaining or even increasing good cholesterol (HDL). These effects contribute to a healthier heart and circulatory system.

Versatile Uses:

Culinary Delight:

Cinnamon is a staple in kitchens around the world, enhancing the flavor of both sweet and savory dishes. It is commonly used in baking, added to desserts, oatmeal, and beverages. Cinnamon's warm and sweet notes make it a versatile spice that complements a wide range of culinary creations.

Caribbean cuisine often incorporates cinnamon for its warm and aromatic flavor. Here are a few recipes that feature cinnamon:

Jamaican Sweet Potato Pudding:

- **Ingredients:**
  - Sweet potatoes
  - Coconut milk
  - Brown sugar
  - Flour
  - Raisins
  - Vanilla extract
  - Nutmeg
  - Cinnamon powder
- **Instructions:**

1. Grate sweet potatoes and mix with coconut milk, brown sugar, flour, raisins, vanilla extract, nutmeg, and cinnamon to form a batter.
2. Pour the batter into a baking dish and bake until the pudding is firm and golden brown.
3. Serve slices of Jamaican Sweet Potato Pudding for a delightful dessert with the warmth of cinnamon.

Jamaican Banana Fritters:

- **Ingredients:**
  - Ripe bananas
  - Flour
  - Sugar
  - Baking powder
  - Cinnamon powder
  - Nutmeg
  - Salt
  - Milk
  - Vanilla extract
  - Vegetable oil (for frying)

- **Instructions:**

1. Mash ripe bananas and mix with flour, sugar, baking powder, cinnamon powder, nutmeg, salt, milk, and vanilla extract to form a thick batter.
2. Heat vegetable oil in a pan and drop spoonfuls of the batter into the hot oil.
3. Fry until golden brown on both sides, then drain on paper towels. Sprinkle with cinnamon and sugar while still warm. Enjoy Jamaican Banana Fritters as a sweet and spiced treat.

These recipes showcase the versatility of cinnamon in Jamaican cuisine, adding a warm and aromatic touch to both savory and sweet dishes.

Cinnamon Apple Oatmeal:

- **Ingredients:**
    - Rolled oats
    - Milk or water
    - Apple, diced
    - Cinnamon powder
    - Honey or maple syrup (optional)
- **Instructions:**

1. Cook rolled oats with milk or water according to package instructions.
2. Stir in diced apples and let them cook until softened.
3. Sprinkle cinnamon powder over the oatmeal and add honey or maple syrup for sweetness if desired. Mix well and enjoy a comforting bowl of Cinnamon Apple Oatmeal.

Cinnamon Honey Glazed Carrots:

- **Ingredients:**
    - Carrots, peeled and sliced
    - Olive oil
    - Honey
    - Ground cinnamon
    - Salt and pepper to taste
- **Instructions:**

1. Preheat the oven to 400°F (200°C).
2. Toss sliced carrots with olive oil, honey, ground cinnamon, salt, and pepper in a bowl.
3. Spread the coated carrots on a baking sheet and roast in the oven until they are tender and caramelized. Serve as a delicious side dish with a touch of cinnamon sweetness.

Cinnamon Swirl Banana Bread:

- **Ingredients:**
    - Ripe bananas, mashed
    - Flour
    - Sugar
    - Eggs

- Butter, melted
- Baking soda
- Vanilla extract
- Ground cinnamon

- **Instructions:**

1. Preheat the oven to 350°F (175°C) and grease a loaf pan.
2. In a bowl, mix mashed bananas, flour, sugar, eggs, melted butter, baking soda, and vanilla extract until well combined.
3. Pour half of the batter into the greased loaf pan, sprinkle with a layer of ground cinnamon, and add the remaining batter on top. Swirl the cinnamon into the batter with a knife.
4. Bake until a toothpick inserted into the center comes out clean. Allow the Cinnamon Swirl Banana Bread to cool before slicing and serving.

These recipes showcase the versatility of cinnamon, adding warmth and depth of flavor to different dishes, from breakfast to side dishes and desserts. Enjoy the delightful aroma and taste of cinnamon in these culinary creations!

Beverage Infusions:

- Cinnamon infusions, commonly known as cinnamon tea, are popular for their comforting and aromatic qualities. Steeping cinnamon sticks or powder in hot water creates a flavorful and soothing beverage that can be enjoyed on its own or blended with other herbal teas.

Health Tonic:

- Some people incorporate cinnamon into their daily routine as a health tonic. This can be achieved by adding a sprinkle of cinnamon to smoothies, yogurt, or even a morning cup of coffee. The potential health benefits make it an easy and delicious addition to a balanced diet.

Aromatherapy and Home Décor:

- Beyond its culinary uses, cinnamon is valued for its aromatic properties. Cinnamon sticks or essential oil can be used for aromatherapy, creating a warm and inviting atmosphere. Additionally, cinnamon-infused potpourri or sachets can add a delightful fragrance to your home.

Cinnamon Leaf Benefits and Usage

Cinnamon leaf, derived from the Cinnamomum verum or Cinnamomum zeylanicum tree, is distinct from cinnamon bark and offers its own set of benefits. Here are few benefits of cinnamon leaf and its common usage:

Antimicrobial Properties:

- Benefits: Cinnamon leaf is known for its potent antimicrobial properties. It contains compounds like eugenol that exhibit antibacterial and antifungal effects. These properties may contribute to inhibiting the growth of harmful microorganisms and supporting overall oral and digestive health.

Anti-Inflammatory Effects:

- Benefits: Cinnamon leaf contains cinnamaldehyde, a compound with anti-inflammatory properties. This can be beneficial in reducing inflammation in the body, potentially aiding in conditions related to inflammation such as arthritis. Incorporating cinnamon leaf into the diet or using it in essential oil form may contribute to managing inflammatory responses.

Skin Health and Acne Control:

- Benefits: Cinnamon leaf essential oil is often used in skincare due to its antimicrobial and anti-inflammatory properties. It may help combat acne by preventing bacterial growth on the skin. However, it's crucial to dilute cinnamon leaf oil with a carrier oil before applying it to the skin to avoid irritation, and a patch test is recommended.

Aromatherapy and Relaxation:

- Benefits: The pleasant and warm aroma of cinnamon leaf makes it a popular choice for aromatherapy. Inhaling the scent of cinnamon leaf essential oil may have relaxing effects, reducing stress and promoting a sense of well-being. Diffusing the oil in living spaces or adding a few drops to a bath can contribute to a calming atmosphere.

Usage:

- **Culinary Uses:** Cinnamon leaf can be used in cooking, particularly in recipes where a milder cinnamon flavor is desired. It is commonly used in curries, stews, and beverages.
- **Essential Oil:** Cinnamon leaf essential oil is extracted from the leaves and twigs. It can be used topically (diluted) for skincare or in aromatherapy diffusers for a pleasant fragrance.
- **Tea Infusion:** Cinnamon leaf can be infused in hot water to create a soothing and aromatic tea. This tea is not only flavorful but may also offer some of the health benefits associated with cinnamon.

Conclusion:

Cinnamon, with its enticing aroma and versatile uses, is more than just a spice; it's a treasure trove of health benefits and culinary delights. Whether sprinkled on your morning oatmeal, infused into a comforting tea, or used to add warmth to your home, cinnamon has stood the test of time as a cherished spice with an array of potential advantages. As with any dietary component, individual responses may vary, and it's advisable to consult with healthcare professionals, especially for those with specific health conditions or concerns. As you savor the sweet and spicy essence of cinnamon, you're not just indulging in flavor – you're embracing a spice that has woven its way into the tapestry of cultures and cuisines across the globe. Back to Table of Contents

Clementines

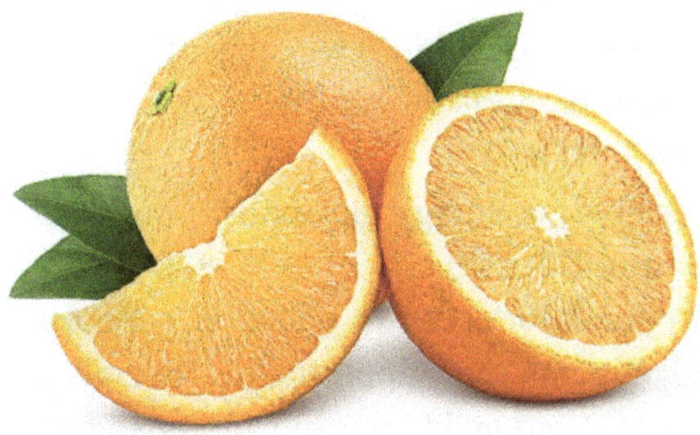

The Bright and Sweet Goodness of Clementines: Benefits and Uses

Clementines, a delightful citrus fruit that belongs to the mandarin orange family, are not only a tasty treat but also a nutritional powerhouse. Bursting with flavor and packed with essential nutrients, clementines have earned their place as a popular and healthy snack option. In this article, we will explore the benefits and versatile uses of clementines.

Nutrient-Rich Goodness:

Clementines are rich in a variety of essential nutrients that contribute to overall health and well-being. Here are some key nutritional components found in clementines:

Vitamin C:

- **Benefits:** Boosts the immune system, supports skin health, acts as an antioxidant, aids in collagen production.

Fiber:

- **Benefits:** Promotes digestive health, helps regulate blood sugar levels, contributes to a feeling of fullness.

Vitamin A:

- **Benefits:** Essential for vision health, supports immune function, and maintains healthy skin.

Potassium:

- **Benefits:** Helps regulate blood pressure, supports heart and muscle function, aids in fluid balance.

Folate (Vitamin B9):

- **Benefits:** Important for DNA synthesis and repair, aids in red blood cell formation.

Calcium:

- **Benefits:** Important for bone health, supports muscle and nerve function.

Phosphorus:

- **Benefits:** Essential for bone and teeth health, involved in energy metabolism.

Magnesium:

- **Benefits:** Important for muscle and nerve function, supports bone health.

Vitamin B6 (Pyridoxine):

- **Benefits:** Important for brain development and function, helps the body convert food into energy, supports the nervous system.

Thiamine (Vitamin B1):

- **Benefits:** Essential for energy metabolism, supports nerve function.

Riboflavin (Vitamin B2):

- **Benefits:** Important for energy production, supports normal vision and skin health.

These vitamins and minerals contribute to the overall health-promoting properties of clementines, making them a nutritious and flavorful addition to a balanced diet. Including a variety of fruits and vegetables in your diet, including clementines, ensures that you benefit from a diverse range of essential nutrients.

Health Benefits:

Immune System Support:

- The high Vitamin C content in clementines supports the immune system, helping the body defend against infections and illnesses.

Heart Health:

- Potassium in clementines contributes to heart health by helping regulate blood pressure and supporting overall cardiovascular function.

Digestive Health:

- The fiber content aids in digestion, promoting a healthy gut and preventing constipation.

Hydration:

- Clementines have a high water content, contributing to hydration and supporting overall health.

Nutritional Content

The nutritional content of clementines can vary slightly based on factors like size and ripeness, but here's an approximate breakdown of the nutrients in 1 cup (about 165 grams) of clementine segments:

- Carbohydrates: Approximately 21 grams
- Protein: Approximately 1 gram
- Fiber: Approximately 3 grams
- Fat: Approximately 0.3 grams
- Sugar: Approximately 16 grams

Deliciously Versatile:

Clementines are not only a convenient and tasty snack on their own, but they can also be incorporated into a variety of culinary creations. Here are some versatile uses:

Fresh Snacking:

- Peel and enjoy clementines as a refreshing and portable snack, providing a natural burst of sweetness.

Salads:

- Add clementine segments to salads for a juicy and citrusy flavor. They pair well with mixed greens, nuts, and vinaigrette dressings.

Smoothies:

- Blend clementines into smoothies for a zesty and vitamin-packed addition. Combine them with other fruits, yogurt, and a liquid of your choice for a delicious beverage.

Desserts:

- Incorporate clementines into desserts such as fruit salads, sorbets, or gelato for a citrusy twist.

Marmalades and Jams:

- Utilize clementines to make homemade marmalades or jams. Their natural sweetness adds a delightful flavor to spreads.

Here are two delicious recipes that incorporate the bright and citrusy flavor of clementines:

Clementine and Avocado Salad:

Ingredients:

- 4 clementines, peeled and segmented
- 2 avocados, diced
- 1 cup cherry tomatoes, halved
- 1/4 red onion, thinly sliced
- 1/4 cup feta cheese, crumbled
- 2 tablespoons fresh mint leaves, chopped
- 2 tablespoons extra-virgin olive oil
- 1 tablespoon balsamic vinegar
- Salt and pepper to taste

Instructions:

1. In a large salad bowl, combine clementine segments, diced avocados, cherry tomatoes, sliced red onion, crumbled feta cheese, and chopped mint leaves.
2. In a small bowl, whisk together the extra-virgin olive oil and balsamic vinegar to create the dressing.

3. Pour the dressing over the salad and gently toss to combine. Season with salt and pepper to taste.
4. Serve the refreshing clementine and avocado salad as a side dish or a light and nutritious lunch.

Clementine and Ginger Glazed Chicken:

Ingredients:

- 4 boneless, skinless chicken breasts
- 4 clementines, juiced
- Zest of 1 clementine
- 2 tablespoons soy sauce
- 1 tablespoon honey
- 1 tablespoon fresh ginger, grated
- 2 cloves garlic, minced
- 1 tablespoon olive oil
- Salt and pepper to taste
- Fresh cilantro for garnish

Instructions:

1. Preheat the oven to 375°F (190°C).
2. Season the chicken breasts with salt and pepper.
3. In a bowl, whisk together clementine juice, clementine zest, soy sauce, honey, grated ginger, and minced garlic to create the glaze.
4. Heat olive oil in an oven-safe skillet over medium-high heat. Brown the chicken breasts on both sides.
5. Pour the clementine and ginger glaze over the chicken.
6. Transfer the skillet to the preheated oven and bake for about 20-25 minutes or until the chicken is cooked through.
7. Garnish with fresh cilantro and serve the clementine and ginger glazed chicken over rice or with your favorite side dishes.

These recipes showcase the versatility of clementines, whether used in a refreshing salad or as a flavorful glaze for chicken. Enjoy the unique and citrusy taste of clementines in these creative and delicious dishes!

In conclusion, clementines offer a delightful combination of flavor and nutrition. Packed with essential vitamins and minerals, these small citrus fruits provide a convenient and healthy option for snacking and culinary exploration. If you have specific health concerns, allergies, or conditions, it's advisable to consult with a healthcare professional or a registered dietitian before making significant changes to your diet.

Whether enjoyed fresh, blended into beverages, or incorporated into various dishes, clementines are a versatile and tasty addition to a well-balanced diet. Embrace the benefits and explore the numerous ways to savor the bright and sweet goodness of clementines in your daily life.

Back to Table of Contents

Clove

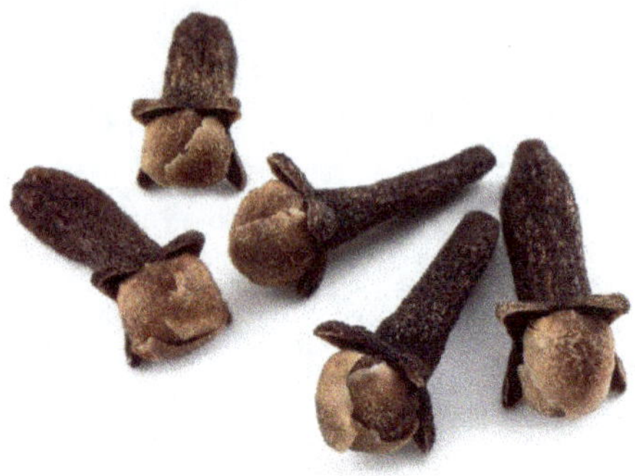

Unveiling the Health and Culinary Marvels

Clove (Syzygium aromaticum) stands as a remarkable herb with a rich history steeped in both culinary traditions and medicinal practices. Native to Indonesia, clove has traversed continents, leaving its aromatic imprint on diverse cultures. This document endeavors to explore the multifaceted benefits of clove, delving into its botanical characteristics, historical significance, culinary applications, and the therapeutic properties that have made it a cherished herb throughout the ages.

Botanical Overview:

Clove, derived from the dried flower buds of the clove tree, belongs to the Myrtaceae family. Known for its strong, warm aroma and distinct flavor, clove has become a staple in global cuisines. The name "clove" is believed to originate from the Latin word "clavus," meaning nail, aptly describing the herb's nail-shaped appearance.

Culinary Applications:

Clove's aromatic and pungent flavor has secured its place in kitchens worldwide. Widely used in both sweet and savory dishes, clove adds depth and warmth to recipes. It is a key ingredient in spice blends such as garam masala and pumpkin spice, as well as in pickling, marinades, and mulled beverages. Clove oil, extracted from the buds, is also employed as a flavoring agent in the food industry.

Here are some ways in which cloves can be prepared:

Clove-Infused Hot Beverage:

Add whole cloves to hot water along with your favorite tea leaves or bags.

Allow the cloves to steep, releasing their warm and aromatic essence.

Optionally, sweeten with honey or add a slice of orange for a flavorful clove-infused hot drink.

Clove-Spiced Rice:

Add whole cloves to rice while cooking for a subtle yet distinctive flavor.

The cloves infuse the rice with a warm and aromatic taste, enhancing the overall dish.

Remove the cloves before serving.

Clove-Orange Marinade for Meat:

Create a marinade by combining crushed cloves with orange juice, soy sauce, garlic, and olive oil.

Marinate meat, such as chicken or pork, in this flavorful mixture before grilling or roasting.

The clove and orange combination adds depth and complexity to the dish.

Clove-Infused Syrup:

Prepare a simple syrup by dissolving sugar in water over heat.

Add whole cloves to the syrup and simmer for a few minutes.

Strain out the cloves, leaving behind a clove-infused syrup that can be used in cocktails, mocktails, or drizzled over desserts.

Clove-Spiced Pickles:

Add whole cloves, along with other spices like cinnamon and mustard seeds, to a jar of pickles.

The cloves contribute a warm and aromatic note to the pickles during the pickling process.

Allow the flavors to meld for a few days before enjoying the clove-spiced pickles.

These diverse preparations highlight the versatility of cloves, offering options for both beverages and savory dishes. Whether used as a subtle spice in rice or a bold flavor enhancer in marinades, cloves bring a unique and aromatic dimension to a variety of culinary creations.

Medicinal Properties:

Clove's medicinal properties have been recognized for centuries, contributing to its prominence in traditional medicine. Some notable benefits include:

Analgesic Properties: Clove is revered for its natural analgesic properties, making it a popular remedy for toothaches and oral discomfort. Clove oil, with its eugenol content, provides a numbing effect.

Antioxidant Richness: High in antioxidants, clove helps combat oxidative stress, potentially reducing the risk of chronic diseases and supporting overall health.

Anti-Inflammatory Effects: Eugenol, a major component of clove, exhibits anti-inflammatory properties, contributing to its traditional use in alleviating inflammatory conditions.

Digestive Aid: Clove has been used to aid digestion, relieve bloating, and soothe gastrointestinal discomfort. It may also support healthy gut function.

Antimicrobial Action: Clove possesses antimicrobial properties, making it effective against bacteria and fungi. It has been utilized historically for its role in preserving food and promoting oral hygiene.

Historical Significance:

Clove has a rich historical background, dating back to ancient civilizations such as the Chinese and Romans. It was highly prized for its medicinal properties, and its scarcity in Europe during the Middle Ages drove exploration and trade. Clove was a coveted commodity in the spice trade routes, contributing to the spice's cultural and economic significance.

Cultivation and Harvesting:

Clove trees thrive in tropical climates and are cultivated primarily in countries like Indonesia, Madagascar, and Sri Lanka. The flower buds are hand-picked before they bloom and are dried to preserve their aromatic and medicinal qualities.

In conclusion, clove herb emerges as a versatile and invaluable botanical treasure, enriching both culinary experiences and holistic well-being. From its culinary prowess in enhancing flavors to its time-honored medicinal applications, clove has carved a niche in diverse cultures globally. The analgesic, antioxidant, and anti-inflammatory properties of clove underscore its potential health benefits, while its historical significance adds a layer of cultural appreciation. As we continue to explore the depths of nature's offerings, clove stands as a testament to the enduring connection between food, medicine, and human history.

If you have specific health concerns, allergies, or conditions, it's advisable to consult with a healthcare professional or a registered dietitian before making significant changes to your diet.

Back to Table of Contents

Cocoa

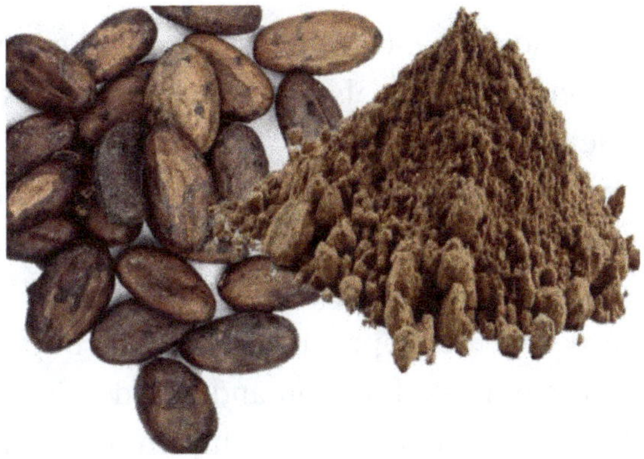

The Versatility and Health Benefits of Cocoa

Cocoa, the primary ingredient in chocolate, has been celebrated not only for its delectable taste but also for its numerous health benefits. Derived from the cacao bean, cocoa has been a cherished ingredient for centuries, dating back to ancient Mesoamerican civilizations. In recent years, scientific research has shed light on the various advantages associated with consuming cocoa, ranging from cardiovascular health to mood enhancement.

Health Benefits of Cocoa:

Rich in Antioxidants:

Cocoa is a powerhouse of antioxidants, such as flavonoids and polyphenols, which help combat oxidative stress in the body. These compounds play a crucial role in neutralizing free radicals, contributing to overall health and well-being.

Flavonoids:

- **Epicatechin:** A powerful flavonoid with antioxidant properties, known for its potential cardiovascular benefits.
- **Catechin:** Another flavonoid associated with various health benefits, including anti-inflammatory effects.

Polyphenols:

- **Procyanidins:** These are a type of condensed tannins found in cocoa that contribute to its antioxidant content. They are believed to have cardiovascular protective effects.
- **Quercetin:** A flavonoid with antioxidant and anti-inflammatory properties found in cocoa, contributing to its potential health benefits.

Theobromine:

- Although not an antioxidant in the traditional sense, theobromine is a stimulant found in cocoa that has been associated with various health benefits. It is known to have mild diuretic effects and may contribute to the mood-enhancing properties of cocoa.

Caffeine:

- While not unique to cocoa, caffeine is present in cocoa beans and contributes to its stimulating effects. Caffeine also has antioxidant properties.

Phenylethylamine (PEA):

- PEA is a compound found in cocoa that acts as a neurotransmitter and is associated with mood enhancement. While not primarily an antioxidant, it contributes to the overall feel-good effects of consuming cocoa.

These antioxidants work together to provide cocoa with impressive health benefits, ranging from cardiovascular support to cognitive function and mood enhancement. It's important to note that the specific antioxidant content can vary based on the type of cocoa product (dark chocolate, cocoa powder, etc.) and the processing methods used. Choosing high-quality, minimally processed cocoa products will likely provide the most antioxidant benefits.

Vitamins and Minerals

Cocoa is a rich source of various vitamins and minerals, though the exact content can vary depending on the type of cocoa product and its processing. Here is a list of some key vitamins and minerals found in cocoa:

Vitamins:

Vitamin B1 (Thiamine):

- Thiamine is essential for energy metabolism and nerve function.

Vitamin B2 (Riboflavin):

- Riboflavin is important for energy production and the metabolism of fats, drugs, and steroids.

Vitamin B3 (Niacin):

- Niacin is crucial for energy metabolism and plays a role in DNA repair.

Vitamin B5 (Pantothenic Acid):

- Pantothenic Acid is involved in the synthesis of fatty acids and is essential for energy production.

Vitamin B6 (Pyridoxine):

- Pyridoxine is important for brain development and function, as well as the metabolism of amino acids.

Folate (Vitamin B9):

- Folate is crucial for DNA synthesis and repair, and it plays a key role in cell division.

Vitamin E (Tocopherols and Tocotrienols):

- Tocopherols and tocotrienols are antioxidants that protect cells from oxidative damage.

Vitamin K:

- Vitamin K is essential for blood clotting and bone health.

Minerals:

Magnesium:

- Magnesium is important for muscle and nerve function, blood sugar control, and bone health.

Iron:

- Iron is essential for the formation of hemoglobin and the transport of oxygen in the blood.

Phosphorus:

- Phosphorus is a vital component of DNA, RNA, and ATP, playing a crucial role in energy metabolism.

Copper:

- Copper is involved in the formation of red blood cells, maintenance of bones and connective tissues, and protection against oxidative stress.

Manganese:

- Manganese is a cofactor for various enzymes involved in bone formation, blood clotting, and reducing oxidative stress.

Zinc:

- Zinc is important for immune function, wound healing, and DNA synthesis.

Potassium:

- Potassium plays a role in maintaining proper fluid balance, nerve signals, and muscle contractions.

Calcium:

- While cocoa is not a particularly high source of calcium, it does contain some. Calcium is crucial for bone health and muscle function.

It's important to note that the amounts of these vitamins and minerals can vary based on the cocoa product and its processing. Additionally, cocoa is often consumed in combination with other ingredients, such as sugar and milk, which can also contribute to the overall nutrient profile of the final product.

Heart Health:

Numerous studies suggest that cocoa may have a positive impact on cardiovascular health. The flavonoids in cocoa have been associated with improvements in blood pressure, cholesterol levels, and overall vascular function. Regular consumption of cocoa has been linked to a reduced risk of heart disease.

Improved Cognitive Function:

Cocoa contains substances that may enhance cognitive function and provide neuroprotective benefits. The flavonoids in cocoa may contribute to improved blood flow to the brain, potentially reducing the risk of age-related cognitive decline.

Mood Enhancement:

Cocoa is known to contain various compounds, including theobromine and phenylethylamine, which can have mood-enhancing effects. Additionally, cocoa stimulates the production of serotonin, a neurotransmitter associated with feelings of happiness and well-being.

Anti-Inflammatory Properties:

Some components of cocoa have demonstrated anti-inflammatory properties, which may help in reducing inflammation in the body. Chronic inflammation is linked to various health issues, including arthritis and certain cardiovascular conditions.

Nutritional Content

The nutritional content of cocoa powder can vary slightly based on brand and processing methods, but here's an approximate breakdown of the nutrients in 1 cup (about 86 grams) of unsweetened cocoa powder:

- Carbohydrates: Approximately 44 grams
- Protein: Approximately 22 grams
- Fiber: Approximately 26 grams
- Fat: Approximately 10 grams
- Sugar: Approximately 1 gram

Keep in mind that these values are estimates and can vary depending on the specific product.

Uses of Cocoa:

Culinary Delight: One of the most well-known uses of cocoa is in the culinary world, particularly in the creation of chocolate. Cocoa is a versatile ingredient that adds depth and richness to various desserts, beverages, and savory dishes. From hot cocoa to chocolate truffles, cocoa is a staple in many kitchens worldwide.

Beverages: Cocoa is a key component in the production of hot chocolate and chocolate milk. Beyond these classics, it is also used in the creation of chocolate-flavored beverages, including smoothies and shakes, providing a delicious and nutritious twist to everyday drinks.

Baking and Cooking: Cocoa is an essential ingredient in baking, contributing to the creation of brownies, cakes, cookies, and other decadent treats. It is also used in savory dishes, adding depth and complexity to mole sauces and chili recipes.

Health Supplements: With the increasing recognition of cocoa's health benefits, it is now available in various supplement forms, such as cocoa powder capsules or extracts. These supplements offer a concentrated dose of cocoa's beneficial compounds for those seeking a convenient way to incorporate it into their diet.

Here are two delicious recipes using cocoa:

Chocolate Avocado Smoothie Bowl

Ingredients:

- 1 ripe avocado
- 1 banana, frozen
- 2 tablespoons cocoa powder
- 1 cup almond milk (or any milk of your choice)
- 1 tablespoon honey or maple syrup (optional, depending on sweetness preference)
- 1/2 teaspoon vanilla extract
- Toppings: sliced strawberries, banana slices, chia seeds, granola, and a drizzle of almond butter

Instructions:

1. In a blender, combine the ripe avocado, frozen banana, cocoa powder, almond milk, honey or maple syrup (if using), and vanilla extract.
2. Blend until smooth and creamy.
3. Pour the chocolate avocado smoothie into a bowl.
4. Arrange the toppings - sliced strawberries, banana slices, chia seeds, granola, and a drizzle of almond butter - on top of the smoothie bowl.
5. Enjoy your nutritious and chocolaty breakfast or snack!

Dark Chocolate Energy Bites

Ingredients:

- 1 cup rolled oats
- 1/2 cup almond butter
- 1/3 cup honey or maple syrup
- 2 tablespoons cocoa powder
- 1 teaspoon vanilla extract
- Pinch of salt
- 1/3 cup dark chocolate chips
- Additional rolled oats or shredded coconut for rolling (optional)

Instructions:

1. In a mixing bowl, combine rolled oats, almond butter, honey or maple syrup, cocoa powder, vanilla extract, and a pinch of salt.
2. Mix well until the ingredients are thoroughly combined.
3. Fold in the dark chocolate chips.
4. Place the mixture in the refrigerator for about 15-30 minutes to firm up.
5. Once the mixture is chilled, take small portions and roll them into bite-sized balls.
6. Optionally, roll the energy bites in additional rolled oats or shredded coconut for added texture.
7. Place the dark chocolate energy bites in an airtight container and store in the refrigerator.

8. Enjoy as a quick energy-boosting snack!

These recipes showcase the versatility of cocoa, from a creamy and nutrient-packed smoothie bowl to a satisfying and wholesome energy bite. Feel free to customize the recipes based on your taste preferences and dietary restrictions.

Conclusion:

Cocoa, once enjoyed primarily for its indulgent taste, has proven to be more than just a treat for the senses. Its rich antioxidant content and associated health benefits make it a valuable addition to a balanced and wholesome diet. Whether enjoyed in a cup of hot cocoa on a chilly day or incorporated into a range of culinary creations, cocoa continues to be a delightful and health-promoting ingredient. As with any food, moderation is key, and individuals with specific health concerns should consult with healthcare professionals before making significant changes to their diet.

Back to Table of Contents

Coconut

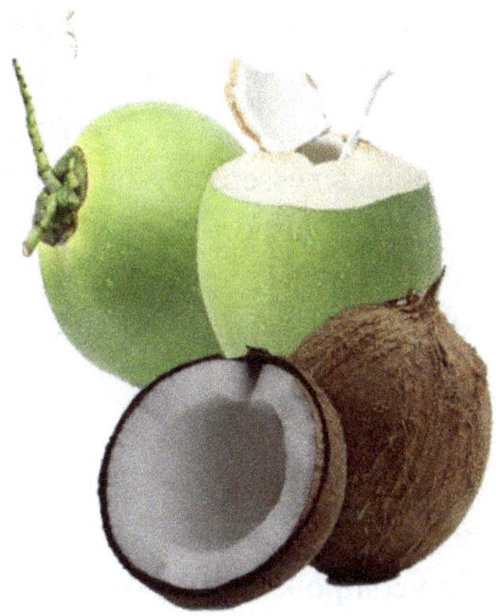

Embracing the Coconut: A Bounty of Benefits and Diverse Uses

The coconut, often referred to as the "tree of life," has been a staple in the diets and lifestyles of various cultures for centuries. This versatile fruit is not only celebrated for its delicious taste but also cherished for its myriad health benefits and diverse range of uses. In this article, we explore the bounty of advantages that coconuts offer and the many ways in which they enrich our lives.

Nutrient-Rich Composition:

Coconuts are a nutritional powerhouse, offering a unique blend of essential nutrients. The coconut kernel is rich in medium-chain triglycerides (MCTs), a type of healthy fat that is easily metabolized by the body for quick energy. Additionally, coconuts are a good source of fiber, vitamins (such as C, E, B vitamins), and minerals (including potassium, magnesium, and phosphorus), making them a well-rounded addition to a balanced diet.

Medium-Chain Triglycerides (MCTs):

- ***Benefit:*** Coconut is rich in MCTs, a type of healthy fat that is easily metabolized by the body. MCTs provide a quick and efficient source of energy, making them beneficial for individuals seeking sustained energy levels. Additionally, MCTs have been associated with potential heart health benefits, including improving lipid profiles and supporting cardiovascular well-being.

Dietary Fiber:

- ***Benefit:*** Coconut contains dietary fiber, which is essential for digestive health. Fiber promotes regular bowel movements, prevents constipation, and supports a healthy gut microbiome. Including coconut-based products in your diet, such as coconut flesh or coconut flour, can contribute to increased fiber intake and overall digestive well-being.

Vitamin E:

- ***Benefit:*** Coconut is a good source of vitamin E, a potent antioxidant that helps protect cells from damage caused by free radicals. Vitamin E is known for its skin-nourishing properties, promoting healthy skin and contributing to overall skin well-being. Additionally, vitamin E supports the immune system and may play a role in reducing inflammation.

Potassium:

- ***Benefit:*** Coconuts are rich in potassium, an essential mineral that plays a crucial role in maintaining proper electrolyte balance. Potassium is important for heart health, as it helps regulate blood pressure and supports cardiovascular function and ensuring proper muscle and nerve function. Including coconut water in your diet can be a refreshing way to replenish potassium levels and stay hydrated.

Phosphorus:

- **Benefit:** Coconut contains phosphorus, an essential mineral that plays a key role in bone health and energy metabolism. Phosphorus is a component of DNA, RNA, and ATP (adenosine triphosphate), the primary energy currency of cells. Adequate phosphorus intake supports bone and teeth formation, as well as the efficient utilization of nutrients for energy production.

Magnesium:

- **Benefit:** Magnesium is found in coconuts and is essential for various physiological functions. Magnesium supports muscle and nerve function, helps regulate blood sugar levels, and contributes to bone health. It also plays a role in energy metabolism and supports the body's stress response. Including coconuts in your diet can be a tasty way to ensure an adequate intake of magnesium.

Copper:

- **Benefit:** Coconuts provide copper, a trace mineral with multiple functions in the body. Copper is involved in the formation of connective tissues, red blood cells, and the absorption of iron. It also acts as an antioxidant, helping to protect cells from oxidative stress. Consuming coconuts as part of a balanced diet contributes to the body's copper needs for overall health and well-being.

Heart Health and MCTs:

The MCTs found in coconut oil have been linked to several heart health benefits. Unlike long-chain fatty acids, MCTs are quickly absorbed and metabolized, providing a readily available source of energy. Some studies suggest that the consumption of coconut oil may contribute to raising levels of HDL (good) cholesterol and promoting a healthier lipid profile, ultimately supporting cardiovascular well-being.

Antioxidant Protection:

Coconuts are rich in antioxidants, including phenolic compounds and vitamin E. These antioxidants help neutralize free radicals in the body, which are known to contribute to aging and various chronic diseases. Regular consumption of coconut-derived products, such as coconut water or coconut oil, can contribute to the body's defense against oxidative stress.

Digestive Health and Fiber:

The coconut's fiber content, found in both the coconut flesh and coconut flour, supports digestive health. Dietary fiber promotes regular bowel movements, prevents constipation, and supports a healthy gut microbiome. Including coconut-based products in your diet can be a tasty way to enhance fiber intake and support overall digestive well-being.

Nutritional Content

The nutritional content of shredded coconut can vary based on factors such as whether it's sweetened or unsweetened, as well as how finely shredded it is. Here's an approximate breakdown of the nutrients in 1 cup (about 80 grams) of unsweetened shredded coconut:

- Carbohydrates: Approximately 12 grams
- Protein: Approximately 2 grams
- Fiber: Approximately 7 grams
- Fat: Approximately 28 grams
- Sugar: Approximately 3 grams

Again, please note that these values are estimates and can vary depending on the specific product. If the coconut is sweetened or in a different form (e.g., coconut flour, coconut milk), the nutritional content may differ.

Versatile Culinary Uses:

Coconut is celebrated in the culinary world for its versatility. Coconut oil, with its high smoke point, is ideal for cooking and baking. Coconut milk adds richness and flavor to both savory and sweet dishes, while coconut water provides a hydrating and refreshing beverage. Coconut flour, derived from dried coconut flesh, is a gluten-free alternative in baking. From curries to desserts, coconuts lend their unique taste and texture to a wide array of dishes.

Coconut Milk:

- ***Preparation:*** Extracting coconut milk involves blending grated coconut with water and then straining the mixture to obtain the liquid. The first extraction results in thick coconut milk, while a second extraction produces a lighter version. Coconut milk is a versatile ingredient used in both savory and sweet dishes, such as curries, soups, smoothies, desserts and Jamaican rice and peas. It adds a rich, creamy texture and imparts a subtle coconut flavor to the dishes.

Toasted Coconut Flakes:

- ***Preparation:*** Toasting coconut flakes enhances their flavor and adds a delightful crunch. Spread unsweetened coconut flakes on a baking sheet and toast them in the oven or on the stovetop until they turn golden brown. Toasted coconut flakes can be used as a topping for oatmeal, yogurt, or desserts, providing a delicious nutty flavor and texture.

Coconut Oil:

- ***Preparation:*** Extracting coconut oil involves pressing the oil from the coconut meat. Coconut oil has a high smoke point, making it suitable for cooking, baking, and frying. Use coconut oil as a flavorful alternative to other cooking oils. It adds a subtle coconut aroma to dishes and is particularly popular in Asian and tropical cuisines. Additionally, coconut oil can be used in skincare routines for moisturizing the skin and conditioning the hair.

Coconut Water Ice Cubes:

- ***Preparation:*** Freeze coconut water in ice cube trays to create coconut water ice cubes. These cubes can be added to beverages like smoothies or iced coffee for a refreshing twist. Coconut water ice cubes not only chill your drinks but also infuse them with a subtle coconut flavor. They're a convenient way to enjoy the hydrating benefits of coconut water in a variety of cold beverages.

Beauty and Skincare:

Coconut oil has gained popularity in the realm of beauty and skincare. Its moisturizing properties make it a natural choice for nourishing the skin and hair. Whether used as a facial moisturizer, hair conditioner, or body lotion, coconut oil provides hydration without clogging pores. Additionally, coconut oil contains antimicrobial properties that can contribute to skin health.

Conclusion:

The coconut's benefits extend far beyond its delicious taste. From promoting heart health and providing antioxidant protection to supporting digestive well-being and enhancing beauty routines, coconuts have rightfully earned their place as a cherished and versatile natural resource. Embrace the coconut in your diet and daily life, savoring its rich flavors and reaping the numerous rewards it brings to your health and well-being.

Back to Table of Contents

Coconut Water

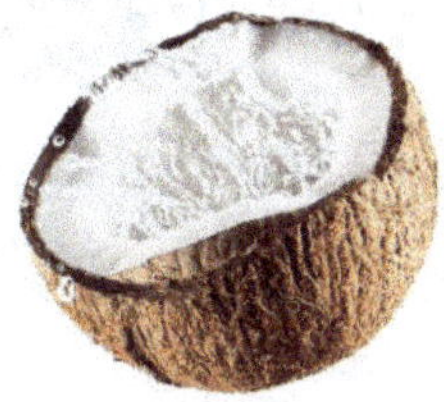

The Refreshing Elixir: The Health Benefits and Culinary Magic of Coconut Water

Coconut water, the clear liquid harvested from young green coconuts, has emerged as a hydrating sensation and nutritional powerhouse in recent years. Beyond its tropical allure and refreshing taste, coconut water is celebrated for its numerous health benefits and versatile uses. Let's dive into the hydrating world of coconut water, exploring its unique qualities and the myriad ways it can enhance both well-being and culinary experiences.

Hydration and Electrolyte Balance:

One of the primary draws of coconut water is its exceptional ability to keep the body hydrated. Packed with electrolytes such as potassium, sodium, magnesium, and calcium, coconut water serves as a natural and replenishing alternative to commercial sports drinks. These electrolytes play a crucial role in maintaining fluid balance, supporting muscle function, and preventing dehydration, making coconut water an ideal choice for staying hydrated, especially after physical activity.

Nutrient-Rich Elixir:

While low in calories and free of fat and cholesterol, coconut water is a nutrient-rich elixir. It contains essential vitamins and minerals, including vitamin C, B-complex vitamins, and antioxidants. The natural sugars found in coconut water provide a quick energy boost, making it an excellent choice for a refreshing beverage that not only hydrates but also nourishes the body.

Vitamins:

Vitamin C: Acts as an antioxidant, supporting the immune system and promoting skin health.

Vitamin B-complex: Includes various B-vitamins such as riboflavin (B2), niacin (B3), pantothenic acid (B5), pyridoxine (B6), and folate (B9). These vitamins play crucial roles in energy metabolism and overall cellular function.

Minerals:

Potassium: An electrolyte that helps regulate fluid balance, supports proper muscle function, and contributes to cardiovascular health.

Sodium: Another electrolyte that, along with potassium, helps maintain fluid balance and supports nerve function.

Calcium: Important for bone health and various cellular processes.

Magnesium: Supports muscle and nerve function, helps maintain steady heart rhythm, and contributes to bone health.

Phosphorus: Essential for bone and teeth formation, as well as energy metabolism.

Antioxidants:

Cytokinins: These plant hormones exhibit antioxidant properties, potentially helping to protect cells from oxidative damage and supporting anti-aging effects.

Flavonoids: Plant compounds with antioxidant and anti-inflammatory properties. They contribute to the overall antioxidant profile of coconut water.

Amino Acids:

Cysteine, Arginine, and Alanine: Coconut water contains various amino acids, which are the building blocks of proteins and play essential roles in the body's structure and function.

Enzymes:

Peroxidase: An enzyme with antimicrobial properties that may contribute to the preservation of coconut water.

It's important to note that the exact nutrient content of coconut water can vary depending on factors such as the age of the coconut, the region it comes from, and how the coconut water is processed. While coconut water is a nutritious and hydrating beverage, it's essential to maintain a balanced diet that includes a variety of foods to ensure a comprehensive intake of all essential nutrients.

Digestive Health and Weight Management:

Coconut water is known for its digestive benefits. The fiber content aids in promoting regular bowel movements and preventing constipation. Additionally, coconut water has been suggested to have a mild diuretic effect, which may help in detoxification and weight management by encouraging the elimination of waste and excess water from the body.

Cardiovascular Health:

The potassium content in coconut water is noteworthy, and maintaining optimal potassium levels is associated with heart health. Potassium helps regulate blood pressure, supports proper heart rhythm, and contributes to overall cardiovascular well-being. Including coconut water in your diet may be a heart-smart choice for those looking to maintain a healthy cardiovascular system.

Nutritional Content

The nutritional content of coconut water can vary slightly depending on factors such as the maturity of the coconut and how it's processed. Here's an approximate breakdown of the nutrients in 1 cup (about 240 grams) of coconut water:

- Carbohydrates: Approximately 9 grams
- Protein: Approximately 2 grams
- Fiber: Approximately 3 grams
- Fat: Approximately 0 grams (negligible amount)
- Sugar: Approximately 6 grams

Please note that these values are estimates and can vary based on factors such as brand and processing methods.

Culinary Uses Beyond Hydration:

Beyond its role as a hydrating beverage, coconut water has found its way into various culinary creations. Here are a few delightful uses:

Smoothies and Shakes:

- Swap regular liquids with coconut water in smoothies and shakes for a tropical twist that adds natural sweetness and electrolytes.

Cocktails and Mocktails:

- Coconut water serves as a refreshing base for cocktails and mocktails, providing a light and hydrating alternative to sugary mixers.

Desserts:

- Incorporate coconut water into desserts such as popsicles, sorbets, and gelatin for a subtle coconut flavor and added nutrients.

Cooking and Baking:

- Use coconut water in cooking rice, quinoa, or grains to infuse a hint of coconut essence. It can also be used in baking to moisten cakes and enhance flavor.

Here are two refreshing and delicious recipes that feature coconut water:

Coconut Water and Pineapple Smoothie:

Ingredients:

- 1 cup coconut water
- 1 cup fresh pineapple chunks
- 1 banana, peeled and sliced

- 1/2 cup Greek yogurt
- 1 tablespoon chia seeds (optional)
- Ice cubes (optional)

Instructions:

1. In a blender, combine the coconut water, fresh pineapple chunks, banana, Greek yogurt, and chia seeds.
2. Blend on high speed until the mixture is smooth and well combined.
3. If a colder consistency is desired, add a handful of ice cubes and blend again until smooth.
4. Pour the smoothie into glasses and garnish with additional pineapple slices or a sprinkle of chia seeds if desired.
5. Serve immediately and enjoy this tropical and hydrating coconut water and pineapple smoothie.

Coconut Water Mojito:

Ingredients:

- 1 cup coconut water
- 1/4 cup fresh lime juice
- 1 tablespoon agave syrup or simple syrup (adjust to taste)
- 8-10 fresh mint leaves
- 1/2 cup club soda
- Ice cubes
- Lime wedges and mint sprigs for garnish

Instructions:

1. In a glass, muddle the fresh mint leaves with lime juice and agave syrup to release the mint flavor.
2. Fill the glass with ice cubes.
3. Pour in the coconut water and club soda.
4. Stir gently to combine the ingredients.
5. Garnish with lime wedges and mint sprigs.
6. Taste and adjust sweetness if needed by adding more agave syrup.
7. Serve immediately and enjoy the refreshing and tropical twist of this coconut water mojito.

These recipes showcase the versatility of coconut water, adding a tropical touch to both smoothies and mocktails. Feel free to customize the recipes based on your preferences and enjoy the natural sweetness and hydration that coconut water brings to these delightful beverages.

Historical uses:

Coconut water has been utilized for various purposes throughout history, beyond its role as a refreshing beverage. Here are two historical uses of coconut water:

Traditional Medicine and Hydration:

- In many tropical regions where coconuts are abundant, traditional healers and communities have long recognized the hydrating properties of coconut water. It has been used as a natural remedy for dehydration and to replenish electrolytes lost due to illnesses such as diarrhea. The electrolyte-rich composition of coconut water, particularly its high potassium content, makes it an effective choice for rehydration. Historical records suggest that coconut water was administered to individuals suffering from fevers or gastrointestinal issues to help restore fluid balance and alleviate symptoms.

Emergency Intravenous Fluid Replacement during World War II:

- During World War II, in the Pacific theater, coconut water gained historical significance as an emergency intravenous fluid replacement. With limited medical supplies, especially in remote and tropical locations, coconut water was used as a sterile and readily available substitute for intravenous fluids. Its natural isotonic properties, similar to human blood plasma, made it a practical solution for providing hydration to wounded soldiers when medical resources were scarce. This historical application of coconut water showcases its adaptability and life-saving potential in challenging circumstances.

These historical uses highlight the practicality and resourcefulness of utilizing coconut water for hydration and medicinal purposes in regions where coconuts have been a traditional part of the landscape. Today, coconut water continues to be valued not only for its historical significance but also for its modern applications as a natural sports drink, a base for refreshing beverages, and a hydrating component in various culinary creations.

Conclusion:

Coconut water is more than just a trendy beverage; it's a hydrating elixir loaded with health benefits and culinary possibilities. Whether sipped straight from the coconut or incorporated into a variety of recipes, this natural thirst-quencher brings a touch of the tropics to your daily routine. If you have specific health concerns, allergies, or conditions, it's advisable to consult with a healthcare professional or a registered dietitian before making significant changes to your diet.

Embrace the benefits of coconut water, stay refreshed, and enjoy the nourishing goodness of this tropical treasure.

Back to Table of Contents

Collard Greens

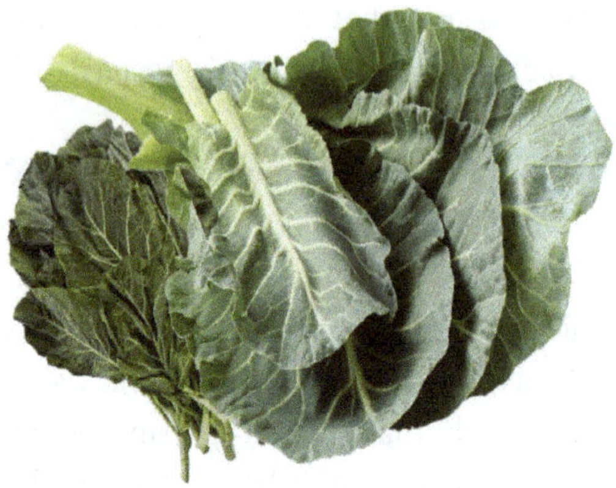

Discovering the Benefits and Culinary Versatility of Collard Greens

Collard greens, a member of the cruciferous vegetable family, are leafy greens that have been cherished for generations in various culinary traditions. Known for their robust flavor and nutritional richness, collard greens are not only a staple in many dishes but also a powerhouse of health benefits. In this article, we'll delve into the numerous advantages and versatile uses of collard greens, showcasing their potential to elevate both the taste and nutrition of your meals.

Nutritional Powerhouse:

Collard greens are a nutritional powerhouse, offering an abundance of essential vitamins, minerals, and phytonutrients. A one-cup (190 grams) serving of cooked collard greens provides:

Vitamin K:

- **Benefits:** Essential for blood clotting and bone health, vitamin K plays a crucial role in preventing excessive bleeding and supporting overall bone density.

Vitamin A:

- **Benefits:** Important for vision, immune function, and skin health, vitamin A in collard greens contributes to maintaining healthy eyes and a strong immune system.

Vitamin C:

- **Benefits:** An antioxidant that supports immune function, vitamin C in collard greens helps protect cells from oxidative stress and promotes the absorption of iron.

Folate (Vitamin B9):

- **Benefits:** Folate is crucial for DNA synthesis and cell division. Adequate folate intake is particularly important during pregnancy to prevent neural tube defects in the developing fetus.

Calcium:

- **Benefits:** Essential for bone health, calcium in collard greens contributes to the formation and maintenance of strong bones and teeth.

Fiber:

- **Benefits:** High in dietary fiber, collard greens support digestive health, regulate blood sugar levels, and contribute to a feeling of fullness, aiding in weight management.

Health Benefits:

Anti-Inflammatory Properties:

- Collard greens contain phytonutrients with anti-inflammatory properties, potentially reducing the risk of chronic diseases associated with inflammation.

Heart Health:

- The high fiber content in collard greens may help lower cholesterol levels, promoting cardiovascular health and reducing the risk of heart disease.

Cancer Prevention:

- The presence of glucosinolates in collard greens has been linked to cancer prevention, particularly in relation to lung, colorectal, and breast cancers.

Blood Sugar Regulation:

- The fiber and antioxidant content in collard greens may contribute to better blood sugar control, making them a suitable choice for individuals managing diabetes.

Nutritional Content

Here's an approximate breakdown of the nutrients in 1 cup (about 36 grams) of cooked collard greens:

Carbohydrates: Approximately 5.4 grams
Protein: Approximately 2.2 grams
Fiber: Approximately 7.6 grams
Fat: Approximately 0.5 grams

These values are based on cooked collard greens without added fats or seasonings. The nutritional content can vary slightly based on factors such as cooking method and specific variety of collard greens.

Culinary Uses:

Sauteed Collard Greens:

- Heat olive oil in a pan, add chopped garlic and red pepper flakes for flavor, then toss in thinly sliced collard greens. Saute until wilted and tender. Finish with a squeeze of lemon juice for brightness.

Collard Green Wraps:

- Use large collard green leaves as a healthy alternative to tortillas. Fill them with your favorite ingredients, such as hummus, lean proteins, and colorful vegetables, for a nutrient-packed wrap.

Collard Green Chips:

- Coat collard green leaves with olive oil, sprinkle with your preferred seasonings, and bake until crispy. Enjoy these collard green chips as a delicious and nutritious snack.

Collard Green Soup:

- Add chopped collard greens to soups or stews for a nutrient boost. Their hearty texture and flavor complement a variety of broths and ingredients.

Here are two delicious and nutritious recipes featuring Collard Greens:

Stuffed Collard Greens Rolls:

Ingredients:

- 10 large collard green leaves, stems removed
- 1 cup quinoa, cooked
- 1 can (15 oz) black beans, drained and rinsed
- 1 cup corn kernels (fresh or frozen)
- 1 cup cherry tomatoes, diced
- 1/2 cup red onion, finely chopped
- 1/4 cup fresh cilantro, chopped
- 1 teaspoon ground cumin
- 1 teaspoon chili powder
- Salt and pepper to taste
- 1 cup salsa for serving

Instructions:

1. Blanch the collard green leaves in boiling water for about 30 seconds. Remove and place them in an ice bath to stop the cooking process. Pat them dry with a towel.
2. In a large bowl, combine cooked quinoa, black beans, corn, cherry tomatoes, red onion, cilantro, cumin, chili powder, salt, and pepper.
3. Lay a collard green leaf flat and spoon the quinoa mixture onto the center. Fold the sides of the leaf over the filling and roll it tightly.
4. Repeat with the remaining collard green leaves.
5. Serve the stuffed collard green rolls with salsa for dipping.

Sautéed Collard Greens with Garlic and Lemon:

Ingredients:

- 1 bunch collard greens, stems removed and leaves chopped
- 2 tablespoons olive oil
- 3 cloves garlic, minced
- 1/2 teaspoon red pepper flakes (optional)

- Salt and pepper to taste
- ***1 lemon, juiced***

Instructions:

1. Heat olive oil in a large skillet over medium heat.
2. Add minced garlic and red pepper flakes (if using) to the skillet and sauté for about 1 minute until fragrant.
3. Add the chopped collard greens to the skillet and toss to coat in the garlic-infused oil. Cook for 5-7 minutes or until the collard greens are wilted and tender.
4. Season with salt and pepper to taste.
5. Squeeze the juice of one lemon over the sautéed collard greens and toss to combine.
6. Serve as a side dish alongside your favorite protein or grains.

These collard greens recipes showcase the versatility of this nutritious leafy green, whether used as a wrap or sautéed for a flavorful and healthy side dish. Incorporate these recipes into your meal rotation for a delicious and wholesome dining experience.

Tips on Growing Collard Greens

Collard greens typically take about 60 to 75 days to reach maturity after being planted. However, this timeline can vary depending on factors such as the specific variety of collard greens, growing conditions (such as temperature and sunlight), and local climate. Some varieties may mature slightly faster or slower than others. Additionally, collard greens can be harvested at different stages of growth depending on the desired size and tenderness of the leaves.

Conclusion:

Collard greens stand out as a versatile and nutritious addition to any diet, offering an array of health benefits and culinary possibilities. Whether enjoyed in traditional Southern dishes, international cuisines, or as a creative substitute in various recipes, collard greens prove that healthy eating can be both delicious and satisfying. If you have specific health concerns, allergies, or conditions, it's advisable to consult with a healthcare professional or a registered dietitian before making significant changes to your diet.

So, embrace the green powerhouse of collard greens and explore the countless ways they can enhance your meals and contribute to your overall well-being.

Back to Table of Contents

Common Wormwood

The Marvels of Common Wormwood

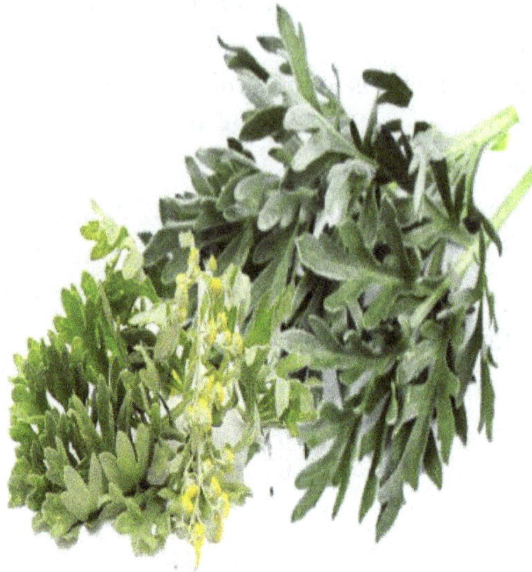

Common Wormwood (Artemisia absinthium), also known simply as wormwood, is an herb with a long history of culinary, medicinal, and cultural significance. Native to Europe, Asia, and North Africa, this perennial plant belongs to the Asteraceae family and is renowned for its distinctive bitter taste and potent properties. While commonly associated with its role in absinthe production, wormwood offers a plethora of benefits and uses beyond its notorious reputation.

Common wormwood contains various vitamins, minerals, and antioxidants that contribute to its potential health benefits. Here's a list of some of the key nutrients found in wormwood and their associated benefits:

Vitamins:

- **Vitamin C:** Acts as an antioxidant, supporting immune function and promoting skin health.
- **Vitamin A:** Essential for vision, immune function, and skin health. It also acts as an antioxidant, protecting cells from damage.
- **Vitamin K:** Important for blood clotting and bone health.

Minerals:

- **Calcium:** Vital for bone and teeth health, muscle function, and nerve transmission.
- **Iron:** Essential for the production of hemoglobin and oxygen transport in the blood.
- **Magnesium:** Involved in over 300 enzymatic reactions in the body, supporting muscle and nerve function, blood sugar regulation, and bone health.
- **Potassium:** Helps regulate fluid balance, muscle contractions, and nerve signals.

Antioxidants:

- **Absinthin:** Found in wormwood, absinthin exhibits antioxidant properties, helping to neutralize free radicals and reduce oxidative stress in the body.
- **Artemisinin:** Known for its potent antimalarial properties, artemisinin also possesses antioxidant activity, which may contribute to its therapeutic effects.
- **Flavonoids:** Wormwood contains various flavonoids, such as quercetin and apigenin, which have antioxidant and anti-inflammatory properties. They may help protect against chronic diseases and support overall wellbeing.

Medicinal Marvels:

For centuries, wormwood has been esteemed for its medicinal properties and therapeutic applications. Here are some of its notable benefits:

- **Digestive Aid**: Wormwood is revered for its ability to stimulate digestion and alleviate gastrointestinal discomfort, including bloating, gas, and indigestion.
- **Antiparasitic Properties**: Certain compounds found in wormwood, such as absinthin and artemisinin, exhibit potent antiparasitic activity, making it a valuable ally in combating intestinal parasites like roundworms and pinworms.
- **Liver Support**: Wormwood is believed to support liver health by stimulating bile production and promoting liver detoxification processes, potentially aiding in the management of liver disorders.
- **Antimicrobial Activity**: Research suggests that wormwood possesses antimicrobial properties, which may help inhibit the growth of harmful bacteria and fungi, thereby supporting overall immune function.

Cultural Significance:

Beyond its culinary and medicinal uses, wormwood holds cultural significance and has been intertwined with folklore and traditional practices:

- **Historical Remedies**: Throughout history, wormwood has been employed in traditional herbal medicine systems worldwide, from ancient Egyptian and Greek civilizations to traditional Chinese and Native American medicine.
- **Absinthe Production**: Wormwood gained infamy in the 19th century as a key ingredient in absinthe, a highly alcoholic and often controversial spirit. Despite its ban in many countries due to concerns over thujone content, absinthe remains an iconic cultural symbol.
- **Herbal Lore**: In folklore and herbal lore, wormwood has been associated with protection, purification, and divination. It was believed to ward off evil spirits, safeguard against illness, and enhance psychic abilities when used in rituals and incantations.

Culinary Delights:

Despite its bitter flavor, wormwood has found its place in the culinary world, adding depth and complexity to various dishes and beverages. Here are some culinary uses of wormwood:

- **Flavoring Agent**: Wormwood's intense bitter taste makes it a prized ingredient in herbal liqueurs, vermouth, and bitters, where it contributes to the overall flavor profile.
- **Aromatic Herb**: In culinary traditions, wormwood leaves are occasionally used to infuse vinegar or added sparingly to marinades and sauces, imparting a unique herbal aroma.
- **Traditional Cuisine**: In certain cuisines, particularly those of Eastern Europe and the Mediterranean, wormwood leaves are occasionally incorporated into savory dishes, such as stews and roasted meats, to add a subtle bitter note.

Wormwood Infused Vermouth:

Ingredients:

- 1 bottle of dry white wine
- 1 cup of brandy or vodka
- 2-3 tablespoons of dried common wormwood leaves
- 1 tablespoon of dried orange peel
- 1 tablespoon of dried lemon peel
- 1 teaspoon of dried gentian root
- 1 teaspoon of dried angelica root
- 1 teaspoon of dried coriander seeds
- 1 teaspoon of dried chamomile flowers
- 1 teaspoon of dried hyssop leaves
- 1 teaspoon of dried juniper berries

Instructions:

1. In a clean glass jar, combine all the dried herbs, including the common wormwood leaves.
2. Pour the brandy or vodka over the herbs, ensuring they are fully submerged.
3. Seal the jar tightly and store it in a cool, dark place for 2-3 weeks, shaking it gently every few days to agitate the mixture.
4. After the infusion period, strain the herb-infused alcohol through a fine-mesh sieve or cheesecloth to remove the solids.
5. In a large glass pitcher or bottle, combine the infused alcohol with the bottle of dry white wine.
6. Add the dried orange and lemon peels to the mixture for additional flavor.
7. Stir the mixture well and let it sit for at least 24 hours to allow the flavors to meld together.
8. Serve the wormwood-infused vermouth chilled or over ice, garnished with a twist of lemon or orange peel.

Wormwood Tonic Syrup:

Ingredients:

- 1 cup of water
- 1 cup of granulated sugar
- 2-3 tablespoons of dried common wormwood leaves
- 1 tablespoon of dried cinchona bark
- 1 teaspoon of dried gentian root
- 1 teaspoon of dried orange peel
- 1 teaspoon of dried lemon peel
- 1 teaspoon of dried juniper berries

Instructions:

1. In a small saucepan, combine the water and granulated sugar, stirring until the sugar is dissolved.
2. Add the dried common wormwood leaves, cinchona bark, gentian root, orange peel, lemon peel, and juniper berries to the saucepan.
3. Bring the mixture to a simmer over medium heat, stirring occasionally.
4. Reduce the heat to low and let the mixture simmer gently for 15-20 minutes, allowing the flavors to infuse.
5. Remove the saucepan from the heat and let the syrup cool to room temperature.
6. Once cooled, strain the syrup through a fine-mesh sieve or cheesecloth to remove the solids.
7. Transfer the wormwood tonic syrup to a clean glass bottle or jar and store it in the refrigerator.
8. To serve, mix the wormwood tonic syrup with sparkling water or soda water in a 1:3 ratio, adjusting to taste.
9. Serve the wormwood tonic over ice, garnished with a sprig of fresh mint or a slice of lemon.

These recipes showcase the unique flavor and versatility of common wormwood, offering creative ways to incorporate this botanical ingredient into your culinary repertoire. Enjoy experimenting with these intriguing flavors!

Historical Uses

Common wormwood, also known as Artemisia absinthium, has a rich history of medicinal use dating back centuries. Here are four historical medicinal uses of common wormwood:

Digestive Aid:

- Common wormwood has traditionally been used to support digestion and alleviate digestive discomfort. It contains bitter compounds that stimulate the production of digestive juices, promoting healthy digestion and appetite. Wormwood tea or tinctures were often consumed before meals to aid digestion and reduce symptoms of bloating, gas, and indigestion.

Vermifuge (Expelling Worms):

- Wormwood has historically been used as a vermifuge, a substance that helps expel parasitic worms from the digestive tract. Its strong, bitter taste and potent properties were believed to be effective against intestinal parasites such as roundworms and pinworms. Wormwood preparations were often administered in conjunction with other herbs to treat worm infestations.

Fever Reducer:

- In traditional herbal medicine, common wormwood was sometimes used to reduce fever and relieve symptoms of feverish illnesses. Its anti-inflammatory properties were thought to help reduce fever by lowering body temperature. Wormwood tea or poultices may have been applied externally to promote sweating and aid in fever reduction.

Menstrual Aid:

- Common wormwood has a history of use in traditional medicine to regulate menstrual cycles and alleviate menstrual discomfort. It was believed to have emmenagogue properties, meaning it could stimulate menstrual flow and relieve symptoms of menstrual cramps and bloating. Wormwood preparations were sometimes used by women to help balance hormones and promote menstrual regularity.

While common wormwood has a long history of medicinal use, it's important to note that some of its constituents, particularly thujone, can be toxic in large doses. As such, wormwood should be used with caution and under the guidance of a qualified healthcare professional. Additionally, pregnant women and individuals with certain medical conditions should avoid the use of wormwood.

Tips on Growing Common Wormwood

Common wormwood (Artemisia absinthium) is a perennial herbaceous plant that grows from seeds or cuttings. Here are the details on how long it takes for common wormwood to grow:

1. **Germination**: Common wormwood seeds typically germinate within 7 to 21 days after sowing, depending on factors such as soil temperature, moisture levels, and seed quality. Germination may occur more rapidly under optimal conditions.
2. **Seedling Stage**: After germination, common wormwood seedlings emerge and begin to grow. During this stage, they require consistent moisture and adequate sunlight or grow lights if grown indoors. Seedlings usually develop true leaves within 2 to 3 weeks after germination.
3. **Establishment**: Once common wormwood seedlings have developed several sets of true leaves and sturdy root systems, they can be transplanted into their final growing location. This can occur within a few weeks to a couple of months after germination, depending on the growth rate of the seedlings and environmental conditions.

4. **Maturity**: Common wormwood plants typically reach maturity within their first year of growth. By the end of the growing season, which can range from 3 to 6 months depending on the climate and growing conditions, common wormwood plants can attain their full size and may be ready for harvest.
5. **Optimal Growth Conditions**: Common wormwood thrives in well-draining soil with full sun exposure. It is drought-tolerant once established but benefits from occasional watering, especially during periods of prolonged dryness. Common wormwood is hardy in USDA zones 4-9.
6. **Propagation**: Common wormwood can also be propagated from stem cuttings, which can root and establish within a few weeks under optimal conditions. This method can expedite the growth process compared to growing from seeds.

Overall, from germination to maturity, common wormwood typically takes several months to grow into a mature plant suitable for harvest. With proper care and attention to its growing needs, common wormwood can thrive and provide a bountiful supply of its aromatic foliage.

Precautions and Considerations:

While wormwood offers a myriad of benefits, it's essential to exercise caution and consult with a healthcare professional before using it, especially if you are allergic or in therapeutic doses or for extended periods. Here are some considerations:

- **Bitterness**: Wormwood's intensely bitter taste may not be palatable to everyone and should be used sparingly in culinary preparations.
- **Thujone Content**: Wormwood contains thujone, a compound that can be toxic in high doses. Excessive consumption or prolonged use of wormwood preparations may lead to adverse effects, including nausea, dizziness, and seizures.
- **Pregnancy and Nursing**: Pregnant and nursing women should avoid wormwood due to its potential to stimulate menstruation and affect uterine contractions, which could pose risks to maternal and fetal health.

In conclusion, common wormwood stands as a testament to the multifaceted nature of botanical treasures. From its role in culinary creations and traditional remedies to its cultural significance and therapeutic potential, wormwood continues to captivate and intrigue. Whether enjoyed in a well-crafted cocktail, embraced for its medicinal virtues, or revered for its cultural heritage, wormwood invites exploration and appreciation for its rich tapestry of benefits and uses, offering a glimpse into the wonders of the natural world.

If you have specific health concerns, allergies, or conditions, it's advisable to consult with a healthcare professional or a registered dietitian before making significant changes to your diet.

Back to Table of Contents

Coriander

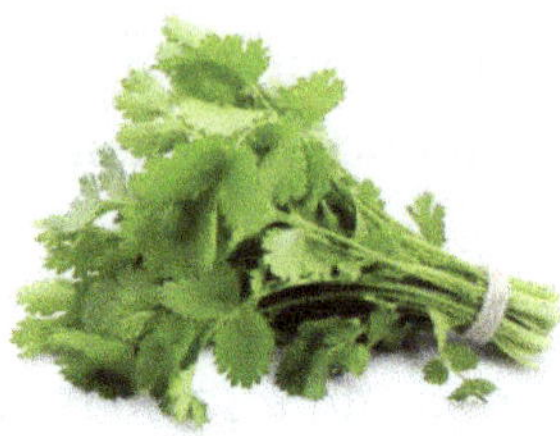

A Flavorful Herb with Remarkable Benefits and Versatility

Coriander, also known as cilantro or Chinese parsley, is a fragrant herb that has been cherished for its culinary and medicinal properties for centuries. Widely used in cuisines around the world, coriander adds a fresh, citrusy flavor and aromatic depth to dishes. Beyond its culinary appeal, coriander boasts a host of health benefits and finds application in traditional medicine and aromatherapy. Let's delve into the fascinating world of coriander, exploring its myriad benefits and diverse uses.

Health Benefits of Coriander

Digestive Aid: Coriander is known for its digestive properties, making it a popular remedy for indigestion, bloating, and gas. It contains natural compounds that help stimulate digestive enzymes and promote gut motility, aiding in the breakdown and absorption of nutrients.

Anti-inflammatory Properties: Coriander possesses anti-inflammatory properties attributed to its high antioxidant content. Regular consumption of coriander may help reduce inflammation in the body, alleviating symptoms of inflammatory conditions such as arthritis and inflammatory bowel diseases.

Cholesterol Management: Studies suggest that coriander may have cholesterol-lowering effects, helping reduce LDL (bad) cholesterol levels while increasing HDL (good) cholesterol levels. These lipid-modulating properties contribute to cardiovascular health and reduce the risk of heart disease.

Blood Sugar Regulation: Coriander may help regulate blood sugar levels and improve insulin sensitivity, making it beneficial for individuals with diabetes or prediabetes. It exerts hypoglycemic effects by enhancing glucose uptake in cells and reducing insulin resistance.

Antimicrobial Activity: Coriander exhibits antimicrobial properties, thanks to its natural compounds like cineole and linoleic acid. These compounds have been shown to inhibit the growth of bacteria and fungi, making coriander a potential ally in combating microbial infections.

Culinary Uses of Coriander

Fresh Herb: Coriander leaves, also known as cilantro, are commonly used as a garnish or flavoring agent in a variety of dishes, including salads, soups, salsas, and curries. The leaves impart a bright, citrusy flavor and aroma that complements both savory and spicy flavors.

Ground Spice: Coriander seeds are dried and ground to produce coriander powder, a staple spice in many cuisines. Ground coriander adds depth and complexity to dishes, enhancing their flavor profile with its warm, citrusy notes. It is commonly used in spice blends, marinades, rubs, and curries.

Pickling: Coriander seeds are often used in pickling recipes to add flavor and aroma to preserved vegetables, fruits, and condiments. The seeds lend a distinctive tanginess and spiciness to pickled foods, balancing their flavors and prolonging their shelf life.

Infusions: Coriander seeds can be used to prepare herbal infusions or teas, which are believed to have digestive benefits and promote overall well-being. Simply steep crushed coriander seeds in hot water for a few minutes to release their flavor and aroma.

Here are two delicious recipes that feature coriander:

Coriander-Lime Grilled Chicken

Ingredients:

- 4 boneless, skinless chicken breasts
- 2 tablespoons olive oil
- 2 cloves garlic, minced
- 1 teaspoon ground coriander
- 1 teaspoon ground cumin
- 1/2 teaspoon smoked paprika
- Zest and juice of 1 lime
- Salt and black pepper to taste
- Fresh coriander leaves (cilantro), chopped, for garnish

Instructions:

1. In a bowl, combine the olive oil, minced garlic, ground coriander, ground cumin, smoked paprika, lime zest, and lime juice. Season with salt and black pepper to taste.
2. Place the chicken breasts in a resealable plastic bag or shallow dish. Pour the marinade over the chicken, making sure it is evenly coated. Marinate in the refrigerator for at least 30 minutes, or up to 4 hours.
3. Preheat your grill to medium-high heat. Remove the chicken from the marinade and discard any excess marinade.
4. Grill the chicken breasts for 6-8 minutes per side, or until cooked through and no longer pink in the center.
5. Remove the chicken from the grill and let it rest for a few minutes before slicing.
6. Garnish the grilled chicken with fresh coriander leaves (cilantro) before serving.

7. Serve the coriander-lime grilled chicken with your favorite side dishes, such as rice, quinoa, or roasted vegetables.
8. Enjoy this flavorful and aromatic dish!

Spicy Coriander and Lime Rice

Ingredients:

- 1 cup basmati rice
- 2 cups water
- 1 tablespoon olive oil
- 2 cloves garlic, minced
- 1 teaspoon ground coriander
- 1/2 teaspoon ground cumin
- 1/4 teaspoon chili powder (adjust to taste)
- Zest and juice of 1 lime
- Salt to taste
- Fresh coriander leaves (cilantro), chopped, for garnish

Instructions:

1. Rinse the basmati rice under cold water until the water runs clear. Drain well.
2. In a saucepan, heat the olive oil over medium heat. Add the minced garlic and cook for 1-2 minutes, or until fragrant.
3. Stir in the ground coriander, ground cumin, and chili powder. Cook for an additional minute, stirring constantly.
4. Add the rinsed basmati rice to the saucepan and stir to coat the rice with the spices.
5. Pour in the water and add the lime zest and lime juice. Season with salt to taste.
6. Bring the water to a boil, then reduce the heat to low. Cover the saucepan and simmer for 15-20 minutes, or until the rice is tender and the liquid is absorbed.
7. Fluff the rice with a fork and transfer it to a serving dish.
8. Garnish the spicy coriander and lime rice with fresh coriander leaves (cilantro) before serving.
9. Serve the rice as a flavorful side dish alongside your favorite main courses, such as grilled chicken, fish, or tofu.
10. Enjoy this zesty and aromatic rice dish!

These recipes showcase the versatility of coriander and how it can enhance the flavor of dishes with its fresh, citrusy notes.

In Conclusion

Coriander, with its enticing flavor and impressive array of health benefits, holds a special place in culinary traditions and herbal medicine practices worldwide. Whether enjoyed as a fresh herb, ground spice, or herbal remedy, coriander continues to captivate taste buds and promote wellness across cultures and cuisines. As we savor its vibrant essence and reap its therapeutic rewards, let us celebrate the enduring legacy of coriander—a humble herb with extraordinary potential to nourish and heal both body and soul.

If you have specific health concerns, allergies, or conditions, it's advisable to consult with a healthcare professional or a registered dietitian before making significant changes to your diet.

- *See Cilantro*

Back to Table of Contents

Corn

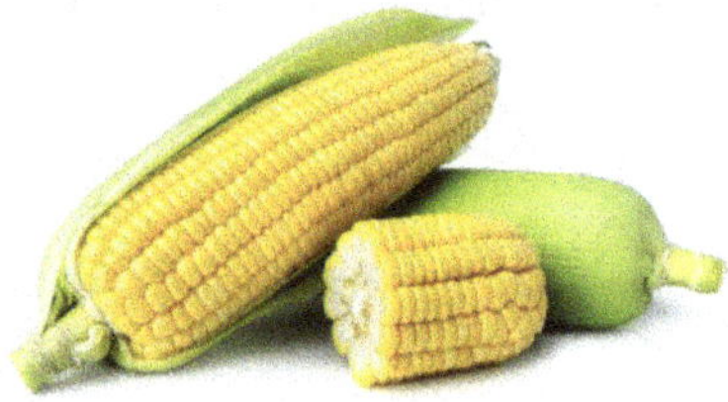

The Golden Grain: Exploring the Benefits and Versatility of Corn

Corn, often referred to as "maize," stands as one of the world's most essential and versatile crops. Originating from the Americas thousands of years ago, corn has become a dietary staple worldwide, offering an array of nutritional benefits and serving as a key ingredient in numerous culinary dishes. Let's delve into the many advantages and uses of this golden grain.

Nutritional Benefits:

Rich in Carbohydrates:

- Corn is a rich source of complex carbohydrates, providing a steady release of energy. It serves as an excellent staple in diets around the globe.

Dietary Fiber:

- Corn contains dietary fiber, aiding in digestion and promoting a healthy digestive system. Fiber helps prevent constipation and supports overall gut health.

Vitamins and Minerals:

Corn is a good source of essential vitamins such as B vitamins, including niacin and folate. It also contains minerals like phosphorus, magnesium, and potassium, contributing to overall health and well-being.

Vitamins:

Vitamin B1 (Thiamine):

- Essential for energy metabolism and nerve function.

Vitamin B2 (Riboflavin):

- Supports energy production, cell growth, and maintenance of healthy skin.

Vitamin B3 (Niacin):

- Plays a role in energy metabolism, skin health, and the functioning of the nervous system.

Vitamin B5 (Pantothenic Acid):

- Important for energy metabolism and the synthesis of various compounds in the body.

Vitamin B6 (Pyridoxine):

- Involved in protein metabolism, immune function, and the formation of red blood cells.

Folate (Vitamin B9):

- Essential for DNA synthesis and cell division, particularly important during pregnancy.

Vitamin C:

- An antioxidant that supports the immune system, collagen synthesis, and overall skin health.

Vitamin E:

- Acts as an antioxidant, protecting cells from oxidative damage.

Minerals:

Magnesium:

- Important for muscle and nerve function, blood glucose control, and bone health.

Phosphorus:

- Vital for bone and teeth formation, energy metabolism, and acid-base balance.

Potassium:

- Critical for maintaining fluid balance, nerve transmission, and muscle contraction.

Zinc:

- Supports immune function, wound healing, and DNA synthesis.

Copper:

- Essential for iron metabolism, connective tissue formation, and antioxidant function.

Iron:

- Necessary for the formation of hemoglobin and oxygen transport in the blood.

Manganese:

- Involved in bone formation, blood clotting, and reducing inflammation.

Selenium:

- Functions as an antioxidant and plays a role in thyroid hormone metabolism.

Calcium:

- Important for bone and teeth health, muscle function, and blood clotting.

Trace Amounts of Other Minerals:

- Corn contains trace amounts of other minerals, including copper, zinc, and selenium.

While corn provides a variety of vitamins and minerals, it's important to note that the nutrient content can vary based on factors such as the type of corn, soil conditions, and cultivation practices. Including a diverse range of foods in your diet ensures a comprehensive intake of essential nutrients.

Antioxidants:

The presence of antioxidants in corn, such as lutein and zeaxanthin, supports eye health and helps protect against age-related macular degeneration.

Lutein:

- A carotenoid antioxidant that is particularly beneficial for eye health. Lutein is known to help prevent age-related macular degeneration.

Zeaxanthin:

- Another carotenoid present in corn, zeaxanthin also contributes to eye health and has antioxidant properties.

Ferulic Acid:

- A phenolic compound with antioxidant properties. Ferulic acid has been associated with various health benefits, including potential anti-inflammatory effects.

Beta-Carotene:

- A precursor to vitamin A, beta-carotene is a carotenoid with antioxidant properties. It supports immune function and skin health.

Anthocyanins:

- Some varieties of corn, particularly purple corn, contain anthocyanins, which are potent antioxidants associated with various health benefits.

Quercetin:

- A flavonoid with antioxidant and anti-inflammatory properties. Quercetin may contribute to heart health and overall well-being.

Kaempferol:

- Another flavonoid found in corn, kaempferol possesses antioxidant and anti-inflammatory properties. It has been studied for its potential health-promoting effects.

Vitamin C:

- While not exclusively an antioxidant found in corn, vitamin C is present in this grain and acts as an antioxidant, supporting the immune system and protecting cells from oxidative stress.

Vitamin E:

- Corn contains various forms of vitamin E, including alpha-tocopherol, which functions as an antioxidant, protecting cell membranes from damage.

Selenium:

- While present in trace amounts, selenium is an essential mineral that also acts as an antioxidant in the body.

It's important to note that the antioxidant content in corn can vary based on factors such as corn variety and growing conditions. Consuming a variety of fruits and vegetables, including corn, can contribute to a well-rounded intake of antioxidants and other beneficial compounds for overall health.

Nutritional Content

Here's an approximate breakdown of the nutrients in 1 cup (about 166 grams) of cooked corn kernels:

- Carbohydrates: Approximately 41 grams
- Protein: Approximately 5 grams
- Fiber: Approximately 4 grams
- Fat: Approximately 2 grams
- Sugar: Approximately 9 grams

Please note that these values are estimates and can vary slightly depending on factors such as the specific variety of corn and how it is prepared. Additionally, if the corn is canned or frozen, the nutritional content may be slightly different compared to fresh corn.

Uses in the Culinary World:

Diverse Corn Products:

- Corn is processed into a myriad of products, including cornmeal, corn flour, corn oil, and corn syrup. These serve as foundational ingredients in baking, cooking, and food manufacturing.

Staple in Diets:

- Corn, in various forms such as corn on the cob, polenta, or grits, is a staple in the diets of many cultures. It serves as a versatile and satisfying component of meals.

Snack Foods:

- Popcorn, a delightful and healthy snack, is a unique variety of corn. Popped corn is not only tasty but also a good source of fiber and antioxidants.

Ethanol Production:

- Corn is a primary source for ethanol production. Ethanol, derived from corn, is commonly used as a biofuel, contributing to the renewable energy sector.

Animal Feed:

- Corn is a crucial component in animal feed, providing necessary nutrients for livestock. Its affordability and nutritional profile make it a preferred choice in the agricultural industry.

Corn Syrup and Sweeteners:

- Corn syrup and corn-based sweeteners are widely used in the food and beverage industry. While controversial in excess, these sweeteners are prevalent in many processed foods.

Here are three delicious recipes that highlight the versatility of corn:

Corn and Black Bean Salad:

Ingredients:

- 2 cups cooked corn kernels (fresh or frozen, thawed)
- 1 can (15 oz) black beans, drained and rinsed
- 1 cup cherry tomatoes, halved
- 1/2 red onion, finely diced
- 1/4 cup fresh cilantro, chopped
- 1 avocado, diced
- Juice of 2 limes
- 2 tablespoons olive oil
- Salt and pepper to taste
- Optional: Jalapeño slices for heat

Instructions:

1. In a large bowl, combine corn, black beans, cherry tomatoes, red onion, and cilantro.
2. In a small bowl, whisk together lime juice, olive oil, salt, and pepper.
3. Pour the dressing over the corn mixture and toss gently to combine.
4. Gently fold in diced avocado.
5. If you like some heat, add jalapeño slices to taste.
6. Serve chilled as a refreshing salad or as a side dish with grilled chicken or fish.

Cheesy Corn Fritters:

Ingredients:

- 2 cups fresh or frozen corn kernels
- 1 cup all-purpose flour
- 1/2 cup cornmeal
- 1 teaspoon baking powder
- 1/2 teaspoon salt
- 1/4 teaspoon black pepper
- 1 cup shredded cheddar cheese
- 2 green onions, finely chopped
- 2 large eggs
- 1/2 cup milk
- Vegetable oil for frying

Instructions:

1. In a large mixing bowl, combine corn kernels, flour, cornmeal, baking powder, salt, and black pepper.
2. Add shredded cheddar cheese and chopped green onions to the mixture.

3. In a separate bowl, whisk together eggs and milk. Pour the wet ingredients into the dry ingredients and stir until well combined.
4. Heat vegetable oil in a skillet over medium heat.
5. Drop spoonfuls of the batter into the hot oil, flattening them slightly with the back of the spoon.
6. Fry until golden brown on both sides, about 3-4 minutes per side.
7. Remove the fritters from the skillet and drain on paper towels.
8. Serve the corn fritters warm with a side of salsa, sour cream, or your favorite dipping sauce.

These recipes showcase the versatility of corn in both salads and savory fritters, offering a burst of flavors and textures. Enjoy these dishes as a delightful addition to your culinary repertoire!

Jamaican Cornmeal Porridge

Jamaican cornmeal porridge is a warm and comforting dish that is often enjoyed as a hearty breakfast or a satisfying snack. Here's a traditional recipe for Jamaican cornmeal porridge:

Ingredients:

- 1 cup fine yellow cornmeal
- 4 cups water
- 1 cinnamon stick
- 4 cups coconut milk (or a combination of coconut milk and cow's milk)
- 1 cup evaporated milk
- 1 cup sweetened condensed milk (adjust to taste)
- 1/2 teaspoon salt
- 1/2 teaspoon vanilla extract
- 1/2 teaspoon grated nutmeg
- 1/4 cup raisins (optional)
- 1/4 cup shredded coconut (optional)
- 1 tablespoon butter (optional)

Instructions:

1. **Mixing the Cornmeal:**
    - In a bowl, mix the cornmeal with 2 cups of water until it forms a smooth, lump-free mixture. Set it aside.
2. **Boiling Water:**
    - In a separate pot, bring the remaining 2 cups of water to a boil. Add the cinnamon stick to infuse flavor.
3. **Adding Cornmeal Mixture:**
    - Slowly pour the cornmeal mixture into the boiling water while stirring continuously to prevent lumps from forming.
4. **Cooking Cornmeal:**
    - Reduce the heat to low and let the cornmeal cook, stirring consistently to prevent sticking. Cook for about 10-15 minutes until the mixture thickens.

5. **Adding Coconut Milk:**
   - Gradually add the coconut milk to the cornmeal mixture, stirring continuously. Allow it to simmer over low heat for an additional 10-15 minutes, or until the cornmeal is fully cooked and has a creamy consistency.
6. **Sweetening the Porridge:**
   - Add the evaporated milk and sweetened condensed milk to the pot. Stir well and adjust the sweetness to your liking.
7. **Seasoning:**
   - Add salt, vanilla extract, and grated nutmeg. Stir to combine.
8. **Optional Ingredients:**
   - If desired, add raisins, shredded coconut, and butter. Continue to simmer for an additional 5-7 minutes, stirring occasionally.
9. **Adjusting Consistency:**
   - If the porridge becomes too thick, you can add more water or milk to reach your desired consistency.
10. **Serve:**
    - Remove the cinnamon stick, and ladle the cornmeal porridge into bowls. Garnish with a sprinkle of nutmeg on top.
11. **Enjoy:**
    - Serve the Jamaican cornmeal porridge hot, and enjoy its comforting and flavorful goodness.

This Jamaican cornmeal porridge recipe provides a delicious and satisfying way to start your day, or it can be enjoyed as a warm and nourishing treat at any time. Adjust the sweetness and optional ingredients to suit your taste preferences.

Cultural Significance:

Culinary Traditions:

- Corn holds cultural significance in many societies, playing a central role in traditional dishes and ceremonies. From corn tortillas in Mexico to cornbread in the Southern United States, it is deeply embedded in culinary traditions.

Ceremonial Uses:

- In various Native American cultures, corn is a sacred symbol, often used in ceremonies and rituals as a representation of life and sustenance.

In conclusion, corn is not merely a grain but a versatile and essential crop that has shaped diets, cultures, and economies around the world. Its nutritional benefits, diverse uses in the culinary world, and cultural significance make it a truly golden grain. If you have specific health concerns, allergies, or conditions, it's advisable to consult with a healthcare professional or a registered dietitian before making significant changes to your diet.

As we continue to explore sustainable agricultural practices, corn remains at the forefront, providing sustenance and contributing to the rich tapestry of global cuisine.

Back to Table of Contents

Costmary

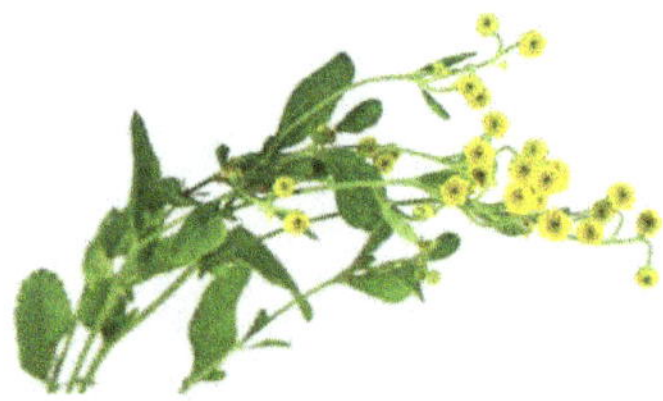

Discovering the Wonders of Costmary: Benefits and Diverse Uses

Costmary, scientifically known as Tanacetum balsamita or Chrysanthemum balsamita, is an aromatic herb that has been cultivated for centuries for both culinary and medicinal purposes. Often referred to as "Bible leaf" or "Alecost," costmary boasts a rich history of traditional uses and a distinctive fragrance that sets it apart. In this article, we will delve into the potential benefits and versatile uses of costmary.

Nutritional Profile:

Costmary is valued not only for its aromatic properties but also for its nutritional content. Rich in essential oils, flavonoids, and other bioactive compounds, costmary contributes to its potential health benefits.

Essential Oils:

- **Benefits:** Costmary is rich in essential oils, including compounds like camphor and menthol. These oils contribute to the herb's aromatic properties and may offer benefits such as soothing digestive discomfort, providing a mild antispasmodic effect, and promoting relaxation when used in aromatherapy.

Flavonoids:

- **Benefits:** Flavonoids are plant compounds with antioxidant properties. In costmary, flavonoids contribute to its potential anti-inflammatory effects, helping to neutralize free radicals and reduce inflammation in the body. Antioxidants play a role in overall health and may contribute to disease prevention.

Vitamins:

- **Benefits:** Costmary may contain vitamins, including vitamin C. Vitamin C is an essential nutrient with antioxidant properties that support immune function, promote skin health, and contribute to the body's ability to repair and maintain tissues.

Minerals:

- **Benefits:** Costmary can provide essential minerals such as potassium. Potassium is crucial for maintaining proper fluid balance, nerve function, and muscle contractions. Adequate potassium intake is associated with cardiovascular health and may help regulate blood pressure.

It's important to note that while costmary may offer certain nutritional benefits, it is often used in culinary and traditional medicinal applications rather than as a primary source of nutrients.

Health Benefits:

Digestive Aid:

- Costmary has been historically used as a digestive aid. The presence of essential oils, such as camphor and borneol, may contribute to its ability to soothe digestive discomfort and alleviate symptoms like bloating and indigestion.

Anti-Inflammatory Properties:

- Some studies suggest that costmary may possess anti-inflammatory properties, which can be attributed to its flavonoid content. These properties may have implications for reducing inflammation and supporting overall health.

Aromatic Relaxation:

- The aromatic compounds in costmary, including camphor and menthol, make it a popular choice for aromatherapy. Inhaling the fragrance of costmary may promote relaxation, alleviate stress, and create a calming atmosphere.

Versatile Uses:

Culinary Delight:

Costmary leaves have a unique, mildly minty flavor with hints of citrus. In culinary applications, costmary can be used to flavor salads, soups, and beverages. It was historically employed to impart a refreshing taste to ale, lending it the moniker "Alecost."

Costmary, with its aromatic leaves, can be prepared in various ways for consumption, both in culinary and herbal applications. Here are three ways costmary can be prepared:

Costmary leaves can be dried and used to prepare herbal tea. The tea is not only flavorful but may offer digestive benefits and a calming effect. Steeping costmary leaves in hot water allows for the extraction of its aromatic and potentially therapeutic compounds.

Herbal Tea:

- **Ingredients:**
    - Fresh or dried costmary leaves
    - Hot water
    - Optional: honey or lemon for flavor
- **Instructions:**

1. Harvest fresh costmary leaves or use dried leaves.
2. Place a teaspoon of fresh leaves or a tablespoon of dried leaves in a teapot or infuser.
3. Pour hot water over the leaves and let them steep for 5-10 minutes.
4. Strain the leaves, and if desired, add honey or lemon for flavor.
5. Enjoy costmary tea as a soothing and aromatic herbal beverage.

Culinary Use in Salads:

- **Ingredients:**
    - Fresh costmary leaves
    - Mixed salad greens
    - Olive oil
    - Balsamic vinegar
    - Salt and pepper to taste
- **Instructions:**

1. Wash and dry fresh costmary leaves.
2. Tear or chop costmary leaves and mix them with other salad greens.
3. Drizzle olive oil and balsamic vinegar over the salad.
4. Season with salt and pepper to taste.
5. Toss the salad, incorporating the aromatic flavor of costmary into a refreshing dish.

Costmary Infused Vinegar:

- **Ingredients:**
    - Fresh costmary leaves
    - White wine vinegar or apple cider vinegar
- **Instructions:**

1. Wash and dry fresh costmary leaves.
2. Fill a clean glass jar with costmary leaves.
3. Heat the vinegar until warm (not boiling).
4. Pour the warm vinegar over the costmary leaves in the jar.
5. Seal the jar and let it sit for a few weeks, allowing the vinegar to absorb the flavor of costmary.
6. Strain the leaves, and you'll have costmary-infused vinegar, perfect for salad dressings or culinary applications.

These preparation methods highlight the versatility of costmary, whether used for its aromatic qualities in teas, as a culinary herb in salads, or infused into vinegar for added flavor in various dishes. Always ensure that costmary is harvested from a safe and pesticide-free source when preparing it for consumption.

Historical Uses:

Costmary has a rich history of traditional uses, often rooted in its aromatic and medicinal properties. Here are a few historical uses of costmary and their associated benefits:

Medicinal Infusions for Digestive Aid:

- **Historical Use:** Costmary has been historically employed as an herbal remedy to soothe digestive discomfort and promote gastrointestinal health. Infusions or teas made from costmary leaves were consumed for their potential ability to ease indigestion, reduce bloating, and alleviate symptoms associated with digestive issues.

- **Benefits:** The essential oils present in costmary, including camphor and menthol, may contribute to its digestive benefits. These compounds are believed to have mild antispasmodic effects, helping to relax the digestive tract and alleviate discomfort.

Aromatic Herb in Potpourri and Sachets:

- **Historical Use:** Due to its pleasant fragrance, costmary has been historically used in potpourri blends and sachets. Dried costmary leaves were often added to mixtures for their aromatic qualities, creating sachets that were placed in living spaces to impart a refreshing and calming scent.
- **Benefits:** The aromatic compounds in costmary, such as camphor, menthol, and borneol, contribute to its historical use in aromatherapy. Inhaling the fragrance of costmary was believed to have a relaxing effect, reducing stress and creating a pleasant atmosphere.

Culinary Uses, Particularly in Brewing Ale:

- **Historical Use:** Costmary earned the nickname "Alecost" due to its historical use in flavoring ale. The herb was added to ale during brewing to impart a mild, minty flavor and enhance the overall taste of the beverage. Costmary was valued for its ability to add a unique aromatic touch to brewed drinks.
- **Benefits:** Beyond its flavor-enhancing properties, costmary's historical use in brewing may have been influenced by the belief that the herb could contribute to digestive health. The aromatic compounds in costmary, when infused in ale, may have provided a mild and pleasing flavor while potentially offering digestive benefits.

Medicinal Infusions:

- Costmary has been used in traditional medicine for various ailments, including respiratory issues and digestive discomfort. Infusions or tinctures made from costmary leaves were historically consumed for their potential health-promoting effects.

Potpourri and Fragrance:

- Dried costmary leaves make an excellent addition to potpourri blends. The herb's fragrance can be harnessed to create sachets, adding a pleasant aroma to living spaces. Costmary can also be used in crafting herbal wreaths or arrangements for decorative and aromatic purposes.

Conclusion:

Costmary, with its aromatic allure and potential health benefits, stands as a versatile herb appreciated in both the kitchen and the realm of traditional medicine. Whether employed to enhance culinary creations, brew a soothing herbal tea, or infuse spaces with its calming fragrance, costmary continues to captivate enthusiasts. As with any herb or plant-based remedy, individuals should exercise moderation and consult with healthcare professionals, especially if they have specific health concerns or conditions. As we rediscover the wonders of costmary, its historical significance and potential applications serve as an invitation to explore the diverse ways in which this herb can contribute to our well-being and sensory experiences.

Back to Table of Contents

Cranberry

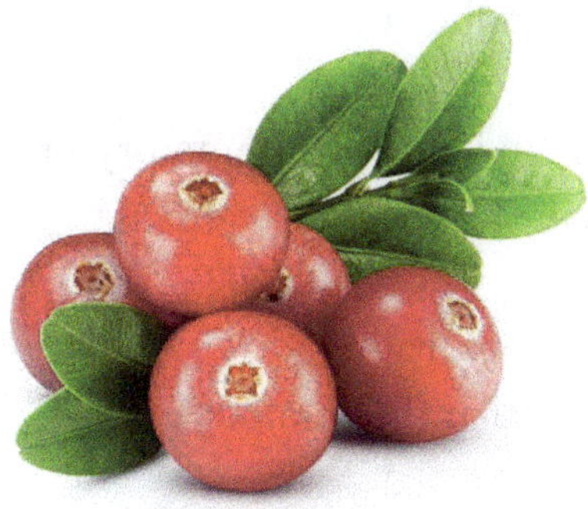

A Tart and Tangy Superfruit with Impressive Benefits

Cranberries, known for their vibrant red color and distinctive tart flavor, are more than just a staple during the holiday season. Packed with nutrients and health-promoting compounds, cranberries offer a range of benefits and versatile uses. From supporting urinary tract health to contributing to antioxidant protection, the small yet powerful cranberry has earned its status as a superfruit.

Nutrient Profile:

Cranberries are rich in essential nutrients, providing a good dose of vitamins, minerals, and antioxidants. Here's a glimpse into the nutrient profile of cranberries:

Vitamin C:

- An antioxidant that supports the immune system.
- Promotes skin health and collagen synthesis.

Fiber:

- Aids in digestion and promotes a feeling of fullness.
- Supports heart health and regulates blood sugar levels.

Manganese:

- Essential for bone health and metabolism.

Vitamin E:

- Acts as an antioxidant, protecting cells from oxidative stress.
- Supports immune function.

Copper:

- Contributes to the formation of red blood cells.
- Supports the nervous system.

Vitamin K:

- Essential for blood clotting and bone health.

Antioxidants:

Proanthocyanidins (PACs):

- Unique to cranberries, these compounds may help prevent urinary tract infections by inhibiting bacteria adhesion.

Quercetin:

- Exhibits antioxidant and anti-inflammatory properties.
- May contribute to cardiovascular health.

Myricetin:

- Functions as an antioxidant.
- May have potential anti-inflammatory effects.

Kaempferol:

- Displays antioxidant and anti-inflammatory properties.
- May contribute to cardiovascular health.

Flavonoids:

- Various flavonoids in cranberries contribute to their antioxidant and anti-inflammatory effects.

Anthocyanins:

- Responsible for the vibrant red color of cranberries.
- Exhibit antioxidant properties and may contribute to overall health.

Resveratrol:

- A polyphenol with antioxidant and anti-inflammatory effects.
- Found in small amounts in cranberries.

Vitamin A (Beta-Carotene):

- Acts as an antioxidant.
- Important for vision and immune function.

Folate (Vitamin B9):

- Essential for DNA synthesis and cell division.

Potassium:

- Regulates fluid balance in the body.
- Supports proper muscle and nerve function.

Phosphorus:

- Essential for bone and teeth formation.
- Involved in energy metabolism.

Selenium:

- Acts as an antioxidant.
- Supports the immune system.

Iron:

- Essential for the formation of hemoglobin, which carries oxygen in the blood.

These vitamins, minerals, and antioxidants contribute to the overall health benefits of cranberries, including their potential to support urinary tract health, provide antioxidant protection, and contribute to heart health. Whether enjoyed fresh, dried, or in various culinary creations, cranberries offer a nutrient-rich addition to a well-balanced diet.

Health Benefits:

Urinary Tract Health:

- Cranberries contain compounds called proanthocyanidins, which may help prevent urinary tract infections by preventing bacteria from adhering to the urinary tract walls.

Antioxidant Protection:

- The antioxidants in cranberries, including vitamin C and polyphenols, help neutralize free radicals in the body, reducing oxidative stress and inflammation.

Heart Health:

- The fiber and antioxidants in cranberries contribute to heart health by reducing the risk factors associated with cardiovascular diseases.

Anti-Inflammatory Properties:

- Some studies suggest that cranberries may have anti-inflammatory effects, potentially benefiting conditions such as inflammatory bowel disease.

Digestive Health:

- The fiber content in cranberries supports digestive health by promoting regular bowel movements and preventing constipation.

Nutritional Content

Here's an approximate breakdown of the nutrients in 1 cup (about 100 grams) of raw cranberries:

- Carbohydrates: Approximately 12 grams
- Protein: Approximately 0.4 grams
- Fiber: Approximately 4.6 grams
- Fat: Approximately 0.1 grams
- Sugar: Approximately 4 grams

These values are based on raw cranberries and may vary slightly depending on factors such as ripeness and variety. Additionally, if the cranberries are sweetened or prepared in other forms (such as dried cranberries or cranberry juice), the nutritional content may be different.

Versatile Uses:

Culinary Delights:

- Cranberries can be used in a variety of culinary creations, from sauces and relishes to baked goods and salads.
- Dried cranberries add a sweet and tangy flavor to trail mixes, oatmeal, and yogurt.

Beverages:

- Cranberry juice is a popular and refreshing beverage choice, known for its vibrant color and tart taste.
- Cranberry tea offers a warm and soothing option, often enjoyed for its potential health benefits.

Condiments:

- Cranberry sauce is a classic accompaniment to holiday meals, complementing the flavors of roasted meats and poultry.
- Cranberry chutney and relishes add a zesty twist to various dishes.

Supplements:

- Cranberry supplements, available in various forms, provide a concentrated dose of cranberry goodness for those seeking specific health benefits.

Here are two delicious and versatile recipes featuring cranberries:

Cranberry Orange Relish:

Ingredients:

- 2 cups fresh or frozen cranberries
- 1 large orange, peeled and segmented
- 1/2 cup granulated sugar (adjust to taste)
- 1/4 cup chopped pecans or walnuts (optional)
- 1 tablespoon orange zest
- 1/4 teaspoon ground cinnamon

Instructions:

1. In a food processor, combine cranberries, orange segments, sugar, orange zest, and cinnamon.
2. Pulse until the mixture reaches your desired consistency (some prefer it chunky, while others prefer it smoother).
3. Taste and adjust the sweetness by adding more sugar if needed.
4. If desired, fold in chopped nuts for added texture.
5. Refrigerate for at least an hour before serving to allow the flavors to meld.
6. Serve as a side dish with turkey, chicken, or as a spread on toast.

Cranberry Almond Energy Bites:

Ingredients:

- 1 cup dried cranberries
- 1 cup old-fashioned rolled oats
- 1/2 cup almond butter

- 1/3 cup honey or maple syrup
- 1/2 cup almond meal
- 1/2 cup chopped almonds
- 1 teaspoon vanilla extract
- Pinch of salt
- Shredded coconut for rolling (optional)

Instructions:

1. In a food processor, combine dried cranberries, rolled oats, almond butter, honey (or maple syrup), almond meal, chopped almonds, vanilla extract, and a pinch of salt.
2. Pulse until the mixture comes together and forms a sticky dough.
3. If the mixture is too dry, you can add a bit more almond butter or honey.
4. With damp hands, roll the mixture into bite-sized balls.
5. If desired, roll each energy bite in shredded coconut for added flavor and texture.
6. Place the energy bites on a parchment-lined tray and refrigerate for at least 30 minutes to set.
7. Store in an airtight container in the refrigerator.

These recipes showcase the versatility of cranberries, whether used in a vibrant relish or incorporated into nutritious energy bites. Feel free to customize these recipes based on your taste preferences and enjoy the delicious and healthful goodness of cranberries!

Cautions and Considerations: While cranberries offer numerous health benefits, individuals taking blood-thinning medications or with a history of kidney stones should exercise caution, as cranberries may interact with these conditions. It's advisable to consult with a healthcare professional for personalized guidance.

Incorporating cranberries into a balanced diet can be a delightful way to enjoy their unique flavor while reaping the health rewards. Whether enjoyed fresh, dried, or as part of various dishes, the cranberry stands out as a versatile and nutritious addition to a vibrant and health-conscious lifestyle.

Back to Table of Contents

Cucumber

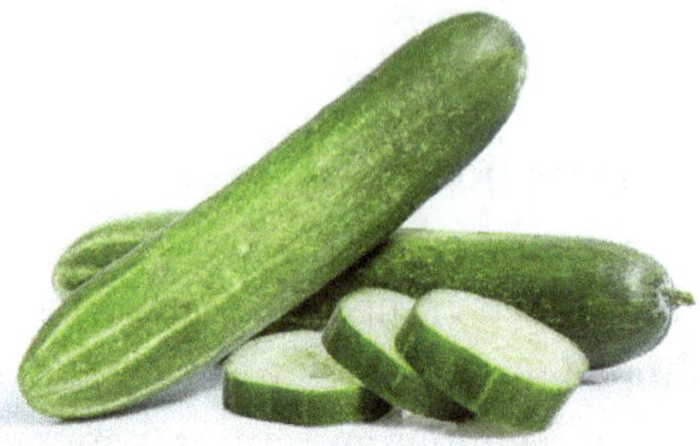

Cucumber (Cucumis sativus) is a widely cultivated plant belonging to the gourd family, Cucurbitaceae. Known for its crisp texture and mild flavor, cucumbers are not only a refreshing addition to various dishes but also pack a nutritional punch with several health benefits. It has a rich history dating back thousands of years. They hold significance in various ancient civilizations, including Egypt, where they were prized for their hydrating properties.

Cucumbers have a high-water content, making them an excellent hydrating food. They are versatile in culinary applications, used both in their raw form and pickled. In addition to their culinary uses, cucumbers offer nutritional benefits, being a good source of vitamins, minerals, and antioxidants. Their hydrating properties, low calorie content, and potential health benefits make cucumbers a popular and healthy choice in many diets around the world.

Nutritional Profile

Cucumbers are low in calories but rich in essential nutrients. The nutritional composition of cucumbers, including vitamins, minerals, and antioxidants. Emphasis will be placed on the following key nutrients:

Water: Cucumbers are composed of about 95% water, making them an ideal hydrating food.

Essential Vitamins

Cucumbers are a good source of vitamins such as vitamin K, vitamin C, and vitamin A. These play crucial roles in bone health, immune function, and vision, respectively.

Vitamin K

Cucumbers are a good source of vitamin K, essential for blood clotting and bone health.

Vitamin C

Cucumbers contain vitamin C, an antioxidant that supports immune function and promotes skin health.

Vitamin A

Cucumbers provide vitamin A, contributing to vision health and immune system support.

Minerals and Antioxidants

Minerals: The mineral content of cucumbers, including potassium, magnesium, and manganese, contributes to various physiological functions such as heart health and metabolism.

Potassium

Cucumbers contain potassium, a mineral crucial for maintaining healthy blood pressure and supporting heart function.

Magnesium

The presence of magnesium in cucumbers contributes to various physiological functions, including muscle and nerve function.

Antioxidants: Cucumbers contain antioxidants like beta-carotene and flavonoids, which help combat oxidative stress and inflammation in the body.

Medicinal Benefits

Hydration and Skin Health: The high-water content in cucumbers aids in hydration, promoting healthy skin and reducing the risk of dehydration-related issues.

Anti-Inflammatory Properties: Cucumbers contain compounds with anti-inflammatory effects, potentially reducing inflammation and the risk of chronic diseases.

Weight Management: With their low calories and high-water content, cucumbers can be a valuable addition to a weight management plan.

Heart Health: Potassium in cucumbers plays a role in regulating blood pressure, supporting cardiovascular health.

Including cucumbers in the diet may contribute to a heart-healthy lifestyle and reduce the risk of hypertension.

Nutritional Content

Here's an approximate breakdown of the nutrients in 1 cup (about 104 grams) of sliced cucumber:

- Carbohydrates: Approximately 3.8 grams
- Protein: Approximately 0.4 grams
- Fiber: Approximately 0.6 grams
- Fat: Approximately 0.2 grams
- Sugar: Approximately 1.8 grams

These values are based on raw cucumber slices and may vary slightly depending on factors such as the specific variety of cucumber and how it is prepared. Cucumbers are low in calories and contain mostly water, making them a refreshing and hydrating snack option.

Culinary Uses and Conclusion

Cucumbers are very versatile in the culinary world. From salads to pickles, cucumbers are used in a variety of dishes globally.

Here are some ways Cucumber can be prepared:

Fresh in Salads

Sliced Cucumber Salad

- Thinly sliced cucumbers combined with tomatoes, red onions, and feta cheese.
  Tossed with olive oil, lemon juice, and fresh herbs for a refreshing salad.

Pickled for Preservation

Classic Dill Pickles

- Cucumbers soaked in a brine of vinegar, water, salt, and dill.
  Left to pickle for several days to develop a tangy flavor and crisp texture.

Blended in Refreshing Beverages

Cucumber Mint Lemonade

- Cucumbers blended with fresh mint, lemon juice, and sugar.
  Diluted with water or sparkling water to create a cooling and hydrating drink.

Stuffed or Rolled in Wraps

Cucumber Roll-Ups

- Cucumber strips filled with cream cheese, smoked salmon, or hummus.
  Rolled up and secured with toothpicks for a light and flavorful appetizer.

Here are two refreshing cucumber-based recipes:

Cucumber Salad with Dill and Feta:

- ***Ingredients:***
  - 2 medium cucumbers, thinly sliced
  - 1/4 cup crumbled feta cheese
  - 2 tablespoons chopped fresh dill
  - 1 tablespoon olive oil
  - 1 tablespoon lemon juice
  - Salt and pepper to taste
- ***Instructions:***
  1. In a bowl, combine the sliced cucumbers, crumbled feta cheese, and chopped fresh dill.
  2. Drizzle with olive oil and lemon juice.
  3. Season with salt and pepper to taste.

4. Toss gently to combine.
5. Serve chilled as a refreshing side dish or light salad.

Cucumber Mint Cooler:

- ***Ingredients:***
    - 1 cucumber, peeled and chopped
    - 1/4 cup fresh mint leaves
    - 2 tablespoons lime juice
    - 2 tablespoons honey or sugar (adjust to taste)
    - 2 cups cold water
    - Ice cubes
- ***Instructions:***
    1. In a blender, combine the chopped cucumber, fresh mint leaves, lime juice, honey or sugar, and cold water.
    2. Blend until smooth.
    3. Strain the mixture through a fine mesh sieve to remove any solids.
    4. Pour the strained liquid into glasses filled with ice cubes.
    5. Garnish with cucumber slices and mint leaves, if desired.
    6. Serve immediately as a refreshing and hydrating drink.

These recipes are perfect for hot summer days or any time you're craving something light and refreshing!

Tips on Growing Cucumber

Cucumbers typically take about 50 to 70 days to grow from planting to harvest, depending on the variety and growing conditions. It's important to note that this is an average timeframe, and the exact duration can vary based on factors such as temperature, sunlight, soil quality, and care practices.

Cucumbers are warm-season vegetables and thrive in temperatures between 70°F to 95°F (21°C to 35°C). They require consistent watering and well-draining soil to grow successfully. Additionally, some cucumber varieties may mature faster than others, so it's essential to check the specific recommendations for the variety you're growing.

In conclusion, cucumbers are not just a refreshing addition to meals but also offer a range of nutritional and medicinal benefits. Understanding and appreciating the holistic nature of this humble vegetable can inspire individuals to make healthier dietary choices.

If you have specific health concerns, allergies, or conditions, it's advisable to consult with a healthcare professional or a registered dietitian before making significant changes to your diet.

Back to Table of Contents

Cumin

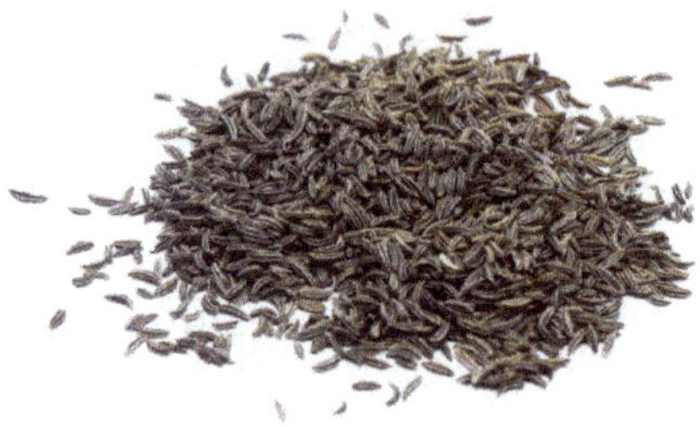

Unveiling the Marvels of Cumin: A Spice with Exceptional Benefits and Versatility

Cumin, with its warm, earthy flavor and aromatic profile, has been a staple in kitchens around the world for centuries. Beyond its culinary prowess, this humble spice boasts a treasure trove of health benefits and versatile uses. From aiding digestion to boosting immune function, cumin stands as a testament to the remarkable intersection of flavor and wellness. Let's explore the wonders of cumin, shedding light on its benefits and diverse applications.

Health Benefits of Cumin

Digestive Aid: Cumin is renowned for its digestive properties, making it a popular remedy for indigestion, bloating, and gas. It stimulates the secretion of digestive enzymes, promotes gut motility, and helps alleviate gastrointestinal discomfort.

Anti-inflammatory Properties: Cumin contains potent antioxidants and anti-inflammatory compounds that help reduce inflammation in the body. Regular consumption of cumin may help mitigate the risk of chronic inflammatory conditions such as arthritis and inflammatory bowel diseases.

Immune Support:

Rich in vitamins and minerals, cumin provides essential nutrients that support immune function and overall health. It contains vitamin C, vitamin E, and iron, which play crucial roles in bolstering the body's defense mechanisms against infections and diseases.

Vitamins:

Vitamin C: While cumin is not a significant source of vitamin C, it still contains small amounts of this antioxidant vitamin. Vitamin C supports immune function, collagen synthesis, wound healing, and iron absorption.

Vitamin B6 (Pyridoxine): Vitamin B6 is present in cumin and is involved in numerous metabolic processes, including carbohydrate and protein metabolism. It also supports brain health and helps in the production of neurotransmitters like serotonin and dopamine.

Minerals:

Iron: Cumin is a good source of iron, an essential mineral involved in the production of hemoglobin, which carries oxygen in the blood. Adequate iron intake helps prevent iron deficiency anemia and supports overall energy levels and vitality.

Calcium: Cumin contains calcium, albeit in small amounts. Calcium is important for bone and teeth health, muscle function, nerve transmission, and blood clotting.

Magnesium: Cumin provides magnesium, a mineral involved in over 300 biochemical reactions in the body. Magnesium supports muscle and nerve function, blood sugar regulation, blood pressure management, and bone health.

Phosphorus: Phosphorus is present in cumin and is important for bone health, energy metabolism, DNA synthesis, and cell signaling.

Potassium: Cumin contains potassium, an electrolyte that helps maintain fluid balance, nerve transmission, muscle function, and blood pressure regulation.

Manganese: Cumin is a good source of manganese, a trace mineral involved in bone formation, cartilage formation, antioxidant defense mechanisms, and metabolism.

Zinc: Cumin contains zinc, an essential mineral with roles in immune function, wound healing, DNA synthesis, and cell division.

Copper: Copper is found in cumin and is necessary for the formation of red blood cells, collagen synthesis, and iron metabolism.

Selenium: Cumin provides trace amounts of selenium, an antioxidant mineral that supports thyroid function, immune function, and reproductive health.

Phytonutrients: Cumin contains various phytonutrients, including flavonoids and phenolic compounds, which have antioxidant, anti-inflammatory, and antimicrobial properties. These compounds contribute to the health-promoting effects of cumin.

While cumin may not be a significant source of all vitamins and minerals, its inclusion in the diet can still contribute to overall nutrient intake and support various aspects of health and well-being.

Blood Sugar Regulation:

Cumin may help regulate blood sugar levels and improve insulin sensitivity, making it beneficial for individuals with diabetes or prediabetes. It exerts hypoglycemic effects by enhancing glucose uptake in cells and reducing insulin resistance.

Cholesterol Management:

Studies suggest that cumin may have cholesterol-lowering effects, helping reduce LDL (bad) cholesterol levels while increasing HDL (good) cholesterol levels. These lipid-modulating properties contribute to cardiovascular health and reduce the risk of heart disease.

Culinary Uses of Cumin

Spice Blends: Cumin is a key ingredient in many spice blends, including curry powder, garam masala, and chili powder. Its distinctive flavor adds depth and complexity to savory dishes, soups, stews, and marinades.

Seasoning: Ground cumin is commonly used as a seasoning for meats, vegetables, rice, and legumes. It pairs well with a wide range of ingredients, enhancing their flavor profiles with its warm, slightly nutty notes.

Tempering: In Indian cuisine, cumin seeds are often tempered in hot oil or ghee to release their aromatic oils before being added to dishes. This tempering technique, known as "tadka" or "tarka," infuses the dish with cumin's distinctive flavor and aroma.

Baking: Cumin seeds can be sprinkled on bread, rolls, or pastries before baking to add a subtle savory flavor and decorative touch. They also complement the sweetness of baked goods like cakes and cookies when used sparingly.

Beverages: Cumin seeds are occasionally used to flavor beverages such as teas, infusions, and cocktails. Cumin-infused drinks are believed to aid digestion and promote overall well-being, particularly after a heavy meal.

Here are two flavorful recipes that feature cumin:

Cumin-Spiced Chickpea Salad

Ingredients:

- 1 can (15 ounces) chickpeas, drained and rinsed
- 1 tablespoon olive oil
- 1 teaspoon ground cumin
- 1/2 teaspoon paprika
- 1/4 teaspoon ground coriander
- Salt and black pepper to taste
- 1 red bell pepper, diced
- 1/2 red onion, finely chopped
- 1/4 cup chopped fresh cilantro
- Juice of 1 lime
- Optional: crumbled feta cheese or avocado slices for serving

Instructions:

1. Preheat your oven to 400°F (200°C).
2. In a bowl, toss the chickpeas with olive oil, ground cumin, paprika, ground coriander, salt, and black pepper until evenly coated.
3. Spread the seasoned chickpeas in a single layer on a baking sheet and roast in the preheated oven for 20-25 minutes, or until crispy, stirring halfway through.
4. In a large bowl, combine the roasted chickpeas, diced red bell pepper, chopped red onion, and chopped cilantro.

5. Squeeze the lime juice over the salad and toss gently to combine.
6. Taste and adjust seasoning if necessary.
7. Serve the cumin-spiced chickpea salad with crumbled feta cheese or avocado slices on top, if desired.
8. Enjoy this flavorful and nutritious salad as a light meal or side dish!

Cumin-Spiced Roasted Carrots

Ingredients:

- 1 pound carrots, peeled and sliced into sticks
- 2 tablespoons olive oil
- 1 teaspoon ground cumin
- 1/2 teaspoon ground coriander
- 1/2 teaspoon smoked paprika
- Salt and black pepper to taste
- Fresh parsley, chopped, for garnish

Instructions:

1. Preheat your oven to 400°F (200°C). Line a baking sheet with parchment paper or aluminum foil.
2. In a large bowl, toss the carrot sticks with olive oil, ground cumin, ground coriander, smoked paprika, salt, and black pepper until well coated.
3. Spread the seasoned carrots in a single layer on the prepared baking sheet.
4. Roast the carrots in the preheated oven for 20-25 minutes, or until tender and caramelized, stirring halfway through.
5. Once roasted, transfer the carrots to a serving platter.
6. Garnish the roasted carrots with chopped fresh parsley before serving.
7. Enjoy these cumin-spiced roasted carrots as a flavorful side dish or snack!

These recipes showcase the versatility of cumin and how it can elevate the flavor of simple ingredients like chickpeas and carrots.

In Conclusion

Cumin, with its multifaceted benefits and culinary versatility, holds a revered position in global gastronomy and traditional medicine. Whether incorporated into savory dishes, spice blends, or herbal remedies, cumin continues to captivate palates and promote wellness across cultures and cuisines. As we savor its rich flavor and reap its healthful rewards, let us celebrate the enduring legacy of cumin—a spice that transcends borders and enlivens the senses with its timeless allure.

If you have specific health concerns, allergies, or conditions, it's advisable to consult with a healthcare professional or a registered dietitian before making significant changes to your diet.

Back to Table of Contents

Essential Nutrients for Optimal Health

Optimal health requires a diverse array of nutrients that support various bodily functions and processes. Here's a comprehensive list of essential nutrients the body needs for optimal health:

Macronutrients:

1. **Carbohydrates:**
    - Provides energy for cellular function, particularly for the brain and muscles.
    - Found in grains, fruits, vegetables, legumes, and dairy products.
2. **Proteins:**
    - Essential for building and repairing tissues, producing enzymes and hormones, and supporting immune function.
    - Found in meat, poultry, fish, eggs, dairy products, legumes, nuts, and seeds.
3. **Fats (Healthy Fats):**
    - Provides energy, support cell structure, assist in nutrient absorption, and help produce hormones.
    - Found in nuts, seeds, avocados, olive oil, fatty fish, and plant-based oils.

Vitamins:

1. **Water-Soluble Vitamins:**
    - Vitamin C: Supports immune function, collagen synthesis, and antioxidant activity.
    - B Vitamins (B1, B2, B3, B5, B6, B7, B9, B12): Essential for energy metabolism, nerve function, and red blood cell production.
2. **Fat-Soluble Vitamins:**
    - Vitamin A: Essential for vision, immune function, and skin health.
    - Vitamin D: Facilitates calcium absorption, supports bone health, and regulates immune function.
    - Vitamin E: Acts as an antioxidant, supports immune function, and protects cell membranes.
    - Vitamin K: Essential for blood clotting and bone metabolism.

Minerals:

1. **Major Minerals:**
    - Calcium: Essential for bone and teeth health, muscle function, and nerve transmission.
    - Magnesium: Supports muscle and nerve function, bone health, and energy metabolism.

- Phosphorus: Important for bone and teeth health, energy metabolism, and cell signaling.

2. **Trace Minerals:**
    - Iron: Necessary for oxygen transport, energy metabolism, and red blood cell production.
    - Zinc: Supports immune function, wound healing, and DNA synthesis.
    - Selenium: Acts as an antioxidant, supports thyroid function, and may reduce the risk of certain cancers.
    - Copper: Essential for iron metabolism, connective tissue formation, and antioxidant defense.

Other Essential Nutrients:

Water:

- Essential for hydration, digestion, nutrient transport, temperature regulation, and overall cellular function.

Fiber:

- Supports digestive health, promotes satiety, regulates blood sugar levels, and may reduce the risk of chronic diseases.

Phytonutrients:

- Found in plant-based foods, phytonutrients have antioxidant, anti-inflammatory, and other health-promoting properties.

Omega-3 Fatty Acids:

- Essential for brain health, heart health, and reducing inflammation.
- Found in fatty fish, flaxseeds, chia seeds, walnuts, and hemp seeds.

Incorporating a balanced diet rich in whole foods is crucial for obtaining these essential nutrients and supporting optimal health and well-being. Additionally, individual nutrient needs may vary based on factors such as age, gender, activity level, and health status. It's important to consult with a healthcare professional or registered dietitian for personalized nutrition recommendations.

Back to Table of Contents

What is Carbohydrate?

Carbohydrates are one of the three macronutrients, along with proteins and fats, that provide energy for the body. Chemically, carbohydrates are made up of carbon, hydrogen, and oxygen atoms, and they come in various forms, including sugars, starches, and fibers. Carbohydrates are found in a wide range of foods, including grains, fruits, vegetables, legumes, and dairy products.

Types of Carbohydrates:

1. **Simple Carbohydrates (Sugars):** These are composed of one or two sugar molecules and are quickly digested and absorbed into the bloodstream. Examples include glucose, fructose, and sucrose (table sugar), which are found in fruits, honey, and sweets.
2. **Complex Carbohydrates (Starches and Fibers):** These are composed of long chains of sugar molecules and take longer to digest, providing a steady source of energy. Examples include starches found in grains, legumes, and starchy vegetables, as well as dietary fibers found in fruits, vegetables, whole grains, and legumes.

Benefits of Carbohydrates:

1. **Energy Source:** Carbohydrates are the body's primary source of energy. When consumed, carbohydrates are broken down into glucose, which is transported to cells and used as fuel for cellular processes, physical activity, and metabolic functions.
2. **Brain Function:** Glucose derived from carbohydrates is the preferred source of energy for the brain. Adequate carbohydrate intake supports cognitive function, concentration, and mental alertness.
3. **Muscle Fuel:** Carbohydrates are essential for supporting muscle function and performance, especially during high-intensity exercise and endurance activities. Glycogen, the stored form of glucose in muscles, serves as a readily available energy source during physical exertion.
4. **Dietary Fiber:** Many carbohydrate-rich foods, such as fruits, vegetables, whole grains, and legumes, are excellent sources of dietary fiber. Fiber promotes digestive health, regulates bowel movements, aids in weight management by promoting satiety, and may reduce the risk of chronic diseases such as heart disease, diabetes, and certain cancers.
5. **Nutrient Dense:** Carbohydrate-rich foods often contain essential vitamins, minerals, and phytonutrients that contribute to overall health and well-being. Choosing whole food sources of carbohydrates, such as whole grains, fruits, and vegetables, provides a wide range of nutrients vital for optimal health.
6. **Blood Sugar Regulation:** Consuming carbohydrates along with fiber, protein, and healthy fats can help slow down the absorption of glucose into the bloodstream, preventing rapid

spikes and crashes in blood sugar levels. This promotes stable energy levels and helps maintain insulin sensitivity.

Overall, carbohydrates play a crucial role in supporting energy production, brain function, muscle health, digestive health, and overall vitality. Including a variety of carbohydrate-rich foods as part of a balanced diet can help meet energy needs and support optimal health and well-being.

Plant-based foods high in Carbohydrates

Carbohydrates are one of the three macronutrients, along with proteins and fats, that provide energy for the body. Chemically, carbohydrates are made up of carbon, hydrogen, and oxygen atoms, and they come in various forms, including sugars, starches, and fibers. Carbohydrates are found in a wide range of foods, including grains, fruits, vegetables, legumes, and dairy products.

Grains and Grain Products:

1. **Bread:** Whole wheat bread, white bread, rye bread, sourdough bread, and multigrain bread.
2. **Cereal:** Oatmeal, granola, cornflakes, bran flakes, and muesli.
3. **Rice:** White rice, brown rice, basmati rice, jasmine rice, and wild rice.
4. **Pasta:** Spaghetti, penne, macaroni, fettuccine, and couscous.
5. **Quinoa:** A pseudo-grain that is high in protein and carbohydrates.
6. **Barley:** Pearl barley, hulled barley, and barley flakes.
7. **Bulgur:** A whole grain made from cracked wheat.
8. **Buckwheat:** Despite its name, buckwheat is not a wheat product and is gluten-free.

Starchy Vegetables:

1. **Potatoes:** Russet potatoes, sweet potatoes, white potatoes, and red potatoes.
2. **Corn:** Fresh corn on the cob, canned corn, and cornmeal.
3. **Peas:** Green peas, split peas, and chickpeas (also known as garbanzo beans).
4. **Winter Squash:** Butternut squash, acorn squash, and pumpkin.
5. **Plantains:** A starchy fruit commonly used in savory dishes.

Legumes:

1. **Beans:** Black beans, kidney beans, pinto beans, navy beans, and cannellini beans.
2. **Lentils:** Green lentils, red lentils, brown lentils, and French lentils.
3. **Chickpeas:** Also known as garbanzo beans, commonly used in dishes like hummus and falafel.
4. **Peas:** Split peas, green peas, and yellow peas.

Fruits:

1. **Bananas:** Known for their high carbohydrate content and potassium.
2. **Apples:** A good source of fiber and natural sugars.
3. **Oranges:** Rich in vitamin C and natural sugars.
4. **Grapes:** Red and green grapes are naturally sweet and contain carbohydrates.
5. **Mangoes:** A tropical fruit high in carbohydrates and vitamin C.
6. **Pineapples:** Sweet and tangy, pineapples are a good source of carbohydrates.

Dairy Products:

1. **Milk:** Cow's milk, soy milk, almond milk, and oat milk.
2. **Yogurt:** Greek yogurt, regular yogurt, and flavored yogurts.
3. **Kefir:** A fermented dairy beverage similar to drinkable yogurt.

These are just some examples of foods high in carbohydrates. Incorporating a variety of these foods into your diet can provide you with the energy and nutrients necessary for optimal health and well-being.

What is Protein?

Protein is one of the three macronutrients essential for human health, alongside carbohydrates and fats. Proteins are made up of amino acids, which are the building blocks of tissues, organs, enzymes, hormones, and various other molecules in the body. Protein is found in a wide range of foods, including animal-based sources such as meat, poultry, fish, eggs, and dairy products, as well as plant-based sources such as legumes, nuts, seeds, and grains.

Benefits of Protein:

1. **Muscle Growth and Repair:** Protein is crucial for building and repairing muscle tissues. During physical activity, muscle fibers undergo microscopic damage, and consuming protein helps repair and rebuild these tissues, leading to muscle growth and recovery.
2. **Supports Immune Function:** Many components of the immune system, including antibodies and immune cells, are made up of proteins. Adequate protein intake is essential for maintaining a strong and healthy immune system, which helps defend the body against infections and illnesses.
3. **Enzyme Function:** Enzymes are proteins that catalyze biochemical reactions in the body, facilitating processes such as digestion, metabolism, and cellular energy production. Without proteins, many essential metabolic reactions would occur at a much slower rate or not at all.
4. **Hormone Regulation:** Proteins play a role in hormone synthesis and signaling, helping regulate various physiological processes such as growth, metabolism, appetite, and mood. Hormones such as insulin, growth hormone, and thyroid hormones are all made up of proteins.
5. **Structural Support:** Proteins provide structural support to cells, tissues, and organs throughout the body. Collagen, for example, is a protein that forms the structural framework of skin, bones, tendons, and ligaments, contributing to their strength and elasticity.
6. **Transport and Storage:** Certain proteins serve as carriers, transporting essential molecules such as oxygen (in the form of hemoglobin) and nutrients (such as iron and vitamin A) throughout the body. Additionally, proteins are involved in storing and releasing nutrients and other molecules for use as energy or building blocks.
7. **Satiety and Weight Management:** Protein is the most satiating macronutrient, meaning it helps promote feelings of fullness and satisfaction after meals. Including protein-rich foods in your diet can help curb hunger, reduce overall calorie intake, and support weight management efforts.
8. **Maintains Hair, Skin, and Nails:** Proteins are vital for maintaining the health and integrity of hair, skin, and nails. Keratin, a structural protein found in these tissues, provides strength and resilience, contributing to healthy hair, skin, and nails.

In summary, protein plays a crucial role in supporting muscle health, immune function, enzyme activity, hormone regulation, structural integrity, nutrient transport, satiety, and overall health and well-being. Including adequate protein sources in your diet is essential for meeting nutrient needs and maintaining optimal health throughout life.

Plant-based foods high in Protein

Protein is one of the three macronutrients essential for human health, alongside carbohydrates and fats. Proteins are made up of amino acids, which are the building blocks of tissues, organs, enzymes, hormones, and various other molecules in the body. Protein is found in a wide range of foods, including animal-based sources such as meat, poultry, fish, eggs, and dairy products, as well as plant-based sources such as legumes, nuts, seeds, and grains.

1. **Legumes:**
    - **Lentils:** Lentils are a rich source of protein, with approximately 18 grams of protein per cooked cup. They are versatile and can be used in soups, salads, stews, and veggie burgers.
    - **Chickpeas:** Also known as garbanzo beans, chickpeas provide about 15 grams of protein per cooked cup. They are commonly used in hummus, curries, salads, and roasted as a crunchy snack.
    - **Black Beans:** Black beans offer approximately 15 grams of protein per cooked cup. They are a staple in Latin American cuisine and can be used in burritos, tacos, soups, and salads.
    - **Kidney Beans:** Kidney beans provide around 15 grams of protein per cooked cup. They are often used in chili, bean salads, soups, and stews.
2. **Soy Products:**
    - **Tofu:** Tofu is made from soybeans and contains about 20 grams of protein per cooked cup. It is a versatile ingredient that can be used in stir-fries, soups, salads, and sandwiches.
    - **Tempeh:** Tempeh is a fermented soy product that offers approximately 30 grams of protein per cooked cup. It has a nutty flavor and can be grilled, sautéed, or crumbled into dishes.
    - **Edamame:** Edamame are young soybeans that provide around 17 grams of protein per cooked cup. They can be boiled or steamed and served as a snack or added to salads, stir-fries, and pasta dishes.
3. **Quinoa:**
    - Quinoa is a pseudo-grain that contains all nine essential amino acids, making it a complete protein source. It offers approximately 8 grams of protein per cooked cup and can be used as a base for salads, stir-fries, pilafs, and breakfast bowls.

4. **Seitan:**
    - Seitan, also known as wheat gluten, is made from wheat protein and provides about 21 grams of protein per cooked 3-ounce serving. It has a meat-like texture and is commonly used in vegetarian and vegan dishes such as stir-fries, sandwiches, and stews.
5. **Nuts and Seeds:**
    - **Almonds:** Almonds offer approximately 6 grams of protein per ounce. They can be eaten as a snack, added to salads, or used to make almond butter.
    - **Chia Seeds:** Chia seeds provide about 5 grams of protein per ounce. They can be sprinkled on yogurt, oatmeal, or salads, or used to make chia pudding.
    - **Hemp Seeds:** Hemp seeds offer approximately 10 grams of protein per ounce. They can be added to smoothies, salads, or granola, or used to make hemp milk.
6. **Green Peas:**
    - Green peas provide around 8 grams of protein per cooked cup. They can be added to soups, salads, stir-fries, or mashed as a side dish.

These plant-based foods are excellent sources of protein and can be incorporated into a balanced diet to meet protein needs and support overall health and well-being.

Back to Table of Contents

Fats - What are Healthy Fats?

Healthy fats, also known as unsaturated fats, are essential components of a balanced diet and play numerous roles in promoting overall health and well-being. Unlike saturated fats and trans fats, which are considered less healthy, healthy fats provide a range of health benefits. Here are some examples of healthy fats and their benefits:

Types of Healthy Fats:

1. **Monounsaturated Fats:**
    - Found in foods such as olive oil, avocado, nuts (e.g., almonds, peanuts, cashews), and seeds (e.g., pumpkin seeds, sesame seeds).
    - Benefits: Monounsaturated fats can help reduce levels of LDL (bad) cholesterol and lower the risk of heart disease. They also provide energy, support cell growth and development, and help maintain healthy skin and hair.
2. **Polyunsaturated Fats:**
    - Includes omega-3 fatty acids and omega-6 fatty acids, both of which are essential fatty acids that the body cannot produce on its own.
    - **Omega-3 Fatty Acids:** Found in fatty fish (e.g., salmon, mackerel, sardines), flaxseeds, chia seeds, walnuts, and hemp seeds.
        - Benefits: Omega-3 fatty acids have anti-inflammatory properties and are crucial for heart health, brain function, and reducing the risk of chronic diseases such as heart disease, stroke, and certain cancers.
    - **Omega-6 Fatty Acids:** Found in vegetable oils (e.g., soybean oil, sunflower oil, corn oil), nuts, seeds, and certain grains.
        - Benefits: Omega-6 fatty acids are important for skin health, hormone production, and immune function. However, excessive consumption of omega-6 fatty acids relative to omega-3s may contribute to inflammation and increase the risk of chronic diseases.

Benefits of Healthy Fats:

Heart Health:

Healthy fats can help improve cholesterol levels by increasing HDL (good) cholesterol and decreasing LDL (bad) cholesterol. They also help reduce triglyceride levels and lower the risk of heart disease, stroke, and hypertension.

Brain Function:

Omega-3 fatty acids, in particular, are essential for brain health and cognitive function. They support the development and maintenance of brain cells, enhance memory and learning, and may reduce the risk of neurodegenerative diseases such as Alzheimer's disease.

Inflammation Reduction:

Omega-3 fatty acids have anti-inflammatory properties that help reduce inflammation in the body, which is associated with various chronic diseases, including heart disease, arthritis, and diabetes.

Skin and Hair Health:

Monounsaturated and polyunsaturated fats help maintain healthy skin and hair by providing essential fatty acids that support cell membranes and promote moisture retention. They also have antioxidant properties that protect against skin damage caused by UV radiation and environmental factors.

Nutrient Absorption:

Healthy fats are essential for the absorption of fat-soluble vitamins (A, D, E, and K) and other fat-soluble nutrients. They help transport these nutrients through the bloodstream and facilitate their uptake into cells.

Satiety and Weight Management:

Including healthy fats in meals can help promote satiety, reduce hunger, and stabilize blood sugar levels, which can aid in weight management efforts by preventing overeating and cravings.

Incorporating sources of healthy fats into your diet, such as olive oil, avocado, fatty fish, nuts, seeds, and plant-based oils, can contribute to overall health and well-being. Aim to include a variety of healthy fats in your meals while being mindful of portion sizes to support optimal health outcomes.

Plant-based foods contain Healthy Fats

Healthy fats, also known as unsaturated fats, are essential components of a balanced diet and play numerous roles in promoting overall health and well-being. Unlike saturated fats and trans fats, which are considered less healthy, healthy fats provide a range of health benefits. Here are some examples of healthy fats and their benefits:

1. **Avocado:**
    - Avocado is one of the richest sources of healthy fats among plant-based foods. It is high in monounsaturated fats, particularly oleic acid.
    - Benefits: Avocado consumption is associated with improved heart health, reduced inflammation, better nutrient absorption, and enhanced skin and hair health.
2. **Nuts:**
    - Various nuts such as almonds, walnuts, cashews, pistachios, and pecans are rich in healthy fats, predominantly monounsaturated and polyunsaturated fats.

- Benefits: Nuts are associated with lower risk of heart disease, improved cholesterol levels, reduced inflammation, and better cognitive function.

3. **Seeds:**
    - Seeds like chia seeds, flaxseeds, hemp seeds, pumpkin seeds, and sunflower seeds are excellent sources of healthy fats, particularly omega-3 fatty acids and monounsaturated fats.
    - Benefits: Seeds contribute to heart health, brain function, reduced inflammation, improved digestion, and enhanced skin health.
4. **Olives:**
    - Olives and olive oil are rich in monounsaturated fats, particularly oleic acid, as well as other beneficial compounds like polyphenols.
    - Benefits: Olive consumption is associated with reduced risk of heart disease, improved cholesterol levels, lower blood pressure, and reduced inflammation.
5. **Coconut:**
    - Coconut, including coconut meat, coconut oil, and coconut milk, contains healthy saturated fats, particularly medium-chain triglycerides (MCTs).
    - Benefits: Coconut consumption is linked to improved heart health, weight management, enhanced brain function, and antimicrobial properties.
6. **Soybeans and Soy Products:**
    - Soybeans and soy-based products like tofu, tempeh, and edamame are good sources of healthy fats, including polyunsaturated and monounsaturated fats.
    - Benefits: Soy consumption is associated with improved heart health, reduced cholesterol levels, better bone health, and reduced risk of certain cancers.
7. **Dark Chocolate:**
    - Dark chocolate with a high cocoa content is a source of healthy fats, particularly monounsaturated fats. It also contains flavonoids with antioxidant properties.
    - Benefits: Dark chocolate consumption is linked to improved heart health, reduced inflammation, better cognitive function, and enhanced mood.

Incorporating these plant-based foods high in healthy fats into your diet can contribute to overall health and well-being. It's important to consume them in moderation as part of a balanced diet to reap their benefits while maintaining a healthy weight and lifestyle.

Other Foods Contain Healthy Fats:

Fatty Fish:

- Fatty fish like salmon, mackerel, sardines, trout, and herring are high in omega-3 fatty acids, particularly EPA and DHA.
- Benefits: Fatty fish consumption is linked to reduced risk of heart disease, improved cognitive function, and better mood.

Back to Table of Contents

Vitamin A

What is Vitamin A?

Vitamin A is a fat-soluble vitamin that plays a critical role in various physiological functions in the human body. It exists in several forms, including retinol, retinal, retinoic acid, and provitamin A carotenoids.

Vitamin A is essential for various functions in the body, including vision, immune function, and skin health. While animal products are rich sources of preformed vitamin A (retinol), some plant-based foods provide provitamin A carotenoids, which the body can convert into active vitamin A.

Vitamin A is essential for:

Vision: One of the most well-known functions of vitamin A is its role in maintaining healthy vision. Retinal, a derivative of vitamin A, is a key component of rhodopsin, a protein found in the retina of the eye that is essential for low-light and color vision. Adequate vitamin A intake helps prevent night blindness and supports overall visual health.

Immune Function: Vitamin A plays a crucial role in supporting the immune system by promoting the production and function of white blood cells, which help the body fight off infections and diseases. It also helps maintain the integrity of mucosal surfaces in the respiratory, digestive, and urinary tracts, which serve as barriers against pathogens.

Skin Health: Vitamin A is involved in the growth and repair of skin cells, making it essential for maintaining healthy skin. It promotes cell turnover, supports the production of collagen, and helps prevent dryness, flakiness, and roughness of the skin. Topical retinoids derived from vitamin A are commonly used in skincare products to treat acne, wrinkles, and other skin conditions.

Reproduction and Growth: Vitamin A is important for reproductive health and fertility in both men and women. It is also necessary for normal growth and development, particularly in children, as it supports bone growth, tissue repair, and overall growth processes.

Gene Expression and Cell Differentiation: Vitamin A regulates gene expression and cell differentiation, influencing the development and function of various tissues and organs throughout the body. It plays a role in embryonic development, organ formation, and the maintenance of tissue integrity.

Vitamin A is found in a variety of foods, including liver, fish liver oils, dairy products, eggs, and fortified foods. It is also abundant in colorful fruits and vegetables, particularly those rich in provitamin A carotenoids such as beta-carotene, which the body can convert into active vitamin A. Consuming a balanced diet that includes a variety of foods rich in vitamin A is essential for maintaining optimal health and preventing deficiency-related health issues.

Plant-based foods high in Vitamin A

Here is a list of plant-based foods high in vitamin A or its precursors:

1. **Sweet Potatoes:**
    - High in beta-carotene, a provitamin A carotenoid.
2. **Carrots:**
    - Rich in beta-carotene, contributing to their orange color.
3. **Butternut Squash:**
    - Contains beta-carotene, providing both vitamin A and antioxidants.
4. **Pumpkin:**
    - Another excellent source of beta-carotene.
5. **Spinach:**
    - Contains beta-carotene and other carotenoids, contributing to its green color.
6. **Kale:**
    - Rich in beta-carotene and other carotenoids.
7. **Broccoli:**
    - Contains beta-carotene and is a good source of various nutrients.
8. **Mango:**
    - Provides beta-carotene, along with a sweet and tropical flavor.
9. **Cantaloupe:**
    - High in beta-carotene and provides a refreshing taste.
10. **Red and Yellow Bell Peppers:**
    - Contain beta-carotene, as well as vitamin C.
11. **Apricots (Dried):**
    - A good source of beta-carotene, especially when dried.
12. **Papaya:**
    - Contains beta-carotene and is rich in vitamin C.
13. **Tomatoes:**
    - Provide beta-carotene and other carotenoids, along with lycopene.
14. **Chili Peppers:**
    - Contain beta-carotene, especially in the red and orange varieties.
15. **Turnip Greens:**

- Rich in beta-carotene, as well as other vitamins and minerals.

It's important to note that while these plant-based foods contain provitamin A carotenoids, the conversion efficiency to active vitamin A (retinol) may vary among individuals. Including a variety of colorful fruits and vegetables in your diet can contribute to overall health and help meet your vitamin A needs.

Vitamin B1 - Thiamine

What is Vitamin B1 (Thiamine)?

Vitamin B1, also known as thiamine, is a water-soluble vitamin that plays a crucial role in energy metabolism and nerve function. It is one of the eight B vitamins that collectively form the vitamin B complex. Thiamine is essential for various physiological processes in the body, including:

1. **Energy Metabolism**: Thiamine is a coenzyme in the metabolism of carbohydrates, fats, and proteins. It helps convert carbohydrates into glucose, the body's primary source of energy. Thiamine is involved in the production of adenosine triphosphate (ATP), a molecule that stores and transports energy within cells.
2. **Nerve Function**: Thiamine is important for maintaining the health and function of the nervous system. It plays a role in the synthesis of neurotransmitters, which are chemical messengers that transmit signals between nerve cells. Thiamine deficiency can lead to nerve damage, resulting in symptoms such as numbness, tingling, muscle weakness, and impaired reflexes.
3. **Heart Health**: Thiamine is necessary for the proper functioning of the heart muscle. It helps regulate the contraction and relaxation of cardiac muscle cells, which is essential for maintaining normal heart rhythm and pumping blood throughout the body. Thiamine deficiency can lead to cardiovascular problems, including heart failure and enlarged heart.
4. **Brain Function**: Thiamine is important for cognitive function and mental health. It is involved in the synthesis of acetylcholine, a neurotransmitter that plays a role in memory, learning, and mood regulation. Thiamine deficiency has been associated with neurological disorders such as Wernicke-Korsakoff syndrome, characterized by confusion, memory loss, and impaired coordination.
5. **Digestive Health**: Thiamine is necessary for the production of stomach acid and the proper functioning of the digestive system. It helps convert carbohydrates into energy and supports

the metabolism of nutrients in the gastrointestinal tract. Thiamine deficiency can lead to digestive issues such as poor appetite, constipation, and bloating.

Good dietary sources of thiamine include whole grains, fortified cereals, legumes, nuts, seeds, pork, beef, poultry, fish, and eggs. Cooking methods such as boiling and milling can deplete thiamine content in foods, so it's important to consume a varied diet that includes a mix of thiamine-rich foods to meet daily requirements. Additionally, certain factors such as alcohol consumption, certain medications, and certain medical conditions can increase the risk of thiamine deficiency, so it's important to be mindful of overall nutritional intake and health status.

Back to Table of Contents

Plant-based foods high in Vitamin B1

Vitamin B1, also known as thiamine, is crucial for energy metabolism and the proper functioning of the nervous system. For individuals following a plant-based or vegan diet, it's important to be aware of plant-based sources of vitamin B1 (thiamine). While animal products are typically rich in this vitamin, several plant-based foods also contain significant amounts of vitamin B1. Here is a list of plant-based foods high in vitamin B1:

Whole Grains:
- Brown rice
- Whole wheat
- Barley
- Quinoa
- Oats

Legumes:
- Lentils
- Black beans
- Kidney beans
- Chickpeas
- Green peas

Nuts and Seeds:
- Sunflower seeds
- Pecans
- Pistachios
- Flaxseeds
- Sesame seeds

Nutritional Yeast:
- Nutritional yeast is a popular ingredient in plant-based diets and is often fortified with vitamin B1 and other B-vitamins.

Fortified Foods:
- Some plant-based foods, especially breakfast cereals and plant-based milk alternatives (like almond, soy, or rice milk), are fortified with vitamin B1.

Whole Wheat Bread and Pasta:
- Choose whole wheat or whole grain bread and pasta for a vitamin B1 boost.

Leafy Greens:
- Spinach
- Kale
- Collard greens
- Swiss chard

Avocado:

- Avocado is not only a good source of healthy fats but also contains vitamin B1.

Dried Fruits:

- Raisins
- Apricots
- Dates

Brown Rice Syrup:

- Brown rice syrup, a sweetener derived from brown rice, can be a source of vitamin B1.

Incorporating a variety of these plant-based foods into your meals can help ensure an adequate intake of vitamin B1. It's essential to maintain a balanced and varied diet to meet overall nutritional needs. If you have specific dietary concerns or are considering a significant change in your diet, consulting with a healthcare professional or a registered dietitian is advisable.

Vitamin B2 - Riboflavin

What is *Vitamin B2 (Riboflavin)?*

Vitamin B2, also known as riboflavin, is an essential water-soluble vitamin that plays a crucial role in energy metabolism and the maintenance of healthy skin, eyes, and nerve functions. It is one of the eight B vitamins that collectively form the vitamin B complex. Riboflavin is involved in numerous biochemical reactions, and its functions include:

Energy Metabolism: Riboflavin serves as a precursor for two important coenzymes involved in energy metabolism: flavin mononucleotide (FMN) and flavin adenine dinucleotide (FAD). These coenzymes participate in the electron transport chain, where they help convert carbohydrates, fats, and proteins into adenosine triphosphate (ATP), the body's primary source of energy.

Antioxidant Defense: Riboflavin functions as an antioxidant, helping to neutralize harmful free radicals and reactive oxygen species (ROS) that can damage cells and contribute to oxidative stress. As part of the antioxidant system, riboflavin helps protect cells and tissues from oxidative damage, which is associated with aging and various chronic diseases.

Cell Growth and Development: Riboflavin is necessary for normal cell growth, development, and repair. It plays a role in the synthesis of DNA, RNA, and proteins, which are essential for cellular processes such as replication, transcription, and translation. Riboflavin also contributes to the maintenance of healthy skin, hair, and nails.

Eye Health: Riboflavin is important for maintaining optimal vision and eye health. It is a component of flavoproteins involved in the production of glutathione, an antioxidant that protects the lens of the eye from oxidative damage. Riboflavin deficiency has been associated with eye disorders such as cataracts and photophobia (sensitivity to light).

Nervous System Function: Riboflavin plays a role in the functioning of the nervous system, including the synthesis of neurotransmitters and the maintenance of myelin sheaths, which protect and insulate nerve fibers. Adequate riboflavin intake is important for normal nerve function and transmission of nerve impulses.

Good dietary sources of riboflavin include dairy products (such as milk, yogurt, and cheese), eggs, lean meats, poultry, fish, nuts, seeds, and fortified cereals and grains. Riboflavin is relatively stable during cooking and food processing, but it can be destroyed by exposure to light. To ensure adequate riboflavin intake, it's important to consume a balanced diet that includes a variety of riboflavin-rich foods. Additionally, certain factors such as alcohol consumption, certain medications, and certain medical conditions can increase the risk of riboflavin deficiency, so it's important to be mindful of overall nutritional intake and health status.

Plant-based foods high in Vitamin B2

Here is a list of plant-based foods that are high in vitamin B2:

1. **Almonds:**
    - Almonds are not only a good source of healthy fats and protein but also contain significant amounts of vitamin B2.
2. **Sunflower Seeds:**
    - Sunflower seeds are rich in various nutrients, including vitamin B2. They make for a nutritious and convenient snack.
3. **Soybeans:**
    - Soybeans and soy-based products, such as tofu and tempeh, provide a substantial amount of vitamin B2 along with other essential nutrients.
4. **Spinach:**
    - Dark leafy greens like spinach are not only high in iron but also contain notable levels of vitamin B2.
5. **Mushrooms:**
    - Mushrooms, especially crimini and shiitake varieties, are good plant-based sources of vitamin B2.
6. **Whole Grains (Brown Rice, Quinoa, and Whole Wheat):**
    - Whole grains are rich in several B-vitamins, including vitamin B2. Opt for whole grains over refined grains for maximum nutritional benefits.
7. **Avocado:**
    - Avocado is a nutrient-dense fruit that contains various vitamins, including vitamin B2.

8. **Asparagus:**
    - Asparagus is a vegetable that not only provides fiber but also contributes to your vitamin B2 intake.
9. **Broccoli:**
    - Broccoli is a cruciferous vegetable that offers a good amount of vitamin B2 along with other vitamins and minerals.
10. **Fortified Plant-Based Milk:**
    - Many plant-based milk alternatives, such as almond milk, soy milk, and oat milk, are fortified with vitamin B2.
11. **Whole Grain Cereals:**
    - Choose whole grain cereals that are fortified with vitamins, including vitamin B2, for a nutritious breakfast option.
12. **Edamame:**
    - Edamame, or young soybeans, is a tasty and vitamin B2-rich snack or addition to salads and stir-fries.

Incorporating these plant-based foods into your diet can help ensure an adequate intake of vitamin B2. A well-balanced and varied plant-based diet provides the necessary nutrients for overall health and well-being.

Vitamin B3 - Niacin

What is Vitamin B3?

Vitamin B3, also known as niacin, is a water-soluble vitamin that plays essential roles in various physiological processes within the body. It is one of the eight B vitamins that collectively form the vitamin B complex. Niacin is involved in numerous biochemical reactions, and its functions include:

Energy Metabolism: Niacin is a precursor for two coenzymes, nicotinamide adenine dinucleotide (NAD) and nicotinamide adenine dinucleotide phosphate (NADP), which are involved in energy metabolism. These coenzymes participate in the conversion of carbohydrates, fats, and proteins into adenosine triphosphate (ATP), the body's primary source of energy.

Cellular Respiration: Niacin plays a critical role in cellular respiration, the process by which cells convert glucose and oxygen into ATP through a series of biochemical reactions. NAD and NADP serve as electron carriers in these reactions, facilitating the transfer of electrons and the production of ATP.

DNA Repair and Synthesis: Niacin is necessary for the repair and synthesis of DNA, the genetic material found in cells. It plays a role in maintaining the integrity of the genome and preventing mutations that can lead to genetic disorders and cancer.

Regulation of Gene Expression: Niacin influences the expression of genes involved in various cellular processes, including metabolism, inflammation, and cell growth. It acts as a signaling molecule that modulates gene transcription and protein synthesis in response to physiological and environmental cues.

Cholesterol and Lipid Metabolism: Niacin has been shown to help regulate cholesterol and lipid levels in the blood. It can increase levels of high-density lipoprotein (HDL) cholesterol, often referred to as "good" cholesterol, while decreasing levels of low-density lipoprotein (LDL) cholesterol and triglycerides. This may help reduce the risk of cardiovascular disease.

Skin Health: Niacin can improve skin health by supporting the production of ceramides, which are lipid molecules that help maintain the skin's barrier function and prevent moisture loss. Niacin supplementation has been shown to benefit individuals with conditions such as acne, eczema, and aging-related skin changes.

Good dietary sources of niacin include meat (such as poultry, beef, and pork), fish, nuts, seeds, legumes, whole grains, and fortified cereals. Niacin can also be synthesized in the body from the amino acid tryptophan, although the conversion rate is relatively low. To ensure adequate niacin intake, it's important to consume a balanced diet that includes a variety of niacin-rich foods. Additionally, certain factors such as alcohol consumption, certain medications, and certain medical conditions can increase the risk of niacin deficiency, so it's important to be mindful of overall nutritional intake and health status.

Plant-based foods high in Vitamin B3 (Niacin)

Here is a list of plant-based foods that are high in Vitamin B3:

1. **Mushrooms:**
    - Mushrooms, especially shiitake and portobello varieties, are a good source of niacin.
2. **Whole Grains:**
    - Whole grains such as brown rice, quinoa, and whole wheat are rich in niacin. Brown rice, in particular, contains more niacin than white rice.
3. **Legumes:**
    - Legumes like lentils, chickpeas, and black beans provide a good amount of niacin. They are also high in protein and fiber.
4. **Nuts and Seeds:**
    - Peanuts, sunflower seeds, and almonds contain niacin. These nuts and seeds are not only a great source of niacin but also provide healthy fats and other essential nutrients.
5. **Fortified Foods:**
    - Some plant-based foods, such as certain fortified cereals and nutritional yeast, are enriched with niacin. Check the product labels for information on added vitamins.
6. **Green Leafy Vegetables:**
    - Certain green leafy vegetables like spinach, kale, and broccoli contain niacin. While the levels may not be as high as in some other foods, they contribute to overall niacin intake.
7. **Avocado:**
    - Avocado is a nutrient-dense fruit that contains small amounts of niacin along with other essential vitamins and minerals.
8. **Sweet Potatoes:**
    - Sweet potatoes are not only rich in niacin but also provide a good dose of other vitamins and minerals.
9. **Bananas:**
    - Bananas contain niacin and are a convenient and portable snack.
10. **Whole Wheat Bread:**
    - Opting for whole wheat bread instead of refined white bread can contribute to your niacin intake.

It's essential to maintain a well-balanced diet that includes a variety of foods to ensure an adequate intake of all essential nutrients, including Vitamin B3. If you have specific dietary concerns or restrictions, consulting with a healthcare professional or a registered dietitian can help you plan a nutritionally balanced plant-based diet.

Vitamin B5 - Pantothenic Acid

What is Vitamin B5?

Vitamin B5, also known as pantothenic acid, is a water-soluble vitamin that plays essential roles in various physiological processes within the body. It is one of the eight B vitamins that collectively form the vitamin B complex. Pantothenic acid is involved in numerous biochemical reactions, and its functions include:

Energy Metabolism: Pantothenic acid is a precursor for coenzyme A (CoA), which is essential for the metabolism of carbohydrates, fats, and proteins. CoA serves as a cofactor in key enzymatic reactions involved in the breakdown of nutrients to produce energy in the form of adenosine triphosphate (ATP).

Synthesis of Fatty Acids: Pantothenic acid is necessary for the synthesis of fatty acids, which are building blocks of cell membranes, hormones, and other lipid molecules. CoA is required for the activation of fatty acids and their incorporation into triglycerides, phospholipids, and cholesterol esters.

Synthesis of Acetylcholine: Pantothenic acid is involved in the synthesis of acetylcholine, a neurotransmitter that plays a role in nerve impulse transmission, muscle contraction, and cognitive function. Acetylcholine is synthesized from acetyl-CoA, a derivative of pantothenic acid.

Synthesis of Steroid Hormones: Pantothenic acid is required for the synthesis of steroid hormones, such as cortisol, aldosterone, and testosterone, which regulate various physiological processes, including metabolism, stress response, fluid balance, and reproductive function.

Detoxification: Pantothenic acid is involved in the detoxification of harmful substances in the body. CoA participates in the metabolism of drugs, alcohol, and environmental toxins, facilitating their breakdown and elimination from the body.

Wound Healing: Pantothenic acid plays a role in wound healing and tissue repair. It is involved in the synthesis of collagen, a protein that provides structure and support to tissues, and in the formation of new blood vessels that deliver oxygen and nutrients to injured tissues.

Good dietary sources of pantothenic acid include meat (such as chicken, beef, and pork), fish, eggs, dairy products (such as milk, yogurt, and cheese), whole grains, legumes, nuts, seeds, and vegetables (such as avocados, broccoli, and sweet potatoes). Pantothenic acid is relatively stable during cooking and food processing, so it is present in a wide variety of foods. To ensure adequate pantothenic acid intake, it's important to consume a balanced diet that includes a variety of pantothenic acid-rich foods. Additionally, certain factors such as alcohol consumption, certain medications, and certain medical conditions can increase the risk of pantothenic acid deficiency, so it's important to be mindful of overall nutritional intake and health status.

Plant-based foods high in Vitamin B5 - Pantothenic Acid

Here is a list of plant-based foods that are high in Vitamin B5:

1. **Mushrooms:**
    - Mushrooms, especially shiitake and portobello varieties, contain pantothenic acid.
2. **Avocado:**
    - Avocado is a nutrient-dense fruit that provides a good amount of Vitamin B5 along with healthy fats.
3. **Sweet Potatoes:**
    - Sweet potatoes are not only rich in Vitamin B5 but also offer a range of other vitamins and minerals.
4. **Legumes:**
    - Lentils, chickpeas, and other legumes are excellent sources of pantothenic acid. They are also rich in protein and fiber.
5. **Whole Grains:**
    - Whole grains such as brown rice, quinoa, and whole wheat contain Vitamin B5. These grains are also valuable sources of other essential nutrients.
6. **Broccoli:**
    - Broccoli is a cruciferous vegetable that provides Vitamin B5 along with a variety of other vitamins and minerals.
7. **Sunflower Seeds:**
    - Sunflower seeds are a nutrient-dense snack that contains Vitamin B5 as well as healthy fats and other essential nutrients.
8. **Cauliflower:**
    - Cauliflower is another cruciferous vegetable that contributes to Vitamin B5 intake.
9. **Potatoes:**
    - Potatoes, especially with the skin on, contain pantothenic acid. They are also a good source of carbohydrates and fiber.
10. **Whole Wheat Bread:**
    - Opting for whole wheat bread instead of refined white bread can contribute to your Vitamin B5 intake.

Including a variety of these plant-based foods in your diet can help ensure an adequate intake of Vitamin B5, supporting energy metabolism and overall health. Keep in mind that a well-balanced and varied diet is essential for meeting all your nutritional needs.

Vitamin B6 - Pyridoxine

What is Vitamin B6?

Vitamin B6, also known as pyridoxine, is a crucial water-soluble vitamin that plays a vital role in various bodily functions, including metabolism, immune function, and neurotransmitter synthesis. It is one of the eight B vitamins that collectively form the vitamin B complex. Pyridoxine is involved in numerous biochemical reactions, and its functions include:

Amino Acid Metabolism: Vitamin B6 is necessary for the metabolism of amino acids, the building blocks of proteins. It is involved in the synthesis and breakdown of amino acids, as well as the conversion of one amino acid into another. Pyridoxine helps ensure that amino acids are available for protein synthesis, as well as for the production of other important molecules such as neurotransmitters, hormones, and enzymes.

Glycogen Metabolism: Pyridoxine plays a role in glycogen metabolism, the process by which glycogen, the storage form of glucose, is broken down into glucose to provide energy for the body. It helps activate enzymes involved in glycogenolysis, the breakdown of glycogen, and gluconeogenesis, the synthesis of glucose from non-carbohydrate sources.

Neurotransmitter Synthesis: Vitamin B6 is involved in the synthesis of several neurotransmitters, including serotonin, dopamine, norepinephrine, and gamma-aminobutyric acid (GABA). These neurotransmitters play important roles in mood regulation, cognition, sleep, and stress response. Pyridoxine helps convert the amino acid tryptophan into serotonin, and it is involved in the synthesis of other neurotransmitters from amino acid precursors.

Hemoglobin Synthesis: Pyridoxine is necessary for the synthesis of hemoglobin, the protein in red blood cells that carries oxygen from the lungs to tissues throughout the body. It helps convert the amino acid glycine into heme, the iron-containing component of hemoglobin. Vitamin B6 deficiency can lead to impaired hemoglobin synthesis and a type of anemia called sideroblastic anemia.

Immune Function: Vitamin B6 plays a role in immune function by supporting the production and activity of immune cells, such as lymphocytes and macrophages. It helps regulate immune responses to infections and inflammation, and it is involved in the production of antibodies that recognize and neutralize pathogens.

Good dietary sources of vitamin B6 include poultry, fish, meat (such as pork and beef), eggs, dairy products, whole grains, nuts, seeds, bananas, avocados, and potatoes. Pyridoxine is relatively stable during cooking and food processing, so it is present in a wide variety of foods. To ensure adequate vitamin B6 intake, it's important to consume a balanced diet that includes a variety of pyridoxine-rich foods. Additionally, certain factors such as alcohol consumption, certain medications, and certain medical conditions can increase the risk of vitamin B6 deficiency, so it's important to be mindful of overall nutritional intake and health status.

Plant-based foods high in Vitamin B6

While animal products are common sources of vitamin B6, there are also plenty of plant-based foods that can help you meet your daily requirements. Here's a list of plant-based foods high in vitamin B6:

1. **Sunflower Seeds:** These tiny seeds are not only rich in vitamin E but also contain a good amount of vitamin B6. They make for a nutritious and crunchy snack.
2. **Pistachio Nuts:** Pistachios are not only delicious but also provide a decent amount of vitamin B6. Snack on them or use them as a topping for salads and desserts.
3. **Bananas:** Along with being a great source of potassium, bananas also contain vitamin B6. They make for a convenient and portable snack.
4. **Avocado:** Avocados are not only creamy and rich in healthy fats but also contain vitamin B6. Enjoy them in salads, sandwiches, or as a topping on toast.
5. **Potatoes:** Potatoes, especially when consumed with the skin, are a good source of vitamin B6. Opt for baked or boiled potatoes for a healthier preparation.
6. **Chickpeas (Garbanzo Beans):** Chickpeas are versatile legumes that can be used in salads, soups, or as the main ingredient in dishes like hummus. They are also a good source of vitamin B6.
7. **Spinach:** Leafy greens like spinach are not only rich in iron but also contain vitamin B6. Add spinach to salads, smoothies, or lightly sauté it as a side dish.
8. **Fortified Plant-Based Milk:** Some plant-based milk alternatives, such as almond, soy, or rice milk, are fortified with vitamins, including B6. Check the labels to ensure they contain added nutrients.
9. **Whole Grains (Brown Rice, Quinoa):** Whole grains like brown rice and quinoa contain vitamin B6. They are excellent additions to a balanced plant-based diet.
10. **Bell Peppers:** Bell peppers, especially the red variety, contain a good amount of vitamin B6. Enjoy them raw in salads or as a crunchy snack.
11. **Watermelon:** This refreshing fruit not only helps keep you hydrated but also provides a small amount of vitamin B6. Enjoy it on its own or add it to fruit salads.
12. **Carrots:** Carrots are not only a good source of vitamin A but also contain vitamin B6. Snack on raw carrot sticks or add them to soups and stews.
13. **Hazelnuts:** Hazelnuts are not only delicious but also contain vitamin B6. Enjoy them as a snack or use them in baking and cooking.
14. **Fortified Cereals:** Many breakfast cereals are fortified with vitamins, including B6. Check the nutritional labels to find fortified cereals that can contribute to your vitamin B6 intake.

Including a variety of these plant-based foods in your diet can help ensure an adequate intake of vitamin B6, supporting overall health and well-being.

What is Vitamin B7 - *Biotin*

Vitamin B7, also known as biotin, is a water-soluble vitamin that plays a key role in energy metabolism and the maintenance of healthy skin, hair, and nails. It is one of the eight B vitamins that collectively form the vitamin B complex. Biotin is involved in numerous biochemical reactions, and its functions include:

Metabolism of Carbohydrates, Fats, and Proteins: Biotin serves as a cofactor for several enzymes involved in the metabolism of macronutrients. It helps convert carbohydrates, fats, and proteins into energy that the body can use for various functions. Biotin assists in the breakdown of glucose for energy production, the synthesis of fatty acids and cholesterol, and the metabolism of amino acids.

Synthesis of Fatty Acids and Gluconeogenesis: Biotin is necessary for the synthesis of fatty acids, which are important components of cell membranes and storage forms of energy. It helps activate enzymes involved in fatty acid synthesis and elongation. Additionally, biotin is involved in gluconeogenesis, the process by which glucose is synthesized from non-carbohydrate sources such as amino acids and glycerol.

Hair, Skin, and Nail Health: Biotin is often referred to as the "beauty vitamin" because of its role in promoting healthy hair, skin, and nails. It contributes to the maintenance of strong and resilient hair follicles, the formation of keratin (the protein that makes up hair and nails), and the renewal of skin cells. Biotin deficiency can lead to symptoms such as thinning hair, brittle nails, and dry, scaly skin.

Regulation of Gene Expression: Biotin influences the expression of genes involved in various cellular processes, including metabolism, cell growth, and differentiation. It acts as a cofactor for enzymes that regulate gene transcription and protein synthesis. Biotin deficiency can disrupt normal gene expression patterns and contribute to metabolic disorders.

Blood Sugar Regulation: Biotin may play a role in regulating blood sugar levels by enhancing insulin sensitivity and glucose uptake in cells. It helps activate enzymes involved in glucose metabolism and insulin signaling pathways. Biotin supplementation has been shown to improve glucose tolerance and reduce insulin resistance in some studies.

Good dietary sources of biotin include egg yolks, liver, nuts (such as almonds, peanuts, and walnuts), seeds (such as sunflower seeds), whole grains, legumes, avocado, sweet potatoes, and certain fruits (such as bananas). Biotin is also produced by bacteria in the gut, although the amount synthesized is thought to be relatively small compared to dietary intake. To ensure adequate biotin intake, it's important to consume a balanced diet that includes a variety of biotin-rich foods. Additionally, certain factors such as pregnancy, breastfeeding, certain medications, and certain medical conditions can increase the need for biotin, so it's important to be mindful of overall nutritional intake and health status.

Plant-based foods high in Vitamin B7

While biotin deficiency is rare, incorporating foods rich in this vitamin into a plant-based diet can contribute to overall well-being. Here is a list of plant-based foods high in vitamin B7 (biotin):

1. **Nuts (especially peanuts and almonds):** Peanuts and almonds are excellent sources of biotin. Snack on them or add them to your salads and meals for a biotin boost.
2. **Seeds (especially sunflower seeds):** Sunflower seeds are rich in biotin and can be sprinkled on salads, yogurt, or enjoyed on their own as a snack.
3. **Legumes (especially lentils):** Lentils, chickpeas, and other legumes are good sources of biotin. Incorporate them into soups, stews, and salads for a nutrient-packed meal.
4. **Whole Grains (especially oats and barley):** Whole grains like oats and barley contain biotin. Enjoy them as part of your breakfast or in various dishes to increase your biotin intake.
5. **Sweet Potatoes:** Sweet potatoes not only provide a healthy dose of biotin but also offer other essential nutrients. Roast, mash, or bake sweet potatoes for a nutritious side dish.
6. **Bananas:** Bananas are not only a convenient and portable snack but also contain biotin. Add them to your smoothies or enjoy them as a quick energy boost.
7. **Avocado:** Avocado is a nutrient-rich fruit that contains biotin. Use it in salads, sandwiches, or as a topping for toast.
8. **Broccoli:** Broccoli is a cruciferous vegetable that is not only high in biotin but also offers various vitamins and minerals. Steam or stir-fry broccoli to retain its nutritional value.
9. **Spinach:** Spinach is a leafy green vegetable that provides biotin along with other essential nutrients. Add spinach to salads, smoothies, or sauté it as a side dish.
10. **Mushrooms:** Certain types of mushrooms, such as shiitake and portobello, contain biotin. Incorporate them into your meals for an umami flavor and a biotin boost.
11. **Tomatoes:** Tomatoes are not only a tasty addition to various dishes but also contain biotin. Include them in salads, sauces, or enjoy them fresh.
12. **Carrots:** Carrots are a good source of biotin and can be enjoyed raw as a snack, in salads, or cooked in various dishes.

Including a variety of these plant-based foods in your diet can help ensure an adequate intake of biotin, supporting the health of your skin, hair, and nails, as well as overall energy metabolism.

Vitamin B9 - Folate or Folic Acid

What is vitamin B9?

Vitamin B9, commonly known as folate or folic acid, is a crucial nutrient for various bodily functions, including DNA synthesis, cell division, and the formation of red blood cells. It is particularly important during pregnancy for fetal development. It is one of the eight B vitamins that collectively form the vitamin B complex. Folate is crucial for several functions, including:

DNA Synthesis and Repair: Folate is essential for the synthesis and repair of DNA, the genetic material found in every cell of the body. It is particularly important during periods of rapid cell division and growth, such as during pregnancy and infancy. Folate helps ensure that cells can replicate and repair their DNA accurately, preventing mutations and abnormalities.

Cell Division and Growth: Folate plays a key role in cell division and growth by supporting the formation of new cells. It is necessary for the production of nucleotides, the building blocks of DNA and RNA, which are required for cell replication and proliferation. Adequate folate intake is important for normal development and growth, especially in fetuses, infants, and children.

Red Blood Cell Formation: Folate is involved in the production of red blood cells, which are responsible for carrying oxygen from the lungs to tissues throughout the body. Folate is necessary for the maturation of red blood cell precursors in the bone marrow and for the synthesis of hemoglobin, the protein that binds and transports oxygen in the blood. Folate deficiency can lead to a type of anemia called megaloblastic anemia, characterized by large, immature red blood cells.

Homocysteine Metabolism: Folate plays a role in the metabolism of homocysteine, an amino acid that can accumulate in the blood if not properly metabolized. High levels of homocysteine are associated with an increased risk of cardiovascular disease, stroke, and other health problems. Folate helps convert homocysteine into methionine, a process that requires vitamin B12 and vitamin B6 as cofactors.

Neurological Function: Folate is important for normal neurological function and brain health. It is involved in the synthesis of neurotransmitters such as serotonin, dopamine, and norepinephrine, which play key roles in mood regulation, cognition, and behavior. Adequate folate intake is important for maintaining mental and emotional well-being.

Good dietary sources of folate include leafy green vegetables (such as spinach, kale, and collard greens), legumes (such as lentils, chickpeas, and black beans), fruits (such as oranges, strawberries, and avocado), fortified grains and cereals, nuts, seeds, and liver. Folate is also available in supplement form, and folic acid is the synthetic form of folate used in fortified foods and supplements. Pregnant women, women of childbearing age, and individuals with certain medical conditions may require additional folate supplementation to meet their needs.

Plant-based foods high in Vitamin B9

Here is a list of plant-based foods high in vitamin B9:

1. **Leafy Greens (Spinach, Kale, Collard Greens):** Leafy greens are rich sources of folate. Add spinach or kale to your salads, smoothies, or stir-fries to boost your folate intake.
2. **Legumes (Lentils, Chickpeas, Black Beans):** Lentils, chickpeas, and black beans are excellent plant-based sources of folate. Incorporate them into soups, stews, and salads for a nutrient-rich meal.
3. **Asparagus:** Asparagus is a tasty vegetable that provides a good amount of folate. Roast or steam asparagus as a side dish or add it to pasta dishes.
4. **Avocado:** Avocado is not only a creamy and nutritious fruit but also contains folate. Enjoy avocado in salads, sandwiches, or as a topping for toast.
5. **Broccoli:** Broccoli is a cruciferous vegetable that offers a significant amount of folate. Include broccoli in your meals by steaming, roasting, or adding it to stir-fries.
6. **Citrus Fruits (Oranges, Grapefruits):** Citrus fruits are known for their vitamin C content, but they also provide folate. Enjoy oranges, grapefruits, or their juices as part of your daily fruit intake.
7. **Brussels Sprouts:** Brussels sprouts are a cruciferous vegetable that contributes to your folate intake. Roast or sauté Brussels sprouts for a flavorful side dish.
8. **Papaya:** Papaya is a tropical fruit that not only provides a burst of sweetness but also contains a good amount of folate. Enjoy fresh papaya or add it to fruit salads.
9. **Sunflower Seeds:** Sunflower seeds are a nutrient-dense snack that contains folate. Sprinkle them on salads, yogurt, or eat them on their own for a crunchy treat.
10. **Edamame:** Edamame, or young soybeans, is a tasty and protein-rich snack that also offers folate. Boil or steam edamame and enjoy them as a snack or appetizer.
11. **Cauliflower:** Cauliflower is a versatile vegetable that can be used in various dishes. Roast, mash, or include cauliflower in curries to increase your folate intake.
12. **Beets:** Beets are not only colorful and flavorful but also provide a good amount of folate. Roast, boil, or grate beets for salads or side dishes.

Incorporating a variety of these plant-based foods into your diet can help ensure an adequate intake of vitamin B9, supporting overall health and well-being. If you are pregnant or planning to become pregnant, it's crucial to consult with a healthcare professional to ensure you meet your folate requirements for optimal fetal development.

Vitamin B12 - Cobalamin

What is Vitamin B12?

Vitamin B12, also known as cobalamin. This plays a crucial role in various bodily functions, including the formation of red blood cells and maintenance of the nervous system. It is one of the eight B vitamins that collectively form the vitamin B complex. Vitamin B12 is crucial for several functions, including:

Red Blood Cell Formation: Vitamin B12 is essential for the production of red blood cells, which are responsible for carrying oxygen from the lungs to tissues throughout the body. B12 is required for the synthesis of DNA and RNA in red blood cell precursors in the bone marrow, as well as for the maturation of red blood cells. Vitamin B12 deficiency can lead to a type of anemia called megaloblastic anemia, characterized by large, immature red blood cells.

Nervous System Function: Vitamin B12 plays a critical role in the functioning of the nervous system. It is involved in the maintenance of myelin, a protective sheath that surrounds and insulates nerve fibers, allowing for efficient transmission of nerve impulses. B12 is also necessary for the synthesis of neurotransmitters such as serotonin, dopamine, and norepinephrine, which play key roles in mood regulation, cognition, and behavior.

DNA Synthesis and Repair: Vitamin B12 is required for the synthesis and repair of DNA, the genetic material found in every cell of the body. It is particularly important during periods of rapid cell division and growth, such as during pregnancy, infancy, and adolescence. B12 helps ensure that cells can replicate and repair their DNA accurately, preventing mutations and abnormalities.

Homocysteine Metabolism: Vitamin B12 is involved in the metabolism of homocysteine, an amino acid that can accumulate in the blood if not properly metabolized. High levels of homocysteine are associated with an increased risk of cardiovascular disease, stroke, and other health problems. B12 helps convert homocysteine into methionine, a process that requires folate and vitamin B6 as cofactors.

Cellular Energy Production: Vitamin B12 plays a role in energy metabolism by aiding in the conversion of certain fatty acids and amino acids into energy. It is involved in the synthesis of succinyl-CoA, a compound that participates in the citric acid cycle, a series of biochemical reactions that generate ATP, the body's primary source of energy.

Good dietary sources of vitamin B12 include animal products such as meat (particularly liver and shellfish), poultry, fish, eggs, dairy products (such as milk, cheese, and yogurt), and fortified foods (such as breakfast cereals, plant-based milk alternatives, and nutritional yeast). Vitamin B12 is not found in plant foods unless they are fortified with the vitamin. Individuals following a vegan or vegetarian diet may need to supplement with vitamin B12 to ensure adequate intake. Additionally, certain factors such as age, digestive disorders, and certain medications can impair the absorption of vitamin B12, so it's important to be mindful of overall nutritional intake and health.

Plant-based foods high in Vitamin B12

It is primarily found in animal products making it challenging for individuals following a strict plant-based diet to obtain adequate amounts. However, there are some plant-based foods that may contain small amounts of B12 or are fortified with synthetic B12. It's important to note that these sources may not provide sufficient B12 for everyone, and supplementation or fortified foods may be necessary. Always consult with a healthcare professional for personalized advice. Here are some plant-based sources of vitamin B12:

1. **Cranberries:**
   - Cranberries may contain trace amounts of vitamin B12, but they are not a reliable source.
2. **Dates:**
   - Dates may contain small amounts of B12, but they are not considered a significant source.
3. **Mulberries:**
   - Mulberries are reported to contain minimal amounts of vitamin B12.

4. **Fortified Foods:**
   - Many plant-based foods are fortified with synthetic vitamin B12, such as:
     - Fortified plant-based milk (soy, almond, coconut, etc.)
     - Fortified breakfast cereals
     - Fortified nutritional yeast
5. **Algae/Spirulina:**
   - Some algae and spirulina products are claimed to contain B12; however, the B12 analogs found in these sources may not be readily absorbed or utilized by the human body. Therefore, they are not considered reliable sources of active B12.
6. **Fortified Plant-Based Meat Alternatives:**
   - Some plant-based meat substitutes are fortified with vitamin B12.
7. **Supplements:**
   - Vitamin B12 supplements are a reliable way for individuals following a plant-based diet to meet their B12 requirements. Always consult with a healthcare professional before starting any supplementation.

It's crucial for individuals following a strict plant-based or vegan diet to monitor their B12 levels regularly and consider supplementation or fortified foods to ensure they meet their nutritional needs. Vitamin B12 is essential for neurological health, red blood cell formation, and overall well-being, and a deficiency can lead to serious health issues over time.

Foods high in Vitamin B12 - Cobalamin

Vitamin B12 is primarily found in animal products, and it plays a crucial role in various bodily functions, including the formation of red blood cells and maintenance of the nervous system. For individuals following a vegetarian or vegan diet, it's essential to obtain vitamin B12 from fortified foods or supplements, as natural sources are limited. Here is a list of foods rich in vitamin B12:

1. **Meat:**
    - Beef
    - Chicken
    - Pork
    - Lamb
2. **Fish:**
    - Salmon
    - Trout
    - Tuna
    - Sardines
    - Mackerel
    - Herring
3. **Shellfish:**
    - Clams
    - Oysters
    - Crab
    - Mussels
4. **Dairy Products:**
    - Milk
    - Cheese
    - Yogurt
5. **Eggs:**
    - Eggs, particularly the yolk
6. **Fortified Plant-Based Foods:**
    - Fortified plant-based milk (soy, almond, coconut, etc.)
    - Fortified breakfast cereals
    - Fortified nutritional yeast
    - Fortified plant-based yogurt

7. **Organ Meats:**
    - Liver (beef, chicken, pork)
8. **Supplements:**
    - Vitamin B12 supplements, available in various forms such as cyanocobalamin or methylcobalamin.

It's important to note that while some plant-based foods may claim to contain B12, the B12 found in these sources is often in the form of analogs, which are structurally similar to B12 but not effectively utilized by the human body. Therefore, individuals following a plant-based or vegan diet should prioritize fortified foods or supplements to ensure adequate B12 intake.

Always consult with a healthcare professional for personalized advice on meeting your nutritional needs, especially if you are following a specific diet or have any health concerns.

Back to Table of Contents

Vitamin C - Ascorbic Acid

What is Vitamin C?

Vitamin C, also known as ascorbic acid, is a water-soluble vitamin and is an essential nutrient that plays a crucial role in various bodily functions, including the formation of collagen, absorption of iron, the immune system, and antioxidant protection. It is a potent antioxidant and is necessary for several functions, including:

Antioxidant Defense: Vitamin C acts as an antioxidant, helping to neutralize harmful free radicals and reactive oxygen species (ROS) that can damage cells and contribute to oxidative stress. As an antioxidant, vitamin C helps protect cells and tissues from oxidative damage caused by environmental toxins, pollutants, UV radiation, and metabolic processes.

Collagen Synthesis: Vitamin C is essential for the synthesis of collagen, a structural protein found in connective tissues, skin, bones, cartilage, and blood vessels. Collagen provides strength and support to tissues, and it is necessary for wound healing, tissue repair, and the maintenance of healthy skin, hair, and nails. Vitamin C plays a critical role in the hydroxylation of proline and lysine residues during collagen synthesis.

Immune Function: Vitamin C is important for supporting the immune system and defending the body against infections and diseases. It enhances the function of various immune cells, including neutrophils, macrophages, and lymphocytes, and it helps promote the production and activity of antibodies that recognize and neutralize pathogens such as bacteria, viruses, and fungi.

Iron Absorption: Vitamin C enhances the absorption of non-heme iron, the form of iron found in plant-based foods and iron supplements. It helps convert ferric iron ($Fe3+$) into ferrous iron ($Fe2+$), which is more readily absorbed in the intestine. By improving iron absorption, vitamin C helps prevent and treat iron deficiency anemia, a common nutritional deficiency worldwide.

Neurotransmitter Synthesis: Vitamin C is involved in the synthesis of neurotransmitters such as serotonin, dopamine, and norepinephrine, which play key roles in mood regulation, cognition, and behavior. It acts as a cofactor for enzymes involved in the conversion of amino acids into neurotransmitters and in the metabolism of catecholamines.

Antiviral Properties: Vitamin C has been shown to exhibit antiviral properties and may help reduce the severity and duration of viral infections such as the common cold, influenza, and COVID-19. It supports the immune response to viral pathogens and may inhibit viral replication and spread.

Good dietary sources of vitamin C include citrus fruits (such as oranges, lemons, and grapefruits), strawberries, kiwi fruit, guava, papaya, pineapple, bell peppers (particularly red and yellow peppers), broccoli, Brussels sprouts, kale, and tomatoes. Vitamin C is also available in supplement form, including ascorbic acid and other vitamin C derivatives. It's important to consume a balanced diet that includes a variety of vitamin C-rich foods to ensure adequate intake of this essential nutrient. Additionally, certain factors such as smoking, alcohol consumption, stress, and certain medical conditions can increase the need for vitamin C, so it's important to be mindful of overall nutritional intake and health status.

Plant-based foods high in Vitamin C

Here is a list of plant-based foods that are high in Vitamin C:

1. **Citrus Fruits:**
    - Oranges
    - Grapefruits
    - Lemons
    - Limes
    - Clementines
2. **Berries:**
    - Strawberries
    - Blueberries
    - Raspberries
    - Blackberries
    - Cranberries
3. **Tropical Fruits:**
    - Pineapple
    - Mango
    - Papaya
    - Guava
    - Kiwi
4. **Melons:**
    - Cantaloupe
    - Honeydew
5. **Citrus-Like Fruits:**
    - Acerola cherries
    - Kiwi (although it's not a citrus fruit, it has a high Vitamin C content)
6. **Cruciferous Vegetables:**
    - Broccoli
    - Brussels sprouts
    - Cauliflower

7. **Leafy Greens:**
    - Kale
    - Spinach
    - Swiss chard
    - Collard greens
8. **Bell Peppers:**
    - Red, green, or yellow bell peppers
9. **Tomatoes:**
    - Fresh tomatoes
    - Tomato juice
    - Tomato sauce
10. **Tropical Root Vegetables:**
    - Sweet potatoes
11. **Berries:**
    - Strawberries
    - Blueberries
    - Raspberries
    - Blackberries
    - Cranberries
12. **Paprika:**
    - This spice, derived from ground peppers, is a potent source of Vitamin C.
13. **Guava:**
    - Guava is an exceptionally rich source of Vitamin C.
14. **Pineapple:**
    - Besides being a tropical delight, pineapple is high in Vitamin C.
15. **Mango:**
    - Mangoes not only offer a sweet taste but also contribute to your Vitamin C intake.

Including a variety of these plant-based foods in your diet can help ensure an adequate intake of Vitamin C, supporting your overall health and well-being.

Back to Table of Contents

Vitamin D

What is Vitamin D?

Vitamin D is a fat-soluble vitamin that plays a crucial role in various physiological processes within the human body. It is unique among vitamins in that it can be synthesized by the body in response to sunlight exposure as well as obtained from dietary sources and supplements. Vitamin D is essential for overall health and is involved in several important functions, including:

1. **Calcium absorption and bone health:** One of the primary functions of vitamin D is its role in promoting the absorption of calcium from the intestines into the bloodstream. Calcium is essential for maintaining strong bones and teeth, and adequate vitamin D levels are necessary for optimal calcium absorption. Vitamin D also helps regulate calcium levels in the blood by promoting calcium reabsorption in the kidneys and supporting bone mineralization.
2. **Bone growth and remodeling:** Vitamin D is important for bone growth and development, particularly during childhood and adolescence. It helps regulate the activity of osteoblasts, the cells responsible for building new bone tissue, and osteoclasts, the cells responsible for breaking down and resorbing old bone tissue. Vitamin D deficiency can lead to impaired bone mineralization, weakened bones, and an increased risk of fractures and bone disorders such as rickets in children and osteomalacia in adults.
3. **Immune function:** Vitamin D plays a role in modulating the immune system and has been shown to have anti-inflammatory and immunomodulatory effects. Adequate vitamin D levels may help reduce the risk of infections, autoimmune diseases, and chronic inflammatory conditions. Vitamin D receptors are found on various immune cells, and vitamin D regulates the expression of genes involved in immune response and inflammation.
4. **Regulation of cell growth and differentiation:** Vitamin D is involved in regulating cell growth, proliferation, and differentiation in various tissues throughout the body. It plays a role in controlling the expression of genes involved in cell cycle regulation, apoptosis (programmed cell death), and differentiation of cells into specialized cell types. Vitamin D may have implications for cancer prevention and treatment, as abnormal cell growth and differentiation are hallmarks of cancer development.
5. **Mood regulation and mental health:** There is growing evidence suggesting a link between vitamin D deficiency and mood disorders such as depression and seasonal affective disorder (SAD). Vitamin D receptors are found in areas of the brain involved in mood regulation, and vitamin D may influence neurotransmitter levels and neuronal function. Adequate vitamin D levels may help support mental well-being and reduce the risk of mood disorders.

Sources of vitamin D include sunlight exposure, dietary sources such as fatty fish (e.g., salmon, mackerel, tuna), fortified foods (e.g., fortified dairy products, breakfast cereals, and orange juice), and vitamin D supplements. However, many people may have difficulty obtaining sufficient vitamin D from sunlight and diet alone, especially during the winter months or in regions with limited sunlight exposure. Therefore, supplementation may be necessary for individuals at risk of vitamin D deficiency, particularly those with limited sun exposure, dark skin, older adults, individuals with certain medical conditions, or those who follow strict vegetarian or vegan diets.

While vitamin D is essential for overall health, it's important to maintain balanced levels, as excessive intake of vitamin D can lead to toxicity, known as hypervitaminosis D, which can cause symptoms such as nausea, vomiting, weakness, and hypercalcemia (elevated calcium levels in the blood). Therefore, it's important to consult with a healthcare professional for personalized guidance on vitamin D supplementation and monitoring of vitamin D levels.

Natural foods high in Vitamin D

Vitamin D is unique because it can be synthesized by the body through exposure to sunlight. However, there are also some foods that naturally contain vitamin D. Here is a list of natural foods high in vitamin D:

1. **Fatty Fish:**
    - Salmon (wild-caught)
    - Mackerel
    - Sardines
    - Herring
    - Trout
    - Tuna (particularly canned in oil)
2. **Cod Liver Oil:**
    - Cod liver oil is an excellent source of vitamin D, but it should be consumed in moderation due to its high vitamin A content.
3. **Egg Yolks:**
    - Egg yolks contain small amounts of vitamin D. Choose eggs from pasture-raised or omega-3 enriched sources for higher vitamin D levels.
4. **Beef Liver:**
    - Beef liver is a good source of vitamin D, but it should be eaten in moderation due to its high vitamin A content.
5. **Mushrooms:**
    - Some mushrooms, when exposed to sunlight or ultraviolet (UV) light during growth, can produce vitamin D2. This includes maitake and UV-exposed portobello mushrooms.
6. **Fortified Foods:**
    - Certain foods are fortified with vitamin D, which means the vitamin is added during processing. This includes:

- Fortified dairy products (milk, yogurt, cheese)
- Fortified plant-based milk (soy, almond, rice, oat)
- Fortified orange juice
- Fortified breakfast cereals

It's essential to note that the amount of vitamin D in food sources can vary, and sunlight exposure remains a crucial factor in maintaining adequate vitamin D levels in the body. The recommended dietary allowance (RDA) for vitamin D can vary based on factors such as age, sex, and individual health conditions. If you have concerns about your vitamin D levels, it's advisable to consult with a healthcare professional for personalized advice.

Vitamin E - Tocopherol

What is Vitamin E?

Vitamin E is a fat-soluble antioxidant that plays essential roles in various physiological processes within the body. It exists in several forms, with alpha-tocopherol being the most biologically active form. Vitamin E acts primarily as an antioxidant, protecting cells and tissues from oxidative damage caused by free radicals and reactive oxygen species. Its functions include:

Antioxidant Protection: Vitamin E scavenges free radicals and reactive oxygen species (ROS) that can damage cell membranes, DNA, proteins, and lipids, leading to oxidative stress and cellular damage. By neutralizing free radicals, vitamin E helps prevent oxidative damage and supports overall health and well-being.

Cell Membrane Stability: Vitamin E helps maintain the integrity and stability of cell membranes by protecting polyunsaturated fatty acids (PUFAs) from lipid peroxidation. It incorporates into cell membranes, where it acts as a lipid-soluble antioxidant, preventing oxidative damage to membrane lipids and preserving membrane structure and function.

Immune Function: Vitamin E supports the function of the immune system by enhancing the activity of immune cells, such as T cells, B cells, natural killer (NK) cells, and macrophages. It helps regulate immune responses to infections, inflammation, and tissue injury, and it plays a role in modulating cytokine production and signaling pathways involved in immune regulation.

Cardiovascular Health: Vitamin E may help protect against cardiovascular disease by reducing oxidative stress, inflammation, and endothelial dysfunction. It inhibits the oxidation of low-density lipoprotein (LDL) cholesterol, a process that contributes to the development of atherosclerosis and coronary artery disease. Vitamin E also helps improve blood vessel function and reduce platelet aggregation and thrombosis.

Skin Health: Vitamin E is often used in skincare products and supplements due to its potential benefits for skin health. It helps protect the skin from UV radiation, environmental pollutants, and oxidative stress, which can cause premature aging, wrinkles, and skin damage. Vitamin E promotes skin hydration, elasticity, and regeneration, and it may help reduce inflammation and promote wound healing.

Neurological Function: Vitamin E plays a role in neurological function and brain health. It protects nerve cells from oxidative damage and supports the integrity of myelin, the fatty substance that insulates nerve fibers and facilitates efficient nerve impulse transmission. Vitamin E may help reduce the risk of neurodegenerative diseases such as Alzheimer's disease and Parkinson's disease.

Good dietary sources of vitamin E include nuts (such as almonds, hazelnuts, and sunflower seeds), seeds (such as pumpkin seeds and flaxseeds), vegetable oils (such as wheat germ oil, sunflower oil, and safflower oil), green leafy vegetables (such as spinach and kale), avocados, and fortified foods (such as cereals and spreads). Vitamin E supplements are also available, but it's important to consult with a healthcare professional before starting supplementation, as excessive intake of vitamin E supplements may have adverse effects in some individuals. Additionally, vitamin E works synergistically with other antioxidants, such as vitamin C, so it's important to consume a balanced diet rich in a variety of antioxidants to support overall health and well-being.

Plant-based foods high in Vitamin E

Here is a list of plant-based foods that are high in vitamin E:

1. **Nuts:**
    - Almonds
    - Sunflower seeds
    - Hazelnuts
    - Pine nuts
    - Brazil nuts
    - Peanuts (and peanut butter)
2. **Seeds:**
    - Sunflower seeds
    - Pumpkin seeds
    - Sesame seeds
3. **Plant Oils:**
    - Sunflower oil
    - Wheat germ oil
    - Olive oil
    - Almond oil
    - Hazelnut oil
4. **Leafy Green Vegetables:**

- Spinach
- Swiss chard
- Kale
- Collard greens
- Turnip greens

5. **Fruits:**
    - Avocado
    - Kiwi
    - Blackberries
    - Blueberries
6. **Fortified Foods:**
    - Some processed and fortified foods, like cereals and plant-based milk, may contain added vitamin E.
7. **Whole Grains:**
    - Wheat germ
    - Brown rice
    - Oats
8. **Legumes:**
    - Chickpeas
    - Lentils

Including a variety of these vitamin E-rich plant-based foods in your diet can contribute to meeting your daily vitamin E needs. Keep in mind that vitamin E is found in different forms, such as tocopherols and tocotrienols, and a diverse diet helps ensure you get a range of these beneficial compounds. As with any nutrient, it's always a good idea to achieve a balance in your diet rather than relying on a single source. If you have specific dietary concerns or conditions, consider consulting with a healthcare professional or a registered dietitian for personalized advice.

Back to Table of Contents

Vitamin K

What is Vitamin K?

Vitamin K is a fat-soluble vitamin that plays essential roles in blood clotting, bone metabolism, and cardiovascular health. There are two main forms of vitamin K: vitamin K1 (phylloquinone) and vitamin K2 (menaquinone).

Blood Clotting: Vitamin K is necessary for the synthesis of clotting factors in the liver, particularly factors II (prothrombin), VII, IX, and X. These clotting factors are essential for the blood coagulation process, which helps stop bleeding when blood vessels are injured. Vitamin K promotes the conversion of precursor proteins into active forms that participate in the clotting cascade, leading to the formation of blood clots.

Bone Metabolism: Vitamin K plays a role in bone metabolism by supporting the activation of osteocalcin, a protein involved in bone mineralization. Osteocalcin helps bind calcium ions to the bone matrix, promoting bone formation and strength. Vitamin K also regulates the activity of matrix Gla protein (MGP), which inhibits the calcification of soft tissues, such as blood vessels and cartilage, thus helping prevent arterial calcification and maintaining cardiovascular health.

Cardiovascular Health: Vitamin K2, in particular, has been associated with cardiovascular health benefits beyond its role in blood clotting. It helps prevent arterial calcification by activating matrix Gla protein (MGP), which inhibits the deposition of calcium in arterial walls and reduces the risk of atherosclerosis and cardiovascular disease. Adequate vitamin K intake has been linked to a lower risk of coronary artery calcification and cardiovascular events.

Brain and Nervous System: Emerging research suggests that vitamin K may play a role in brain and nervous system health. Vitamin K-dependent proteins are found in the brain, where they may contribute to neuronal function and protect against neurodegenerative diseases such as Alzheimer's disease. Further studies are needed to elucidate the specific mechanisms by which vitamin K influences brain health.

Immune Function: Vitamin K may modulate immune function by regulating the production of cytokines and inflammatory mediators. Some studies suggest that vitamin K deficiency may impair immune responses and increase susceptibility to infections and inflammatory diseases. However, more research is needed to fully understand the role of vitamin K in immune function.

Good dietary sources of vitamin K1 include green leafy vegetables (such as kale, spinach, collard greens, and Swiss chard), broccoli, Brussels sprouts, cabbage, and other cruciferous vegetables. Vitamin K2 is found in fermented foods (such as natto, a traditional Japanese dish made from fermented soybeans), cheese, egg yolks, and animal products (such as meat and liver).

Additionally, vitamin K is synthesized by bacteria in the gut, but the extent of absorption varies among individuals. Adequate vitamin K intake is important for overall health and well-being, and deficiencies can lead to bleeding disorders, osteoporosis, and other health problems.

Plant-based foods high in Vitamin K

Here is a list of plant-based foods that are high in vitamin K:

1. **Leafy Greens:**
    - Kale
    - Spinach
    - Swiss chard
    - Collard greens
    - Mustard greens
    - Turnip greens
    - Beet greens
2. **Cruciferous Vegetables:**
    - Broccoli
    - Brussels sprouts
    - Cabbage
    - Cauliflower
3. **Herbs:**
    - Parsley
    - Basil
    - Thyme
    - Cilantro
    - Sage
4. **Lettuce Varieties:**
    - Romaine lettuce
    - Iceberg lettuce
    - Green leaf lettuce
5. **Green Vegetables:**
    - Asparagus
    - Green beans
    - Peas
    - Zucchini
6. **Natto:**
    - Natto, a traditional Japanese dish made from fermented soybeans, is particularly high in vitamin K2
    -

7. **Seaweed:**
    - Nori
    - Kelp
    - Wakame
8. **Avocado:**
    - Avocado provides a moderate amount of vitamin K.
9. **Brussels Sprouts:**
    - These cruciferous vegetables deserve a separate mention due to their notable vitamin K content.
10. **Kiwi:**
    - Kiwi fruit contains a modest amount of vitamin K.

Remember that vitamin K is fat-soluble, so consuming these foods with a source of healthy fat may enhance its absorption. Including a variety of these plant-based foods in your diet can help ensure an adequate intake of vitamin K, promoting overall health and well-being. Always consult with a healthcare professional or nutritionist to determine your specific nutritional needs.

Essential Minerals

What are Minerals?

Minerals are naturally occurring inorganic substances that are essential for various physiological functions in the human body. These substances cannot be synthesized by the body and must be obtained from dietary sources. Minerals play crucial roles in processes such as bone formation, nerve transmission, muscle function, fluid balance, and energy metabolism.

There are two main categories of minerals:

Macrominerals: These are minerals that are required by the body in larger amounts. Common macrominerals include calcium, phosphorus, magnesium, sodium, potassium, chloride, and sulfur. These minerals are vital for maintaining healthy bones, teeth, muscles, and electrolyte balance.

Microminerals (Trace Minerals): Microminerals are required by the body in smaller amounts compared to macrominerals. Examples of trace minerals include iron, zinc, copper, selenium, iodine, manganese, chromium, and molybdenum. Despite their lower concentration in the body, trace minerals play crucial roles in enzyme function, hormone synthesis, immune function, and antioxidant defense.

Minerals are found in a variety of foods, including fruits, vegetables, whole grains, legumes, nuts, seeds, dairy products, and lean meats. The bioavailability of minerals can vary depending on factors such as the form of the mineral, the presence of other nutrients, and individual factors such as age and health status.

Here is a comprehensive list of crucial minerals that our body needs, along with their respective functions:

1. **Calcium:**
    - Functions: Bone and teeth health, blood clotting, nerve function, and muscle contraction.
2. **Phosphorus:**
    - Functions: Bone health, energy metabolism, and DNA and RNA synthesis.
3. **Potassium:**
    - Functions: Fluid balance, nerve function, muscle contraction, and blood pressure regulation.
4. **Sodium:**
    - Functions: Fluid balance, nerve function, muscle contraction, and blood pressure regulation.

5. **Magnesium:**
    - Functions: Muscle and nerve function, bone health, energy metabolism, and DNA synthesis.
6. **Sulfur:**
    - Functions: Component of certain amino acids and vitamins, supports protein structure.
7. **Iron:**
    - Functions: Oxygen transport (hemoglobin), energy metabolism, and immune function.
8. **Zinc:**
    - Functions: Immune function, wound healing, DNA synthesis, and cell division.
9. **Copper:**
    - Functions: Red blood cell formation, connective tissue health, and enzyme activity.
10. **Manganese:**
    - Functions: Bone formation, blood clotting, and antioxidant defense.
11. **Selenium:**
    - Functions: Antioxidant activity, thyroid function, and immune response.
12. **Iodine:**
    - Functions: Essential for thyroid hormone synthesis, which regulates metabolism.
13. **Fluoride:**
    - Functions: Dental health, prevents tooth decay, and strengthens tooth enamel.
14. **Chromium:**
    - Functions: Enhances insulin activity, supports glucose metabolism.
15. **Molybdenum:**
    - Functions: Enzyme activity, including those involved in amino acid metabolism.
16. **Cobalt:**
    - Functions: Component of vitamin B12, involved in red blood cell formation.
17. **Nickel:**
    - Functions: Enzyme activity, though its essential role in humans is not well-established.

These minerals are crucial for a wide range of physiological functions, and maintaining an adequate intake is essential for overall health. A balanced and varied diet that includes nutrient-dense foods is the best way to ensure proper mineral intake. If there are concerns about mineral levels or specific health conditions, consulting with a healthcare professional can provide personalized guidance.

Back to Table of Contents

Calcium

What is Calcium?

Calcium is a chemical element with the symbol Ca and atomic number 20. It is an essential mineral that plays a crucial role in various physiological processes within the human body. Calcium is the most abundant mineral in the body, with about 99% of it stored in bones and teeth, where it provides strength and structure. The remaining 1% of calcium circulates in the bloodstream and is involved in numerous vital functions, including:

Bone Health: Calcium is a key component of bone tissue, contributing to bone density and strength. Adequate calcium intake during childhood and adolescence is crucial for optimal bone development and growth. Throughout adulthood, calcium helps maintain bone mass and prevents osteoporosis, a condition characterized by weakened and porous bones.

Teeth Health: Calcium is also essential for dental health, as it helps build and maintain the structure of tooth enamel, the outer layer of the teeth. Tooth enamel is primarily composed of hydroxyapatite, a calcium phosphate mineral that provides protection against decay and erosion.

Muscle Contraction: Calcium ions play a central role in muscle contraction, including both skeletal muscle (voluntary muscle) and smooth muscle (involuntary muscle). When stimulated by nerve impulses, calcium is released from storage sites within muscle cells, triggering a series of biochemical reactions that result in muscle contraction.

Nerve Function: Calcium ions are involved in nerve transmission and signaling. They help regulate the release of neurotransmitters, which are chemical messengers that transmit signals between nerve cells. Calcium ions also participate in the generation and propagation of action potentials, the electrical impulses that allow nerve cells to communicate with each other.

Blood Clotting: Calcium is essential for the process of blood clotting (coagulation), which helps prevent excessive bleeding when blood vessels are injured. Calcium ions interact with various proteins and enzymes involved in the coagulation cascade, leading to the formation of fibrin, a fibrous protein that forms blood clots and stops bleeding.

Cell Signaling: Calcium ions serve as universal signaling molecules within cells, regulating a wide range of cellular processes, including gene expression, enzyme activity, hormone secretion, and cell proliferation. Calcium signaling pathways are involved in the control of cell growth, differentiation, and apoptosis (programmed cell death).

Good dietary sources of calcium include dairy products (such as milk, cheese, and yogurt), fortified plant-based milk alternatives (such as almond milk and soy milk), leafy green vegetables (such as kale, broccoli, and collard greens), tofu, sardines, salmon, almonds, and calcium-fortified foods (such as breakfast cereals and orange juice). In addition to dietary sources, calcium supplements may be recommended for individuals who have difficulty meeting their calcium needs through diet alone. However, it's important to consult with a healthcare professional before starting any supplement regimen, as excessive calcium intake can have adverse effects.

Plant-based foods high in Calcium

Calcium is an essential mineral for bone health, muscle function, and nerve transmission. While dairy products are a well-known source of calcium, there are plenty of plant-based foods that provide this vital nutrient. Here is a list of plant-based foods that are high in calcium:

1. **Leafy Green Vegetables:**
   - Kale
   - Collard greens
   - Turnip greens
   - Bok choy
   - Broccoli
2. **Fortified Plant Milks:**
   - Soy milk (fortified)
   - Almond milk (fortified)
   - Oat milk (fortified)
   - Coconut milk (fortified)
   - Rice milk (fortified)
3. **Tofu and Tempeh:**
   - Tofu, especially firm or extra-firm varieties
   - Tempeh
4. **Nuts and Seeds:**
   - Almonds
   - Chia seeds
   - Sesame seeds
   - Poppy seeds
5. **Legumes:**
   - Chickpeas
   - Lentils
   - Black beans
   - White beans
6. **Whole Grains:**
   - Amaranth
   - Quinoa
   - Oats (especially fortified oatmeal)
   - Teff

7. **Fortified Foods:**
    - Certain plant-based foods are fortified with calcium. Check labels for added calcium in products like breakfast cereals, energy bars, and plant-based yogurt.
8. **Dried Fruits:**
    - Figs (dried)
    - Apricots (dried)
9. **Seaweed:**
    - Wakame and hijiki seaweed are good sources of calcium. However, their consumption should be moderated due to their iodine content.
10. **Oranges and Figs:**
    - Oranges and figs contain some calcium and can contribute to your overall intake.

Remember that the absorption of calcium can be influenced by other nutrients in your diet. Consuming foods rich in vitamin D, magnesium, and vitamin K, as well as maintaining a well-balanced diet, can optimize calcium absorption. If you have specific dietary concerns or restrictions, it's advisable to consult with a healthcare professional or a registered dietitian for personalized advice on meeting your calcium needs.

Magnesium

What is Magnesium?

Magnesium is a chemical element with the symbol Mg and atomic number 12. It is a vital mineral that plays numerous essential roles in the human body. Magnesium is involved in over 300 biochemical reactions, making it crucial for various physiological functions. Some key functions of magnesium include:

Muscle Function: Magnesium is necessary for proper muscle function, including muscle contraction and relaxation. It works in concert with calcium to regulate muscle contractions by activating and deactivating muscle proteins.

Nerve Function: Magnesium plays a role in nerve transmission and neuromuscular conduction. It helps regulate the flow of calcium ions across nerve cell membranes, which is essential for transmitting nerve impulses.

Energy Metabolism: Magnesium is involved in the production and utilization of ATP (adenosine triphosphate), the primary energy currency of cells. It participates in various enzymatic reactions involved in carbohydrate, protein, and fat metabolism.

Protein Synthesis: Magnesium is required for the synthesis of proteins, including enzymes and structural proteins. It helps stabilize the structure of ribosomes, the cellular machinery responsible for protein synthesis.

DNA and RNA Synthesis: Magnesium is essential for the replication and transcription of DNA and RNA. It facilitates the binding of enzymes involved in DNA replication and repair, as well as the assembly of ribonucleotides into RNA molecules.

Bone Health: Magnesium is a component of bone tissue and contributes to bone density and strength. It works synergistically with calcium and vitamin D to support bone mineralization and prevent osteoporosis.

Cardiovascular Health: Magnesium plays a role in maintaining normal heart rhythm and function. It helps regulate the contraction and relaxation of the heart muscle and supports the function of the cardiovascular system.

Blood Pressure Regulation: Magnesium helps regulate blood pressure by relaxing blood vessels and improving blood flow. It inhibits the constriction of blood vessels and counteracts the effects of calcium, which can promote vasoconstriction.

Good dietary sources of magnesium include green leafy vegetables (such as spinach, kale, and Swiss chard), nuts and seeds (such as almonds, pumpkin seeds, and sunflower seeds), legumes (such as beans, lentils, and chickpeas), whole grains (such as brown rice, quinoa, and oats), avocados, bananas, and dark chocolate. In addition to dietary sources, magnesium supplements are available and may be recommended for individuals who have difficulty meeting their magnesium needs through diet alone. However, it's important to consult with a healthcare professional before starting any supplement regimen, as excessive magnesium intake can have adverse effects, particularly in individuals with kidney problems.

Plant-based foods high in Magnesium

Magnesium is an essential mineral that plays a crucial role in various bodily functions, including muscle and nerve function, blood sugar regulation, and bone health. Here is a list of plant-based foods that are high in magnesium:

1. **Leafy Green Vegetables:**
    - Spinach
    - Swiss chard
    - Kale
    - Collard greens
    - Turnip greens
2. **Nuts and Seeds:**
    - Almonds
    - Cashews
    - Pumpkin seeds
    - Sunflower seeds
    - Flaxseeds
    - Chia seeds
3. **Whole Grains:**
    - Brown rice
    - Quinoa
    - Oats
    - Buckwheat
    - Barley
    - Whole wheat
4. **Legumes:**
    - Black beans
    - Chickpeas
    - Lentils
    - Kidney beans
    - Edamame
5. **Fruits:**
    - Bananas
    - Avocados
    - Figs
    - Prunes
    - Raisins

6. **Vegetables:**
    - Potatoes (with skin)
    - Sweet potatoes
    - Broccoli
    - Brussels sprouts
    - Zucchini
7. **Tofu:**
    - Tofu and other soy products can be good sources of magnesium.
8. **Dark Chocolate:**
    - Dark chocolate with a high cocoa content is not only a delicious treat but also contains magnesium.
9. **Whole Plant Foods:**
    - Eating a variety of whole, plant-based foods in your diet ensures a balanced intake of magnesium. Include a colorful array of fruits, vegetables, nuts, seeds, and whole grains to meet your nutritional needs.

It's important to note that the magnesium content in foods can vary based on factors such as soil quality and processing methods. Additionally, some plant-based foods contain compounds that may affect magnesium absorption. Consuming a diverse and balanced plant-based diet is key to obtaining not only magnesium but also a wide range of essential nutrients for overall health. If you have specific dietary concerns or health conditions, consider consulting with a healthcare professional or a registered dietitian.

Back to Table of Contents

Phosphorus

What is Phosphorus?

Phosphorus is a chemical element with the symbol P and atomic number 15. It is an essential mineral that plays critical roles in various biological processes within the human body. Phosphorus is the second most abundant mineral in the body, after calcium, and is primarily found in bones and teeth, where it provides structural support and strength. Some key functions of phosphorus include:

Bone and Teeth Health: Phosphorus is a major component of bone mineral hydroxyapatite, along with calcium. It contributes to bone density, strength, and rigidity, making it essential for bone formation and maintenance. Phosphorus is also present in tooth enamel, where it helps protect against decay and erosion.

Energy Metabolism: Phosphorus is a crucial component of adenosine triphosphate (ATP), the primary energy currency of cells. ATP is involved in various cellular processes that require energy, including muscle contraction, nerve transmission, and biochemical reactions involved in metabolism.

Cellular Structure and Function: Phosphorus is a key structural component of cell membranes, where it forms phospholipids, a type of lipid molecule. Phospholipids help maintain the integrity and fluidity of cell membranes and play roles in cell signaling, transport, and cell-to-cell communication.

DNA and RNA Synthesis: Phosphorus is an essential component of nucleic acids, including DNA (deoxyribonucleic acid) and RNA (ribonucleic acid). It forms the backbone of the nucleic acid molecules, providing structural stability and serving as a template for genetic information.

Buffering System: Phosphorus participates in the body's acid-base balance as a component of buffer systems, such as phosphate buffers. Buffer systems help maintain the pH (acidity or alkalinity) of bodily fluids within a narrow range, which is essential for proper cellular function and physiological processes.

Cellular Signaling and Communication: Phosphorus-containing molecules, such as phosphorylated proteins and second messengers like cyclic adenosine monophosphate (cAMP) and inositol triphosphate (IP3), play crucial roles in cellular signaling pathways. They regulate various cellular processes, including gene expression, enzyme activity, hormone secretion, and cell growth and differentiation.

Good dietary sources of phosphorus include dairy products (such as milk, cheese, and yogurt), meat, poultry, fish, eggs, nuts, seeds, legumes (such as beans and lentils), whole grains (such as wheat, oats, and barley), and fortified foods (such as breakfast cereals and beverages). Most people obtain an adequate amount of phosphorus through a balanced diet, and deficiencies are rare in healthy individuals. However, excessive phosphorus intake from phosphorus-rich processed foods and additives may contribute to health issues, particularly in individuals with kidney problems or certain medical conditions.

Plant-based foods high in Phosphorus

Phosphorus is an essential mineral that plays a crucial role in various bodily functions, including bone and teeth health, energy metabolism, and kidney function. While animal products are often rich sources of phosphorus, several plant-based foods also contain significant amounts of this essential nutrient. Here is a list of plant-based foods high in phosphorus:

1. **Sunflower Seeds:**
   - Sunflower seeds are not only a tasty snack but also a good source of phosphorus. They can be sprinkled on salads, yogurt, or enjoyed on their own.
2. **Pumpkin Seeds:**
   - Pumpkin seeds, also known as pepitas, are rich in phosphorus and make a nutritious addition to salads, granola, or trail mix.
3. **Soybeans:**
   - Soybeans and soy-based products, such as tofu and tempeh, contain significant amounts of phosphorus. Incorporate soy-based foods into your diet for a plant-based phosphorus boost.
4. **Lentils:**
   - Lentils are a versatile legume that provides not only protein and fiber but also phosphorus. They can be used in soups, stews, salads, or as a side dish.
5. **Chickpeas:**
   - Chickpeas, whether cooked and tossed into salads or blended into hummus, are a good plant-based source of phosphorus.
6. **Quinoa:**
   - Quinoa, a protein-rich pseudo-grain, contains phosphorus. It can be used as a base for salads, bowls, or served as a side dish.
7. **Nuts (Almonds, Cashews, Walnuts):**
   - Various nuts, including almonds, cashews, and walnuts, contain phosphorus. Enjoy them as a snack or incorporate them into your meals and desserts.
8. **Whole Grains (Brown Rice, Oats):**
   - Whole grains such as brown rice and oats provide not only complex carbohydrates but also phosphorus. They can be used in a variety of dishes, from breakfast porridge to savory meals.
9. **Spinach:**
   - Leafy greens like spinach contain phosphorus, along with other essential nutrients. Add spinach to salads, smoothies, or sauté it as a side dish.
10. **Broccoli:**

- Broccoli is a cruciferous vegetable that is not only rich in vitamins but also contains phosphorus. Include broccoli in stir-fries, salads, or as a side dish.

11. **Brussels Sprouts:**
    - Brussels sprouts are another cruciferous vegetable that contributes to your phosphorus intake. Roast or sauté them for a delicious side dish.
12. **Sweet Potatoes:**
    - Sweet potatoes provide not only a healthy dose of beta-carotene but also contain phosphorus. Bake or roast sweet potatoes for a nutritious side dish.

It's important to note that the phosphorus content in plant-based foods may vary, and factors like cooking methods can influence nutrient availability. Maintaining a well-balanced and varied plant-based diet can help ensure an adequate intake of essential nutrients, including phosphorus. If you have specific dietary concerns or conditions, it's advisable to consult with a healthcare professional or a registered dietitian.

Sodium

What is Sodium?

Sodium is a chemical element with the symbol Na and atomic number 11. It is an essential mineral that plays crucial roles in various physiological processes within the human body. Sodium is primarily known for its role in regulating fluid balance, blood pressure, and nerve function. Some key functions of sodium include:

Fluid Balance: Sodium is one of the main electrolytes in the body and plays a central role in maintaining fluid balance. It works in conjunction with other electrolytes, such as potassium and chloride, to regulate the distribution of water inside and outside of cells. Sodium helps maintain proper hydration levels and prevents dehydration by facilitating the movement of water across cell membranes through osmosis.

Blood Pressure Regulation: Sodium plays a key role in regulating blood pressure by controlling blood volume and fluid balance. It helps maintain the proper concentration of electrolytes in the blood and extracellular fluid, which influences blood volume and vascular tone. High sodium intake can lead to increased blood volume and fluid retention, raising blood pressure and increasing the risk of hypertension and cardiovascular disease.

Nerve Function: Sodium ions are essential for the generation and propagation of nerve impulses (action potentials) along nerve cells (neurons). When stimulated, sodium channels in the cell membrane open, allowing sodium ions to flow into the cell and depolarize the membrane. This depolarization triggers an action potential, which is transmitted along the length of the neuron to communicate signals between cells.

Muscle Contraction: Sodium ions also play a role in muscle contraction, particularly in skeletal muscle (voluntary muscle) and smooth muscle (involuntary muscle). During muscle contraction, sodium ions enter muscle cells, triggering the release of calcium ions from intracellular stores and initiating the contraction process.

Acid-Base Balance: Sodium bicarbonate ($NaHCO_3$) is an important buffer in the body that helps regulate acid-base balance. It acts as a base to neutralize excess acids in the blood and maintain the pH (acidity or alkalinity) within a narrow range. Sodium bicarbonate is produced by the kidneys and helps prevent acidosis (excess acidity) by removing hydrogen ions from the bloodstream.

Good dietary sources of sodium include table salt (sodium chloride), processed foods (such as canned soups, snack foods, condiments, and ready-to-eat meals), cured meats (such as bacon and ham), cheese, pickled foods, and restaurant meals. While sodium is essential for health, excessive sodium intake can have adverse effects on blood pressure and cardiovascular health. Therefore, it's important to consume sodium in moderation and to choose whole, unprocessed foods whenever possible.

Plant-based foods Contain Sodium

While excessive sodium intake is generally discouraged due to its association with health issues like high blood pressure, some plant-based foods naturally contain sodium. It's important to note that the sodium content in plant-based foods is typically lower compared to processed and animal-based products. Here are some plant-based foods that naturally contain sodium:

1. **Vegetables:**
    - Many vegetables contain small amounts of sodium. Examples include:
        - Spinach
        - Beets
        - Celery
        - Carrots
        - Tomatoes
2. **Legumes:**
    - Legumes are a good source of plant-based protein and may contain some sodium. Examples include:
        - Lentils
        - Chickpeas
        - Black beans
        - Kidney beans
3. **Whole Grains:**
    - Some whole grains naturally contain small amounts of sodium. Examples include:
        - Quinoa
        - Brown rice
        - Oats
4. **Nuts and Seeds:**
    - Nuts and seeds may contain trace amounts of sodium. Examples include:
        - Almonds
        - Sunflower seeds
        - Chia seeds
5. **Fruits:**
    - While fruits are generally low in sodium, certain fruits like avocados may contain small amounts.
6. **Seaweed:**
    - Seaweed, such as nori or dulse, naturally contains sodium due to its marine environment.
7. **Plant-Based Condiments:**
    - Some plant-based condiments and seasonings can contribute sodium to your diet. Examples include:
        - Soy sauce (choose low-sodium options if available)

- Tamari
- Miso paste
- Pickles

It's important to emphasize that while these plant-based foods contain some sodium, they are generally much lower in sodium than processed foods and animal products. For individuals aiming to reduce their sodium intake, focusing on a diet rich in whole, minimally processed plant-based foods is a recommended approach. Always consult with a healthcare professional or nutritionist for personalized dietary advice.

Potassium

What is Potassium?

Potassium is a chemical element with the symbol K and atomic number 19. It is an essential mineral that plays numerous critical roles in various physiological processes within the human body. Potassium is one of the most abundant electrolytes in the body and is primarily found inside cells, where it helps maintain fluid balance, regulate muscle function, and support nerve transmission. Some key functions of potassium include:

Fluid Balance: Potassium is a major intracellular cation and plays a crucial role in maintaining fluid balance inside cells. It works in conjunction with sodium, another electrolyte, to regulate osmotic pressure and water distribution across cell membranes. Potassium helps prevent cellular dehydration and maintains proper hydration levels, which is essential for cell function and overall health.

Nerve Function: Potassium is essential for nerve transmission and impulse conduction. It helps regulate the electrical excitability of nerve cells (neurons) by maintaining the resting membrane potential and repolarizing the cell membrane after an action potential. Potassium ions move across nerve cell membranes through specialized channels, contributing to the generation and propagation of nerve impulses.

Muscle Contraction: Potassium plays a crucial role in muscle function, including skeletal muscle (voluntary muscle) and smooth muscle (involuntary muscle). It helps regulate muscle contraction by controlling the resting membrane potential and action potential in muscle cells. Potassium ions flow into muscle cells during repolarization, allowing muscles to relax after contraction.

Heart Function: Potassium is essential for maintaining normal heart rhythm and function. It plays a key role in regulating the electrical activity of cardiac muscle cells (cardiomyocytes) and coordinating the contraction and relaxation of the heart muscle. Potassium ions contribute to the generation of action potentials in cardiac cells and help propagate electrical impulses throughout the heart, ensuring coordinated heartbeats.

Blood Pressure Regulation: Potassium helps regulate blood pressure by counteracting the effects of sodium on blood volume and vascular tone. High potassium intake can help lower blood pressure by promoting sodium excretion through the kidneys and relaxing blood vessel walls (vasodilation). Adequate potassium intake is associated with a reduced risk of hypertension and cardiovascular disease.

Good dietary sources of potassium include fruits (such as bananas, oranges, kiwi, and avocados), vegetables (such as potatoes, sweet potatoes, spinach, and broccoli), legumes (such as beans, lentils, and peas), nuts, seeds, whole grains, dairy products, and fish. Most people obtain adequate potassium through a balanced diet rich in fruits, vegetables, and whole foods. However, certain medical conditions, medications, and dietary factors can affect potassium levels in the body, so it's important to consult with a healthcare professional for personalized guidance on potassium intake and supplementation.

Plant-based foods high in Potassium

Potassium is an essential mineral that plays a crucial role in maintaining proper heart, muscle, and nerve function. Including potassium-rich foods in your diet is important for overall health. Here is a list of plant-based foods that are high in potassium:

1. **Bananas:**
    - Bananas are perhaps one of the most well-known potassium-rich fruits. They are convenient and make for a great portable snack.
2. **Sweet Potatoes:**
    - Sweet potatoes are not only delicious but also packed with potassium. Roasted, baked, or mashed, they offer a versatile and nutritious addition to your meals.
3. **Spinach:**
    - Dark leafy greens, such as spinach, are excellent sources of potassium. Whether eaten raw in salads or cooked in various dishes, spinach is a nutrient powerhouse.
4. **Avocado:**
    - Avocado is not only a good source of healthy fats but also contains a substantial amount of potassium. Enjoy it sliced on toast, in salads, or as guacamole.
5. **Oranges:**
    - Oranges and other citrus fruits like grapefruits and mandarins are not only rich in vitamin C but also provide a decent amount of potassium.
6. **Potatoes:**
    - Potatoes, whether white or sweet, are reliable sources of potassium. Be sure to eat the skin, as it contains additional nutrients.
7. **Beans and Lentils:**
    - Legumes, including kidney beans, black beans, lentils, and chickpeas, are excellent plant-based sources of potassium. They are also high in fiber and protein.
8. **Tomatoes and Tomato Products:**
    - Tomatoes, tomato sauce, and tomato paste are good sources of potassium. They can be included in a variety of dishes, from salads to sauces.
9. **Coconut Water:**
    - Coconut water is not only a hydrating beverage but also contains potassium. It's a natural and refreshing option to help meet your potassium needs.
10. **Mushrooms:**
    - Mushrooms, especially white button mushrooms and shiitake mushrooms, contain potassium and can be a tasty addition to various dishes.
11. **Cantaloupe:**

- Cantaloupe and other melons, such as honeydew, provide a sweet and hydrating way to increase potassium intake.

12. **Broccoli:**
    - Broccoli is a nutrient-rich vegetable that contains potassium along with vitamins, fiber, and other minerals.

Including a variety of these potassium-rich plant-based foods in your diet can contribute to maintaining a healthy balance of electrolytes and supporting overall well-being. As with any dietary changes, it's advisable to consult with a healthcare professional, especially if you have specific health concerns or conditions.

Chloride

What is Chloride?

Chloride is an essential mineral and an electrolyte that plays important roles in various physiological processes within the human body. It is an anion, meaning it carries a negative electrical charge, and is often found in the form of chloride ions (Cl-) dissolved in bodily fluids. Chloride is the major negatively charged ion in extracellular fluid, working in tandem with other electrolytes like sodium and potassium to maintain fluid balance, regulate pH, and support nerve function. Some key functions of chloride include:

Fluid Balance: Chloride ions help maintain the balance of fluids inside and outside of cells. Together with sodium, chloride regulates osmotic pressure and water distribution across cell membranes. This balance is critical for proper cell hydration and overall cellular function.

Acid-Base Balance: Chloride ions are involved in the body's acid-base balance, helping to regulate pH levels in bodily fluids. Chloride serves as a component of the bicarbonate buffer system, which helps neutralize excess acids or bases in the blood and maintain the body's pH within a narrow, optimal range.

Digestion: Chloride ions play a role in the production of hydrochloric acid (HCl) in the stomach. Hydrochloric acid is essential for the breakdown of food in the stomach, aiding in digestion and the absorption of nutrients such as proteins, minerals, and vitamins.

Nerve Function: Chloride ions contribute to the transmission of nerve impulses (action potentials) along nerve cells (neurons). They help maintain the resting membrane potential and regulate the excitability of nerve cells, influencing nerve signaling and communication throughout the nervous system.

Electrolyte Balance: Chloride ions, along with sodium and potassium, help maintain the balance of electrolytes in the body. These electrolytes play critical roles in cellular function, muscle contraction, nerve transmission, and fluid balance, among other physiological processes.

Good dietary sources of chloride include table salt (sodium chloride), seaweed, olives, celery, tomatoes, lettuce, and other vegetables. Chloride is also present in many processed foods, as salt (sodium chloride) is commonly used as a flavoring and preservative. Most people obtain adequate chloride through their diet, and deficiencies are rare in healthy individuals. However, excessive intake of sodium chloride (salt) can contribute to health issues such as high blood pressure and cardiovascular disease, so it's important to consume salt in moderation and to focus on a balanced diet rich in whole, unprocessed foods.

Plant-based foods Contain Chloride

Plant-based foods that contain chloride include:

1. **Celery:** Celery is a crunchy vegetable that contains a moderate amount of chloride.
2. **Tomatoes:** Tomatoes are a versatile fruit (often consumed as a vegetable) that contain chloride.
3. **Lettuce:** Various types of lettuce, such as romaine, iceberg, and leaf lettuce, contain chloride.
4. **Olives:** Olives, whether green or black, are a source of chloride.
5. **Seaweed:** Certain types of seaweed, such as nori, kombu also known as Kelp, and wakame, contain chloride.
6. **Spinach:** Spinach is a leafy green vegetable that contains chloride, among other nutrients.
7. **Swiss Chard:** Swiss chard, a leafy green vegetable similar to spinach, contains chloride.
8. **Kale:** Kale, a nutrient-rich leafy green vegetable, contains chloride.
9. **Arugula:** Arugula, also known as rocket or rucola, contains chloride and other essential nutrients.
10. **Cabbage:** Various types of cabbage, including green cabbage, red cabbage, and Napa cabbage, contain chloride.

These plant-based foods provide a variety of essential nutrients, including chloride, as part of a balanced diet. Incorporating a diverse range of fruits, vegetables, whole grains, legumes, nuts, and seeds into meals can help ensure adequate intake of essential minerals like chloride, along with other vitamins, minerals, fiber, and phytonutrients.

Iron

What is Iron?

Iron is a crucial mineral that plays a vital role in various physiological processes within the human body. It is classified as a trace mineral because the body requires it in relatively small amounts compared to other nutrients, but its importance cannot be overstated. Iron is essential for the formation of hemoglobin, a protein found in red blood cells that is responsible for transporting oxygen from the lungs to the rest of the body's tissues and organs. Additionally, iron is a key component of myoglobin, a protein found in muscles that helps store and transport oxygen for muscle function.

There are two main forms of dietary iron: heme iron and non-heme iron. Heme iron is found in animal-based foods, such as meat, poultry, and fish, and is more easily absorbed by the body. Non-heme iron is found in plant-based foods, such as beans, lentils, fortified grains, and leafy green vegetables, but it is not as readily absorbed by the body as heme iron.

Iron deficiency is one of the most common nutritional deficiencies worldwide and can lead to a condition known as iron deficiency anemia. Symptoms of iron deficiency anemia may include fatigue, weakness, pale skin, shortness of breath, dizziness, headaches, and cold hands and feet. It is particularly prevalent among pregnant women, infants, young children, adolescents, menstruating individuals, and individuals following vegetarian or vegan diets.

To prevent iron deficiency, it is important to consume an adequate amount of iron-rich foods in your diet. Additionally, consuming vitamin C-rich foods alongside iron-rich foods can enhance the absorption of non-heme iron. In cases of severe iron deficiency or anemia, supplementation with iron supplements may be necessary under the guidance of a healthcare professional.

In summary, iron is an essential mineral that plays a critical role in oxygen transport, energy production, and overall health. Consuming a balanced diet that includes iron-rich foods is essential for preventing iron deficiency and maintaining optimal health and well-being.

Plant-based foods high in Iron

Iron is also involved in energy metabolism, DNA synthesis, and the production of neurotransmitters. Some key benefits of iron are Oxygen Transport, Energy Metabolism, Immune Function, Cognitive Function, Muscle Function, Healthy Pregnancy, Healthy Skin, Hair and Nails.

Here is a list of plant-based foods that are high in iron:

1. **Legumes:**

- Lentils
- Chickpeas (garbanzo beans)
- Black beans
- Kidney beans
- Soybeans (including tofu and tempeh)
- Peas (green peas, split peas)

2. **Leafy Greens:**
    - Spinach
    - Kale
    - Swiss chard
    - Collard greens
    - Beet greens
3. **Seeds:**
    - Pumpkin seeds (pepitas)
    - Sesame seeds (including tahini)
    - Hemp seeds
    - Flaxseeds
4. **Nuts:**
    - Cashews
    - Pine nuts
    - Almonds
    - Pistachios
5. **Whole Grains:**
    - Quinoa
    - Oats (including oatmeal)
    - Brown rice
    - Amaranth
    - Buckwheat
6. **Fortified Foods:**
    - Fortified breakfast cereals
    - Fortified plant-based milk (such as almond milk, soy milk, or oat milk)
    - Fortified tofu
7. **Dried Fruits:**
    - Apricots
    - Raisins
    - Prunes
    - Dates
8. **Herbs and Spices:**
    - Thyme
    - Cumin

- Parsley
- Turmeric
- Coriander

Incorporating these iron-rich plant-based foods into your diet can help meet your daily iron needs and support overall health. Pairing iron-rich foods with sources of vitamin C can enhance iron absorption, so consider including citrus fruits, bell peppers, strawberries, or tomatoes in your meals to maximize iron absorption. Additionally, soaking, sprouting, fermenting, or cooking certain plant-based foods can help improve the bioavailability of iron. If you have concerns about your iron intake or suspect iron deficiency, consult with a healthcare professional for personalized advice.

Zinc

What is Zinc?

Zinc is an essential mineral that is vital for numerous physiological functions in the human body. It plays a crucial role in various enzymatic reactions, immune function, protein synthesis, wound healing, DNA synthesis, and cell division. Zinc is classified as a trace mineral, meaning that the body requires only small amounts of it for optimal health, but its importance cannot be understated.

One of the primary functions of zinc is its role as a cofactor for over 300 enzymes involved in various biochemical processes. These enzymes are involved in tasks such as metabolism, digestion, and the synthesis of DNA and proteins. Zinc also plays a key role in maintaining the integrity of cell membranes and supporting the function of the immune system, helping to defend the body against infections and diseases.

Zinc deficiency is relatively common, particularly in populations with inadequate dietary intake or impaired absorption of zinc. Symptoms of zinc deficiency may include impaired growth and development, delayed wound healing, hair loss, skin rashes, loss of appetite, and weakened immune function. Severe zinc deficiency can lead to more serious health problems, including immune system dysfunction and impaired neurological function.

Good dietary sources of zinc include meat, poultry, seafood (especially oysters), dairy products, nuts, seeds, and whole grains. Plant-based sources of zinc, such as legumes and grains, contain phytates, which can inhibit the absorption of zinc. However, soaking, sprouting, or fermenting these foods can help reduce phytate levels and enhance zinc absorption.

In some cases, supplementation with zinc may be necessary to address deficiency or support specific health conditions. However, excessive intake of zinc can lead to adverse effects, including nausea, vomiting, diarrhea, and impaired immune function. Therefore, it's important to consult with a healthcare professional before starting any zinc supplementation regimen.

In conclusion, zinc is an essential mineral that plays a vital role in numerous physiological processes in the body. Consuming a balanced diet that includes zinc-rich foods is crucial for maintaining optimal health and well-being, while supplementation may be necessary in cases of deficiency or certain health conditions, under the guidance of a healthcare professional.

Plant-based foods high in Zinc

Zinc is an essential mineral that plays a crucial role in various physiological processes, including immune function, wound healing, and DNA synthesis. While animal products like meat and seafood are rich sources of zinc, there are also several plant-based foods that provide this important nutrient. Here are some plant-based foods that are relatively high in zinc:

Legumes:

1. **Chickpeas (Garbanzo Beans):** Chickpeas are an excellent source of zinc, providing approximately 2.5 milligrams of zinc per 1 cup serving when cooked. They are versatile legumes commonly used in salads, stews, curries, and hummus.
2. **Lentils:** Lentils are rich in zinc, offering around 2 milligrams of zinc per 1 cup serving when cooked. They come in various colors, including green, brown, red, and black, and can be used in soups, stews, salads, and side dishes.
3. **Black Beans:** Black beans contain a moderate amount of zinc, providing approximately 1.8 milligrams of zinc per 1 cup serving when cooked. They are commonly used in Latin American, Caribbean, and Tex-Mex cuisines, in dishes such as black bean soup, burritos, and salads.
4. **Kidney Beans:** Kidney beans are another legume with a decent zinc content, offering around 1.5 milligrams of zinc per 1 cup serving when cooked. They are often used in chili, bean salads, bean dips, and casseroles.
5. **White Beans (Navy Beans/Cannellini Beans):** White beans are relatively high in zinc, providing approximately 1.4 milligrams of zinc per 1 cup serving when cooked. They have a mild flavor and creamy texture, making them suitable for soups, stews, casseroles, and salads.
6. **Adzuki Beans:** Adzuki beans contain a moderate amount of zinc, offering approximately 1.2 milligrams of zinc per 1 cup serving when cooked. They are commonly used in Asian cuisine, particularly in sweet red bean paste for desserts, as well as in savory dishes like soups and stews.
7. **Soybeans (Edamame):** Soybeans are rich in zinc, providing approximately 1.1 milligrams of zinc per 1 cup serving when cooked. They are used to make various soy products, including tofu, tempeh, soy milk, and edamame, and are also used in Asian dishes such as stir-fries and salads.

Seeds:

1. **Pumpkin Seeds (Pepitas):** Pumpkin seeds are one of the best plant-based sources of zinc. They provide approximately 7.5 milligrams of zinc per 1 ounce (28 grams) serving. Pumpkin seeds are versatile and can be enjoyed roasted as a snack, added to salads, soups, granola, or used as a topping for yogurt or oatmeal.
2. **Hemp Seeds:** Hemp seeds are rich in zinc, providing around 5 milligrams of zinc per 3 tablespoon serving. These nutritious seeds have a slightly nutty flavor and can be sprinkled on salads, blended into smoothies, or incorporated into baked goods like bread and muffins.
3. **Sesame Seeds:** Sesame seeds contain a good amount of zinc, offering approximately 2.8 milligrams of zinc per 1 ounce (28 grams) serving. They are commonly used in Asian, Middle Eastern, and Mediterranean cuisines to add flavor and texture to dishes like tahini (sesame seed paste), hummus, salads, stir-fries, and baked goods.
4. **Sunflower Seeds:** Sunflower seeds are a decent source of zinc, providing around 1.5 milligrams of zinc per 1 ounce (28 grams) serving. They can be enjoyed roasted as a snack, added to salads, trail mix, granola, or used as a garnish for soups and stir-fries.
5. **Flaxseeds:** Flaxseeds contain a moderate amount of zinc, offering approximately 1.2 milligrams of zinc per 2 tablespoon serving. These tiny seeds are rich in omega-3 fatty acids and fiber, and they can be ground and added to smoothies, yogurt, oatmeal, or used in baking recipes like bread, muffins, and cookies.
6. **Chia Seeds:** Chia seeds contain a small amount of zinc, providing around 1 milligram of zinc per 1 ounce (28 grams) serving. These nutritious seeds are high in fiber, protein, and omega-3 fatty acids, and they can be soaked in water or milk to make chia pudding, added to smoothies, yogurt, oatmeal, or used as an egg substitute in baking.

Nuts:

1. **Cashews:** Cashews are one of the best plant-based sources of zinc among nuts. They provide approximately 1.6 milligrams of zinc per 1 ounce (28 grams) serving. Cashews are creamy and versatile, making them a popular snack on their own or used in recipes like cashew cheese, sauces, and desserts.
2. **Pine Nuts:** Pine nuts contain a good amount of zinc, offering approximately 1.3 milligrams of zinc per 1 ounce (28 grams) serving. They have a sweet, buttery flavor and are commonly used in Mediterranean and Middle Eastern cuisines in dishes like pesto, salads, pilafs, and baked goods.
3. **Almonds:** Almonds are a decent source of zinc, providing around 0.9 milligrams of zinc per 1 ounce (28 grams) serving. They are crunchy and nutritious, making them a popular snack and ingredient in recipes like almond butter, almond milk, granola, and baked goods.
4. **Brazil Nuts:** Brazil nuts contain a moderate amount of zinc, offering approximately 0.8 milligrams of zinc per 1 ounce (28 grams) serving. They are also rich in selenium, another essential mineral with antioxidant properties. Brazil nuts have a rich, creamy flavor and can be enjoyed on their own or added to trail mix, salads, and desserts.

5. **Pecans:** Pecans contain a small amount of zinc, providing around 0.7 milligrams of zinc per 1 ounce (28 grams) serving. They have a sweet, buttery flavor and are commonly used in baked goods like pies, cookies, and bars, as well as salads and savory dishes.

Whole Grains:

1. **Wheat Germ:** Wheat germ is one of the best whole grain sources of zinc. It provides approximately 4.7 milligrams of zinc per 100 grams. Wheat germ can be sprinkled on yogurt, oatmeal, or smoothies, or used as an ingredient in baked goods like bread, muffins, and pancakes.
2. **Quinoa:** Quinoa contains a decent amount of zinc, providing around 2 milligrams of zinc per 100 grams. It is a versatile whole grain that can be used as a base for salads, pilafs, stir-fries, and breakfast porridge. Quinoa is also gluten-free and high in protein, making it a popular choice among health-conscious individuals.
3. **Oats:** Oats contain a moderate amount of zinc, offering approximately 3 milligrams of zinc per 100 grams. They are a nutritious whole grain that can be enjoyed as oatmeal, granola, overnight oats, or added to baked goods like cookies, bread, and muffins.
4. **Brown Rice:** Brown rice contains a small amount of zinc, providing around 1.2 milligrams of zinc per 100 grams. It is a whole grain alternative to white rice and can be used in various dishes, including stir-fries, pilafs, casseroles, and sushi rolls.
5. **Barley:** Barley contains a modest amount of zinc, offering approximately 1.1 milligrams of zinc per 100 grams. It is commonly used in soups, stews, salads, and risottos, and can also be ground into flour for baking or used as a substitute for rice or pasta.

Tofu: Tofu, made from **soybeans**, is a good source of zinc. It is also a versatile ingredient that can be used in a variety of dishes, including stir-fries, soups, and sandwiches.

Tempeh: Tempeh, another soy-based product, is high in zinc. It is a fermented food that offers protein, probiotics, and other nutrients along with zinc.

Vegetables: Some vegetables contain small amounts of zinc, although they are not as high as other plant-based foods. Examples include **spinach, kale, peas**, and **Brussels sprouts**. While these vegetables may not be significant sources of zinc individually, they can contribute to overall zinc intake when consumed regularly as part of a balanced diet.

Incorporating a variety of these plant-based foods into meals and snacks can help individuals following a vegetarian or vegan diet meet their zinc requirements. It's important to note that plant-based sources of zinc may have lower bioavailability compared to animal sources, so consuming a diverse range of zinc-rich foods and including sources of vitamin C, which enhances zinc absorption, can help optimize zinc intake from plant-based sources.

Back to Table of Contents

Copper

What is Copper?

Copper is an essential trace mineral that plays a crucial role in various physiological processes within the human body. It is involved in the formation of red blood cells, maintenance of connective tissues, energy production, and functioning of the nervous and immune systems. Copper is also a cofactor for several enzymes involved in antioxidant defense, iron metabolism, and the synthesis of neurotransmitters and collagen.

One of the primary functions of copper is its role in the synthesis of hemoglobin, the protein in red blood cells that carries oxygen from the lungs to the body's tissues and organs. Copper is also involved in the production of collagen and elastin, which are essential for the formation and maintenance of connective tissues, such as bones, cartilage, and skin.

In addition to its structural and enzymatic roles, copper plays a key role in antioxidant defense. Copper-containing enzymes, such as superoxide dismutase (SOD), help neutralize harmful free radicals and protect cells from oxidative damage. This antioxidant activity is essential for maintaining cellular health and reducing the risk of chronic diseases associated with oxidative stress, such as cardiovascular disease, cancer, and neurodegenerative disorders.

Copper deficiency is relatively rare but can occur in individuals with inadequate dietary intake, malabsorption disorders, or excessive zinc intake, which can interfere with copper absorption. Symptoms of copper deficiency may include anemia, fatigue, weakness, impaired immune function, bone abnormalities, and neurological disturbances.

On the other hand, excessive intake of copper can lead to toxicity, resulting in symptoms such as nausea, vomiting, diarrhea, abdominal pain, liver damage, and neurological symptoms. Chronic copper toxicity can also lead to Wilson's disease, a rare genetic disorder characterized by the accumulation of copper in the liver, brain, and other organs.

Good dietary sources of copper include organ meats (such as liver), shellfish (such as oysters and crab), nuts, seeds, whole grains, legumes, and dark leafy greens. Consuming a balanced diet that includes copper-rich foods is essential for maintaining optimal health and well-being.

In summary, copper is an essential trace mineral that plays a crucial role in numerous physiological processes within the body. Consuming a balanced diet that includes copper-rich foods is important for ensuring adequate intake of this vital nutrient and supporting overall health and well-being. However, excessive intake of copper should be avoided to prevent toxicity and adverse health effects.

Plant-based foods high in Copper

While copper is predominantly found in animal-based foods like liver and shellfish, several plant-based foods also contain significant amounts of this mineral. Here is a list of plant-based foods that are high in copper:

1. **Nuts and Seeds:**
    - Sunflower seeds
    - Sesame seeds
    - Pumpkin seeds (Pepitas)
    - Cashews
    - Almonds
    - Pine nuts
    - Hemp seeds
    - Flaxseeds
2. **Legumes:**
    - Lentils
    - Chickpeas (Garbanzo beans)
    - Soybeans
    - Black beans
    - Lima beans
    - Navy beans
    - Pinto beans
3. **Whole Grains:**
    - Quinoa
    - Buckwheat
    - Oats
    - Barley
    - Brown rice
    - Wild rice
4. **Leafy Greens and Vegetables:**
    - Spinach
    - Kale
    - Swiss chard
    - Asparagus
    - Mushrooms (especially shiitake mushrooms)
    - Sweet potatoes
    - Avocado
5. **Dried Fruits:**
    - Dried apricots
    - Prunes (Dried plums)
    - Raisins

- Dates

6. **Cocoa and Dark Chocolate:**
    - Cocoa powder
    - Dark chocolate (with high cocoa content)
7. **Tofu:**
    - Firm tofu
    - Silken tofu
8. **Whole Grains:**
    - Whole wheat
    - Spelt
    - Millet

Incorporating these plant-based foods into your diet can help ensure an adequate intake of copper, supporting overall health and well-being. It's essential to consume a variety of nutrient-rich foods to meet your body's copper requirements and maintain optimal health.

Selenium

What is Selenium?

Selenium is a trace mineral that is essential for human health. It acts primarily as an antioxidant, helping to protect cells from damage caused by free radicals and oxidative stress. Selenium is also involved in various physiological processes, including thyroid function, immune system regulation, and reproduction.

One of the key functions of selenium is its role in the production of selenoproteins, a group of proteins that contain selenium in the form of the amino acid selenocysteine. These selenoproteins play important roles in antioxidant defense, thyroid hormone metabolism, DNA synthesis and repair, and immune function.

As an antioxidant, selenium helps neutralize harmful free radicals and reduce oxidative stress, which can damage cells and contribute to chronic diseases such as heart disease, cancer, and neurodegenerative disorders. Selenium works in concert with other antioxidants, such as vitamin E, to protect cells and tissues from oxidative damage.

Selenium is also important for thyroid function, as it is required for the conversion of the inactive thyroid hormone thyroxine (T4) to the active form triiodothyronine (T3). Adequate selenium levels are essential for maintaining proper thyroid hormone levels and supporting metabolic function, energy production, and overall health.

In addition, selenium plays a role in immune system regulation by modulating inflammation and promoting immune cell function. It helps regulate the production of cytokines, which are signaling molecules involved in the immune response, and supports the activity of white blood cells, which are responsible for fighting off infections and pathogens.

Selenium deficiency is relatively rare in healthy individuals, as selenium is widely distributed in foods and is present in trace amounts in many soils. However, certain factors, such as poor dietary intake, gastrointestinal disorders, and soil depletion, can increase the risk of deficiency. Symptoms of selenium deficiency may include fatigue, weakness, hair loss, poor immune function, and cognitive impairment.

Conversely, excessive intake of selenium can lead to toxicity, known as selenosis, which can cause symptoms such as nausea, vomiting, diarrhea, hair loss, brittle nails, and neurological abnormalities. Chronic selenium toxicity can also lead to more serious health problems, including liver and kidney damage.

Good dietary sources of selenium include seafood (such as fish, shellfish, and seaweed), Brazil nuts, organ meats (such as liver and kidney), whole grains, eggs, poultry, and dairy products. Consuming a balanced diet that includes selenium-rich foods is important for maintaining optimal selenium levels and supporting overall health and well-being.

In summary, selenium is an essential trace mineral that plays important roles in antioxidant defense, thyroid function, immune regulation, and overall health. Consuming a varied diet that includes selenium-rich foods is essential for ensuring adequate selenium intake and supporting optimal health and well-being. However, excessive intake of selenium should be avoided to prevent toxicity and adverse health effects.

Plant-based foods high in Selenium

Selenium is an essential mineral that plays a critical role in various bodily functions, including thyroid function, antioxidant defense, and immune system health. While selenium is primarily found in animal-based foods like seafood, there are several plant-based sources available. Here are some plant-based foods high in selenium:

1. **Brazil Nuts:**
    - Brazil nuts are one of the richest sources of selenium. Just one or two nuts can provide your daily recommended intake of selenium.
2. **Sunflower Seeds:**
    - Sunflower seeds are a nutritious snack and a good source of selenium. They can be enjoyed on their own, added to salads, or incorporated into baked goods.
3. **Chia Seeds:**
    - Chia seeds are not only high in fiber and omega-3 fatty acids but also contain selenium. They can be added to smoothies, yogurt, oatmeal, or used as an egg substitute in baking.
4. **Flaxseeds:**
    - Flaxseeds are rich in alpha-linolenic acid (ALA) and also contain selenium. They can be ground and added to baked goods, sprinkled over salads, or mixed into smoothies.
5. **Mushrooms (especially Shiitake Mushrooms):**
    - Certain varieties of mushrooms, such as shiitake mushrooms, contain selenium. Incorporating mushrooms into stir-fries, soups, or pasta dishes can boost your selenium intake.
6. **Whole Grains (especially Whole Wheat Bread and Brown Rice):**
    - Whole grains like whole wheat bread, brown rice, oats, and barley contain small amounts of selenium. Enjoying whole grain foods as part of your meals can contribute to your selenium intake.
7. **Legumes (especially Lentils and Chickpeas):**
    - Legumes such as lentils, chickpeas, and kidney beans contain selenium. They are versatile ingredients that can be used in soups, stews, salads, or as a base for vegetarian patties or burgers.
8. **Spinach:**

- Spinach is a nutrient-rich leafy green vegetable that contains selenium. Enjoy spinach raw in salads, cooked in stir-fries, soups, or as a side dish.

Incorporating these plant-based foods high in selenium into your diet can help ensure you meet your daily selenium needs and support overall health and wellbeing. Remember to consume a varied and balanced diet to obtain a wide range of essential nutrients.

Iodine

What is Iodine?

Iodine is a chemical element that is essential for human health. It is primarily known for its role in the production of thyroid hormones, which are critical for regulating metabolism, growth, and development. The human body does not produce iodine on its own, so it must be obtained from dietary sources.

The thyroid gland, located in the neck, absorbs iodine from the bloodstream and uses it to produce thyroid hormones, primarily thyroxine (T4) and triiodothyronine (T3). These hormones play a crucial role in regulating various metabolic processes, including energy production, temperature regulation, heart rate, and digestion. They are also important for proper growth and development, particularly during infancy and childhood.

Iodine deficiency can lead to inadequate production of thyroid hormones, resulting in a condition known as hypothyroidism. Symptoms of hypothyroidism may include fatigue, weight gain, cold intolerance, dry skin, hair loss, constipation, and cognitive impairment. Severe iodine deficiency during pregnancy can also lead to developmental abnormalities in the fetus, including intellectual disabilities and impaired growth.

To prevent iodine deficiency, it is important to consume an adequate amount of iodine-rich foods in the diet. Good dietary sources of iodine include iodized salt, seafood (such as fish, shellfish, and seaweed), dairy products, eggs, and fortified foods. In regions where iodine deficiency is common, iodine supplementation may be recommended, particularly for pregnant women and infants.

While iodine deficiency is a concern in certain parts of the world, excessive iodine intake can also have adverse health effects. Chronic excessive intake of iodine, known as iodine toxicity, can lead to thyroid dysfunction, autoimmune thyroid disease, and other health problems. Therefore, it is important to consume iodine in moderation and avoid excessive intake from supplements or iodine-rich foods.

In summary, iodine is an essential mineral that plays a critical role in thyroid function and overall health. Consuming a balanced diet that includes iodine-rich foods is important for preventing iodine deficiency and supporting optimal thyroid function. However, excessive intake of iodine should be avoided to prevent adverse health effects.

Plant-based foods Contain Iodine

While iodine is most commonly associated with seafood and dairy products, there are some plant-based sources available. Here are some plant-based foods that are relatively high in iodine:

1. **Seaweed (Nori, Kelp, Wakame, Dulse):**
   - Seaweed is one of the richest sources of iodine, with some varieties containing exceptionally high levels. Nori, commonly used in sushi rolls, and kelp are particularly iodine-rich. Seaweed can be incorporated into soups, salads, stir-fries, or used as a seasoning in dishes.
2. **Iodized Salt:**
   - Some brands of table salt are fortified with iodine to help prevent iodine deficiency. Using iodized salt in cooking or seasoning food can contribute to your iodine intake.
3. **Potatoes (with skin):**
   - Potatoes, especially when consumed with the skin, contain moderate levels of iodine. Enjoy baked potatoes, mashed potatoes, or roasted potatoes as part of your meals to add a source of iodine.
4. **Cranberries:**
   - Cranberries are a good source of iodine and can be enjoyed fresh, dried, or in juice form. They can be added to salads, smoothies, oatmeal, or used to make sauces and jams.
5. **Strawberries:**
   - Strawberries contain small amounts of iodine and can be enjoyed fresh as a snack or added to salads, yogurt, smoothies, or desserts.
6. **Organic Soy Products:**
   - Some organic soy products, such as tofu and soy milk, may contain higher levels of iodine compared to conventional varieties. Incorporating organic soy products into your diet can provide a source of iodine.
7. **Lima Beans:**
   - Lima beans are a legume rich in various nutrients, including iodine. Enjoy lima beans cooked and added to soups, stews, salads, or served as a side dish.
8. **Prunes:**
   - Prunes, also known as dried plums, contain small amounts of iodine and can be enjoyed as a snack or added to baked goods, salads, or oatmeal.

While these plant-based foods can contribute to iodine intake, it's essential to consume them as part of a balanced diet to ensure adequate nutrition. If you have specific concerns about iodine intake, consult with a healthcare professional or registered dietitian for personalized advice.

Manganese

What is Manganese?

Manganese is an essential trace mineral that plays a vital role in numerous physiological processes within the human body. It is required for the functioning of various enzymes and is involved in processes such as metabolism, bone formation, wound healing, and the synthesis of connective tissues. Manganese also acts as an antioxidant, helping to protect cells from oxidative stress and damage caused by free radicals.

One of the primary functions of manganese is its role as a cofactor for several enzymes involved in carbohydrate, amino acid, and lipid metabolism. These enzymes help convert food into energy and support the proper functioning of various metabolic pathways in the body.

Manganese is also important for bone health, as it is involved in the formation and maintenance of healthy bones and cartilage. It helps stimulate the production of osteoblasts, the cells responsible for building new bone tissue, and plays a role in the synthesis of collagen, a protein that provides structural support to bones and other connective tissues.

In addition, manganese is essential for the synthesis of glycosaminoglycans (GAGs), a type of carbohydrate molecule found in connective tissues such as cartilage, tendons, and ligaments. GAGs help maintain the structure and function of these tissues and are important for joint health and mobility.

Manganese also acts as an antioxidant, helping to neutralize harmful free radicals and protect cells from oxidative damage. It works in concert with other antioxidants, such as vitamin C, vitamin E, and selenium, to maintain cellular health and reduce the risk of chronic diseases associated with oxidative stress, such as cardiovascular disease, cancer, and neurodegenerative disorders.

While manganese deficiency is relatively rare, it can occur in individuals with certain medical conditions, such as malabsorption disorders or liver disease, or in those with poor dietary intake. Symptoms of manganese deficiency may include impaired growth and development, skeletal abnormalities, reproductive issues, and neurological symptoms.

On the other hand, excessive intake of manganese can lead to toxicity, known as manganism, which can cause symptoms such as tremors, muscle stiffness, cognitive impairment, and psychiatric disturbances. Chronic manganese toxicity is rare and is more commonly associated with occupational exposure, such as in industries involving mining or welding.

Good dietary sources of manganese include nuts, seeds, whole grains, legumes, leafy green vegetables, tea, and pineapple. Consuming a balanced diet that includes manganese-rich foods is important for ensuring adequate manganese intake and supporting overall health and well-being.

Plant-based foods high in Manganese

Manganese is an essential mineral that is naturally present in many foods and is also found in the environment, including soil, water, and air. It is considered a trace mineral because the body requires it in small amounts, but it plays a crucial role in various physiological processes, including metabolism, bone health, and antioxidant defense. Here are some plant-based foods that are high in manganese:

1. **Nuts and Seeds:**
    - Pumpkin seeds
    - Sesame seeds
    - Sunflower seeds
    - Pine nuts
    - Almonds
    - Pecans
    - Walnuts
2. **Whole Grains:**
    - Brown rice
    - Quinoa
    - Oats
    - Barley
    - Buckwheat
    - Spelt
    - Amaranth
3. **Legumes:**
    - Soybeans
    - Lentils
    - Chickpeas (garbanzo beans)
    - Black beans
    - Lima beans
    - Navy beans

- Pinto beans

4. **Leafy Green Vegetables:**
    - Spinach
    - Kale
    - Swiss chard
    - Collard greens
    - Beet greens
    - Mustard greens
    - Turnip greens
5. **Other Vegetables:**
    - Sweet potatoes
    - Peas
    - Brussels sprouts
    - Broccoli
    - Cauliflower
    - Green beans
    - Asparagus
6. **Fruits:**
    - Pineapple
    - Raspberries
    - Strawberries
    - Blueberries
    - Avocado
    - Bananas
    - Kiwi

Incorporating these plant-based foods into your diet can help ensure an adequate intake of manganese, supporting overall health and wellbeing. Remember to consume a varied and balanced diet to obtain a wide range of essential nutrients.

Back to Table of Contents

What is Fluoride?

Fluoride is a naturally occurring mineral found in water, soil, rocks, and various foods. It is also commonly added to drinking water, toothpaste, and dental products for its dental health benefits. Fluoride plays a crucial role in dental health by helping to prevent tooth decay and cavities.

When fluoride is consumed, it becomes incorporated into the structure of tooth enamel, the outer layer of the teeth. Fluoride helps strengthen tooth enamel and makes it more resistant to acid erosion caused by bacteria and sugars in the mouth. This protective effect helps prevent the formation of cavities and slows down the progression of existing dental decay.

In addition to its topical benefits when applied directly to the teeth, fluoride also has systemic effects when ingested. Drinking fluoridated water or consuming foods and beverages containing fluoride can help provide systemic protection against tooth decay by increasing the fluoride concentration in saliva and dental plaque.

Fluoride is particularly beneficial during childhood when teeth are developing and becoming more susceptible to decay. The Centers for Disease Control and Prevention (CDC) and the American Dental Association (ADA) recommend community water fluoridation as one of the most effective and cost-effective public health measures for preventing dental caries.

While fluoride is generally considered safe and effective for preventing tooth decay when used appropriately, excessive fluoride intake can lead to potential side effects and adverse health effects. Some of the side effects of fluoride include:

1. Dental fluorosis: Dental fluorosis is a condition characterized by changes in the appearance of tooth enamel, such as white or brown discoloration, mottling, or pitting. Dental fluorosis typically occurs during tooth development in childhood and is more common when children consume excessive amounts of fluoride from multiple sources, such as fluoridated water, toothpaste, and supplements.
2. Skeletal fluorosis: Skeletal fluorosis is a bone disorder that occurs due to excessive accumulation of fluoride in the bones. In mild cases, skeletal fluorosis may cause stiffness and joint pain, while severe cases can lead to skeletal deformities, decreased bone density, and an increased risk of fractures. Skeletal fluorosis is more commonly associated with long-term exposure to high levels of fluoride, particularly from drinking water with naturally high fluoride levels.
3. Thyroid dysfunction: Some research suggests that excessive fluoride intake may interfere with thyroid function and contribute to thyroid dysfunction, including hypothyroidism (underactive thyroid) or hyperthyroidism (overactive thyroid). However, more studies are needed to fully understand the relationship between fluoride exposure and thyroid health.
4. Neurological effects: Some studies have suggested a potential link between fluoride exposure and adverse effects on neurological development and cognitive function, particularly in children. However, the evidence is limited and conflicting, and further research is needed to determine the potential neurological effects of fluoride exposure.

5. Allergic reactions: In rare cases, individuals may experience allergic reactions or skin irritation in response to fluoride-containing dental products, such as toothpaste or mouthwash. Symptoms may include rash, itching, swelling, or difficulty breathing. If you experience any allergic reactions to fluoride products, discontinue use and consult with a healthcare professional.

It's important to note that the risk of experiencing adverse effects from fluoride is generally low when fluoride-containing products are used appropriately and as directed. Additionally, the benefits of fluoride in preventing tooth decay and promoting dental health typically outweigh the potential risks, especially when fluoride exposure is carefully monitored.

In addition to its dental health benefits, fluoride has also been shown to have positive effects on bone health. Fluoride helps increase bone density and reduce the risk of osteoporosis and fractures, particularly in older adults.

Overall, fluoride is an important mineral for maintaining dental health and preventing tooth decay. It can be obtained from fluoridated water, fluoride-containing dental products, and certain foods and beverages. However, it's important to use fluoride-containing products as directed and to consult with a dentist or healthcare provider about appropriate fluoride intake, especially for young children.

Plant-based foods Contain Fluoride

Fluoride is a mineral that occurs naturally in various foods and water sources, although the levels can vary significantly depending on factors such as soil composition and water fluoridation practices. While fluoride is most commonly associated with dental health, it also plays a role in bone health and preventing tooth decay. Here are some plant-based foods that contain fluoride:

1. **Tea:**
    - Tea leaves naturally accumulate fluoride from the soil, particularly green and black tea. Drinking tea, whether hot or cold, can contribute to fluoride intake.
2. **Spinach:**
    - Spinach is a leafy green vegetable that contains some fluoride, albeit in lower amounts compared to tea. Including spinach in salads, soups, stir-fries, or smoothies can provide a modest amount of fluoride.
3. **Kale:**
    - Kale, another leafy green vegetable, contains small amounts of fluoride. Enjoy kale raw in salads, sautéed as a side dish, or blended into smoothies.
4. **Cabbage:**

- Cabbage, including green cabbage and red cabbage, contains trace amounts of fluoride. Incorporating cabbage into coleslaw, stir-fries, salads, or soups can contribute to fluoride intake.

5. **Parsley:**
   - Parsley, an herb commonly used as a garnish or flavoring agent, contains fluoride. Adding fresh parsley to salads, soups, sauces, or dips can provide a source of fluoride.
6. **Cilantro (Coriander):**
   - Cilantro, another herb used in various cuisines, contains small amounts of fluoride. Including fresh cilantro in salads, salsas, marinades, or as a garnish can add flavor and a touch of fluoride.
7. **Almonds:**
   - Almonds are a nut rich in various nutrients, including fluoride. Snacking on almonds, adding them to salads, oatmeal, or trail mixes can contribute to fluoride intake.
8. **Potatoes:**
   - Potatoes, especially when consumed with the skin, contain small amounts of fluoride. Enjoy baked potatoes, mashed potatoes, or roasted potatoes as part of your meals to add a source of fluoride.

It's important to note that the fluoride content of plant-based foods can vary depending on factors such as growing conditions, soil composition, and processing methods. Additionally, fluoride intake from plant-based foods is typically lower compared to other sources such as fluoridated water or dental products. If you have specific concerns about fluoride intake, consult with a healthcare professional or dentist for personalized advice.

Chromium

What is *Chromium?*

Chromium is an essential trace mineral that plays a crucial role in various physiological processes within the human body. It is required in small amounts for normal carbohydrate, fat, and protein metabolism, as well as for maintaining proper glucose metabolism and insulin sensitivity.

One of the primary functions of chromium is its role in enhancing the action of insulin, a hormone produced by the pancreas that helps regulate blood sugar levels. Chromium helps insulin transport glucose from the bloodstream into cells, where it can be used for energy production. This process is particularly important for individuals with insulin resistance or type 2 diabetes, as chromium supplementation may help improve insulin sensitivity and glucose control.

In addition to its role in glucose metabolism, chromium is also involved in lipid metabolism, where it helps regulate the synthesis, storage, and breakdown of fats in the body. Chromium may help lower levels of LDL ("bad") cholesterol and triglycerides while increasing levels of HDL ("good") cholesterol, which can reduce the risk of cardiovascular disease.

Chromium is also believed to play a role in maintaining proper weight management and body composition. Some studies suggest that chromium supplementation may help reduce food cravings, suppress appetite, and promote fat loss while preserving lean body mass. However, more research is needed to fully understand the effects of chromium on weight loss and body composition.

While chromium deficiency is rare, certain factors such as poor diet, aging, pregnancy, and certain medical conditions may increase the risk of deficiency. Symptoms of chromium deficiency may include impaired glucose tolerance, insulin resistance, elevated blood sugar levels, fatigue, and weight changes.

Good dietary sources of chromium include meats, poultry, fish, whole grains, nuts, seeds, fruits, and vegetables. However, the chromium content of foods can vary depending on factors such as soil quality and processing methods.

In summary, chromium is an essential trace mineral that plays important roles in glucose metabolism, insulin sensitivity, lipid metabolism, and weight management. Consuming a balanced diet that includes chromium-rich foods is important for ensuring adequate intake of this vital nutrient and supporting overall health and well-being. Additionally, chromium supplementation may be beneficial for individuals with insulin resistance, type 2 diabetes, or certain other health conditions, under the guidance of a healthcare professional.

Plant-based foods Contain Chromium

Chromium is a trace mineral that plays a role in glucose metabolism and insulin sensitivity. While chromium is primarily found in animal-based foods, there are also some plant-based sources available. Here are some plant-based foods that contain chromium:

1. **Broccoli:**
    - Broccoli is a cruciferous vegetable that contains small amounts of chromium. Enjoy broccoli steamed, roasted, or stir-fried as a side dish or incorporated into salads, soups, and casseroles.
2. **Green Beans:**
    - Green beans, also known as string beans or snap beans, contain trace amounts of chromium. Incorporate green beans into stir-fries, salads, or as a side dish for added nutrition.
3. **Whole Grains (especially Whole Wheat and Barley):**
    - Whole grains such as whole wheat and barley contain small amounts of chromium. Enjoy whole wheat bread, barley salads, or barley porridge as part of your meals to add a source of chromium.
4. **Oats:**
    - Oats are a nutritious whole grain that contains some chromium. Start your day with a bowl of oatmeal topped with fresh fruit and nuts for a wholesome breakfast rich in chromium.
5. **Potatoes (with skin):**
    - Potatoes, especially when consumed with the skin, contain trace amounts of chromium. Enjoy baked potatoes, mashed potatoes, or roasted potatoes as part of your meals to add a source of chromium.
6. **Green Leafy Vegetables (such as Spinach and Kale):**
    - Green leafy vegetables like spinach and kale contain small amounts of chromium. Incorporate these nutrient-rich greens into salads, smoothies, soups, or stir-fries for added health benefits.
7. **Tomatoes:**
    - Tomatoes contain trace amounts of chromium and can be enjoyed fresh in salads, sandwiches, or as a base for sauces and soups.
8. **Romaine Lettuce:**
    - Romaine lettuce is a variety of lettuce that contains some chromium. Use romaine lettuce as a base for salads, wraps, or sandwiches for a refreshing and nutritious meal.

While these plant-based foods can contribute to chromium intake, it's essential to consume them as part of a balanced diet to ensure adequate nutrition. If you have specific concerns about chromium intake, consult with a healthcare professional or registered dietitian for personalized advice.

Molybdenum

What is Molybdenum?

Molybdenum is a trace mineral that is essential for human health. It is found naturally in many foods and is also available as a dietary supplement. Molybdenum plays a crucial role in various physiological processes within the body, including metabolism, detoxification, and the functioning of certain enzymes.

One of the primary functions of molybdenum is its role as a cofactor for several enzymes involved in the metabolism of carbohydrates, fats, and proteins. These enzymes, known as molybdoenzymes, catalyze important chemical reactions in the body, including the conversion of sulfite to sulfate, the metabolism of sulfur-containing amino acids, and the breakdown of certain toxins and drugs.

Molybdenum is also involved in the synthesis of purines and pyrimidines, which are essential components of DNA and RNA. It plays a role in the formation of uric acid, a waste product that is excreted from the body through urine. Additionally, molybdenum is important for the proper functioning of the nervous system and may play a role in preventing neurodegenerative disorders.

Dietary sources of molybdenum include legumes (such as beans, lentils, and peas), nuts, seeds, whole grains, leafy green vegetables, and certain animal products (such as liver and kidney). The molybdenum content of plant-based foods can vary depending on factors such as soil quality and growing conditions.

Molybdenum deficiency is rare in humans, as the mineral is found in many common foods and is required in only small amounts. However, certain medical conditions or dietary factors may increase the risk of deficiency. Symptoms of molybdenum deficiency may include fatigue, weakness, loss of appetite, and neurological symptoms.

On the other hand, excessive intake of molybdenum is also rare and is more likely to occur through occupational exposure or from high-dose supplements. Chronic excessive intake of molybdenum may interfere with copper metabolism and lead to copper deficiency, which can cause anemia, neurological symptoms, and other health problems.

In summary, molybdenum is an essential trace mineral that plays important roles in metabolism, detoxification, enzyme function, and neurological health. Consuming a balanced diet that includes molybdenum-rich foods is important for ensuring adequate intake of this essential nutrient and supporting overall health and well-being. If you have concerns about molybdenum intake or deficiency, it's important to consult with a healthcare professional for personalized guidance and recommendations.

Plant-based foods Contain Molybdenum

Molybdenum is a trace mineral that plays a crucial role in various physiological processes, including enzyme function and metabolism. While molybdenum is found in relatively small amounts in plant-based foods compared to animal-based sources, there are still several plant-based options that contain this essential mineral. Here are some plant-based foods that are sources of molybdenum:

1. **Legumes (Beans, Lentils, Peas):**
    - Legumes are excellent sources of molybdenum. Beans (such as black beans, kidney beans, and navy beans), lentils, and peas contain significant amounts of this mineral. Enjoy them in soups, stews, salads, or as a side dish to boost your molybdenum intake.
2. **Whole Grains (Barley, Oats, Quinoa):**
    - Whole grains like barley, oats, and quinoa also contain molybdenum. Incorporate these grains into your meals as a source of complex carbohydrates, fiber, and molybdenum. Enjoy them as porridge, salads, pilafs, or in baked goods.
3. **Leafy Green Vegetables (Spinach, Kale):**
    - Leafy green vegetables like spinach and kale contain small amounts of molybdenum. Include these nutrient-rich greens in salads, smoothies, stir-fries, or soups to add molybdenum to your diet.
4. **Nuts and Seeds (Sunflower Seeds, Sesame Seeds):**
    - Certain nuts and seeds, such as sunflower seeds and sesame seeds, are good sources of molybdenum. Snack on them raw or roasted, sprinkle them over salads or oatmeal, or use them in homemade energy bars or granola for a molybdenum boost.
5. **Cruciferous Vegetables (Broccoli, Cauliflower):**
    - Cruciferous vegetables like broccoli and cauliflower contain small amounts of molybdenum. Enjoy them steamed, roasted, or stir-fried as part of your meals to reap their nutritional benefits, including molybdenum.
6. **Soy Products (Tofu, Tempeh, Edamame):**
    - Soy products, such as tofu, tempeh, and edamame, contain molybdenum. Incorporate these plant-based protein sources into stir-fries, curries, salads, or grain bowls to add molybdenum to your diet.
7. **Potatoes (with skin):**
    - Potatoes, especially when consumed with the skin, contain small amounts of molybdenum. Enjoy baked potatoes, mashed potatoes, or roasted potatoes as part of your meals to add a source of molybdenum.

Including a variety of these plant-based foods in your diet can help ensure you meet your molybdenum needs and support overall health and wellbeing. If you have specific concerns about molybdenum intake, consult with a healthcare professional or registered dietitian for personalized advice.

What is Choline?

Choline is an essential nutrient that plays several important roles in the body. It is often grouped with the B vitamins, although it's not officially classified as one. Choline is crucial for various bodily functions, including:

Cell structure: Choline is a component of phospholipids, which are essential for the structure and function of cell membranes. It helps maintain cell integrity and facilitates cell communication.

Neurotransmission: Choline is a precursor to acetylcholine, a neurotransmitter involved in muscle control, memory, and cognitive function. Sufficient choline intake is necessary for optimal brain function.

Fat metabolism: Choline is involved in the transport and metabolism of fats and cholesterol. It helps prevent the accumulation of fats in the liver and promotes the export of fats from the liver.

DNA synthesis: Choline is required for the synthesis of phosphatidylcholine, a component of DNA and a precursor to cell membranes.

Methylation reactions: Choline is involved in methylation reactions, which are essential for regulating gene expression and various metabolic processes.

Good dietary sources of choline include eggs, meat, poultry, fish, dairy products, nuts, and certain vegetables like broccoli and Brussels sprouts. In some cases, dietary intake may not be sufficient, and choline supplements may be recommended, especially for pregnant and breastfeeding women to support fetal brain development. However, it's essential to consult with a healthcare professional before starting any supplement regimen.

Plant-based foods high in Choline

Choline is an essential nutrient that plays a crucial role in various bodily functions, including liver health, brain development, and muscle function. While animal products are often rich sources of choline, there are plant-based foods that also provide this nutrient. Here is a list of plant-based foods high in choline:

1. **Broccoli:**
    - Broccoli is a cruciferous vegetable that contains a moderate amount of choline. It's also rich in other vitamins and minerals, making it a nutritious addition to your diet.
2. **Brussels Sprouts:**
    - Brussels sprouts are another cruciferous vegetable that contains a good amount of choline. They are also high in fiber and vitamin C.
3. **Quinoa:**
    - Quinoa is a grain that contains a decent amount of choline. It is also a complete protein, providing all nine essential amino acids.
4. **Peanuts:**
    - Peanuts and peanut butter are good sources of choline. They are also rich in healthy fats and protein.
5. **Soy Products (Tofu, Tempeh):**
    - Soy-based products such as tofu and tempeh are good sources of choline. They are versatile ingredients in vegetarian and vegan diets.
6. **Chickpeas:**
    - Chickpeas, also known as garbanzo beans, contain a moderate amount of choline. They are a great plant-based protein source.
7. **Baked Potatoes:**
    - Potatoes, especially when baked with the skin on, contain a reasonable amount of choline. Ensure you eat the skin to maximize the choline content.
8. **Spinach:**
    - Spinach and other leafy greens provide some choline. They are also rich in iron, calcium, and other essential nutrients.
9. **Almonds:**
    - Almonds are nuts that contains a moderate amount of choline. They are also a good source of healthy fats, protein, and vitamin E.
10. **Flaxseeds:**
    - Flaxseeds, including flaxseed meal, contain a moderate amount of choline. They are also rich in omega-3 fatty acids and fiber.

It's important to note that while these plant-based sources contain choline, the levels may vary. A well-balanced diet that includes a variety of these foods can contribute to meeting your choline requirements, especially for individuals following vegetarian or vegan lifestyles.

Here is a list of animal-based foods high in choline:

Animal-based Sources:

1. **Eggs:**
    - Eggs are one of the richest sources of choline. The yolk, in particular, contains a significant amount.
2. **Beef Liver:**
    - Beef liver is exceptionally high in choline. However, it's important to consume liver in moderation due to its high vitamin A content.
3. **Chicken Liver:**
    - Like beef liver, chicken liver is a potent source of choline.
4. **Salmon:**
    - Salmon is a fatty fish that provides a good amount of choline along with omega-3 fatty acids.
5. **Chicken Breast:**
    - Chicken breast is a lean source of choline and protein.
6. **Pork:**
    - Various cuts of pork, such as pork chops or pork loin, contain choline.
7. **Shrimp:**
    - Shellfish, including shrimp, is a seafood source of choline.

Including a variety of these foods in your diet can contribute to meeting your choline requirements, supporting overall health and well-being.

Water

What is Water?

Water is a transparent, tasteless, and odorless chemical substance composed of two hydrogen atoms bonded to one oxygen atom, with the chemical formula H_2O. It is the most abundant molecule on Earth and is essential for life. Water plays numerous vital roles in the human body, and its benefits include:

1. **Hydration:** Water is crucial for maintaining proper hydration levels in the body. It serves as a medium for transporting nutrients to cells, regulating body temperature through sweating and respiration, and removing waste products through urine and perspiration.
2. **Lubrication:** Water lubricates joints, tissues, and organs, helping to reduce friction and facilitate smooth movement. Adequate hydration is essential for maintaining joint health and preventing conditions like arthritis.
3. **Digestion:** Water aids in the digestion and absorption of nutrients by breaking down food particles, assisting in the production of digestive enzymes, and promoting the movement of food through the digestive tract. Drinking water before meals can also help reduce appetite and support weight management.
4. **Detoxification:** Water helps flush toxins and waste products from the body through urine, sweat, and bowel movements. Staying hydrated supports proper kidney function and prevents the buildup of waste substances that can harm health.
5. **Skin Health:** Drinking enough water helps keep the skin hydrated and moisturized, promoting elasticity, suppleness, and a healthy complexion. Proper hydration can also reduce the risk of skin problems like dryness, acne, and premature aging.
6. **Cognitive Function**: Adequate hydration is essential for maintaining optimal cognitive function, including concentration, alertness, and memory. Even mild dehydration can impair cognitive performance and mood.
7. **Energy Levels:** Water plays a crucial role in energy metabolism, as it is involved in the production of adenosine triphosphate (ATP), the body's primary energy currency. Staying hydrated can help prevent fatigue and support physical performance and endurance.
8. **Immune Function:** Drinking water helps support the immune system by maintaining proper lymphatic function, which is essential for transporting immune cells and fighting off infections and illnesses.
9. **Weight Management**: Water has zero calories and can help promote feelings of fullness when consumed before or with meals, leading to reduced calorie intake and supporting weight loss or weight maintenance efforts.
10. **Regulation of Body Temperature:** Water helps regulate body temperature by absorbing and releasing heat through perspiration and evaporation. Staying hydrated is particularly

important during hot weather or physical activity to prevent dehydration and heat-related illnesses.

Overall, staying adequately hydrated by drinking water throughout the day is essential for maintaining optimal health and well-being. The exact water intake needs vary depending on factors like age, sex, body weight, activity level, climate, and overall health status, but a general recommendation is to drink about 8 glasses (64 ounces) of water per day, or more if needed.

Fiber

What is Fiber?

Fiber, also known as dietary fiber or roughage, refers to the indigestible portion of plant foods. It is found in fruits, vegetables, grains, nuts, seeds, and legumes. There are two main types of fiber:

1. **Soluble Fiber:** This type of fiber dissolves in water to form a gel-like substance. It can help lower cholesterol levels and regulate blood sugar levels by slowing down the absorption of sugar into the bloodstream. Foods rich in soluble fiber include oats, barley, beans, lentils, fruits (such as apples, oranges, and berries), and vegetables (such as carrots and broccoli).
2. **Insoluble Fiber**: This type of fiber does not dissolve in water and adds bulk to the stool, helping to promote regular bowel movements and prevent constipation. It also helps to prevent hemorrhoids and diverticulosis. Foods rich in insoluble fiber include whole grains (such as wheat bran, brown rice, and whole wheat bread), nuts, seeds, and the skins of fruits and vegetables.

The benefits of fiber include:

Improved Digestive Health:

Fiber adds bulk to the stool, softens it, and helps move it through the digestive tract more efficiently, reducing the risk of constipation, hemorrhoids, and diverticulosis.

Weight Management:

High-fiber foods are often lower in calories and can help you feel full longer, reducing overall calorie intake and aiding in weight management.

Heart Health: Soluble fiber can help lower LDL cholesterol levels (the "bad" cholesterol), thereby reducing the risk of heart disease and stroke.

Blood Sugar Control:

Soluble fiber can slow down the absorption of sugar into the bloodstream, helping to regulate blood sugar levels and reduce the risk of type 2 diabetes.

Improved Gut Health:

Fiber acts as a prebiotic, providing fuel for beneficial bacteria in the gut, which can promote a healthy gut microbiome and improve overall gut health.

Reduced Risk of Certain Diseases:

A high-fiber diet has been associated with a reduced risk of certain diseases, including colorectal cancer, breast cancer, and cardiovascular disease.

It's recommended to consume a variety of high-fiber foods as part of a balanced diet to reap the many health benefits that fiber offers. The daily recommended intake of fiber varies depending on age, gender, and other factors, but most adults should aim for at least 25-30 grams of fiber per day.

Phytonutrients

What are Phytonutrients?

Phytonutrients, also known as phytochemicals, are natural compounds found in plants that have various health-promoting properties. These compounds are responsible for the vibrant colors, flavors, and aromas of fruits, vegetables, herbs, spices, nuts, seeds, and whole grains. While they are not essential nutrients like vitamins and minerals, phytonutrients have been shown to provide numerous health benefits. Some common types of phytonutrients include:

1. **Carotenoids:** These pigments give fruits and vegetables their yellow, orange, and red colors. Examples include beta-carotene (found in carrots, sweet potatoes, and pumpkin), lycopene (found in tomatoes and watermelon), and lutein (found in leafy greens like spinach and kale). Carotenoids act as antioxidants, helping to protect cells from damage caused by free radicals, and they may also support eye health and reduce the risk of certain cancers.
2. **Flavonoids**: This large class of phytonutrients includes compounds like quercetin (found in apples, onions, and citrus fruits), catechins (found in green tea), and anthocyanins (found in berries and red cabbage). Flavonoids have antioxidant and anti-inflammatory properties, and they may help reduce the risk of heart disease, improve blood vessel function, and support brain health.
3. **Polyphenols**: Polyphenols are found in a wide variety of plant foods, including cocoa, grapes, berries, tea, and nuts. They have antioxidant and anti-inflammatory effects, and

research suggests they may help reduce the risk of chronic diseases such as heart disease, cancer, and neurodegenerative disorders.

4. **Sulfur**-containing compounds: Phytonutrients like glucosinolates (found in cruciferous vegetables like broccoli, cabbage, and Brussels sprouts) and allyl sulfides (found in garlic and onions) have been shown to have anti-cancer properties and may help support detoxification pathways in the body.
5. **Phytoestrogens:** These compounds, found in soybeans, flaxseeds, and other legumes, have a structure similar to estrogen and may have hormone-balancing effects. They have been studied for their potential role in reducing the risk of hormone-related cancers and managing symptoms of menopause.

The benefits of phytonutrients include:

- **Antioxidant activity:** Phytonutrients help protect cells from oxidative damage caused by free radicals, thereby reducing the risk of chronic diseases like cancer, heart disease, and diabetes.
- **Anti-inflammatory effects:** Many phytonutrients have anti-inflammatory properties, which can help reduce inflammation in the body and lower the risk of inflammatory diseases.
- **Immune support:** Some phytonutrients have been shown to support immune function and help the body defend against infections and diseases.
- **Hormone balance:** Certain phytonutrients may have hormone-balancing effects, which can be beneficial for reproductive health and managing symptoms of hormonal imbalances.
- **Detoxification support:** Phytonutrients like glucosinolates help support the body's natural detoxification pathways, aiding in the elimination of toxins and harmful substances.

Including a variety of colorful fruits, vegetables, herbs, spices, nuts, seeds, and whole grains in your diet is an excellent way to ensure you're getting a wide range of phytonutrients and reaping their many health benefits.

Back to Table of Contents

Omega-3 Fatty Acids

What is Omega-3 Fatty Acids?

Omega-3 fatty acids are a group of essential polyunsaturated fatty acids that are important for maintaining overall health. They are considered essential because the body cannot produce them on its own, so they must be obtained through diet. There are three main types of omega-3 fatty acids:

1. **Alpha-linolenic acid (ALA):** This is found in plant sources such as flaxseeds, chia seeds, walnuts, and hemp seeds.
2. **Eicosapentaenoic acid (EPA): This** is found mainly in fatty fish such as salmon, mackerel, sardines, and trout.
3. **Docosahexaenoic acid (DHA):** This is also found in fatty fish and is particularly abundant in seafood.

Sources of Omega -3 Fatty acid

1. **Dietary Sources**: The primary source of omega-3 fatty acids is through the consumption of foods rich in these nutrients. Sources include:
    - ALA: Found in plant-based foods such as flaxseeds, chia seeds, hemp seeds, walnuts, and soybeans.
    - EPA and DHA: Found primarily in fatty fish such as salmon, mackerel, sardines, herring, and trout. These marine sources of omega-3 fatty acids are particularly rich in EPA and DHA.
2. **Conversion of ALA to EPA and DHA**: While ALA is the most common omega-3 fatty acid found in plant-based foods, the body can convert a portion of ALA into EPA and DHA. However, this conversion process is inefficient, and only a small amount of ALA is converted into EPA and DHA. Therefore, it's important to consume adequate sources of EPA and DHA from marine sources or supplements, especially for individuals following a vegetarian or vegan diet.
3. **Supplements**: Omega-3 fatty acid supplements, such as fish oil capsules or algae oil capsules, are available and can provide a concentrated source of EPA and DHA. These supplements can be particularly beneficial for individuals who do not consume enough fatty fish or who have specific dietary restrictions.

In summary, the body obtains omega-3 fatty acids through dietary sources, primarily from fatty fish rich in EPA and DHA, as well as from plant-based sources rich in ALA. Consuming a balanced diet that includes a variety of omega-3-rich foods is important for ensuring an adequate intake of these essential nutrients and supporting overall health and well-being.

The benefits of omega-3 fatty acids include:

Heart Health:

Omega-3 fatty acids have been shown to help reduce the risk of heart disease by lowering triglyceride levels, reducing inflammation, improving blood vessel function, and lowering blood pressure. They may also help prevent the formation of blood clots and reduce the risk of stroke.

Brain Health:

DHA, in particular, is important for brain development and function. It is a major component of the brain and plays a crucial role in cognitive function, memory, and learning. Omega-3 fatty acids may also help reduce the risk of age-related cognitive decline and Alzheimer's disease.

Eye Health:

DHA is also found in high concentrations in the retina of the eye, where it helps support healthy vision and may reduce the risk of age-related macular degeneration.

Joint Health:

Omega-3 fatty acids have anti-inflammatory properties that can help reduce joint pain and stiffness in conditions like rheumatoid arthritis and osteoarthritis.

Mental Health:

Some research suggests that omega-3 fatty acids may help improve mood and reduce symptoms of depression and anxiety. They may also have a protective effect against other mental health disorders such as schizophrenia and bipolar disorder.

Pregnancy and Infant Development:

Omega-3 fatty acids are important for fetal brain and eye development during pregnancy. They may also help reduce the risk of preterm birth and may be beneficial for infant development and cognitive function.

Skin Health: Omega-3 fatty acids may help maintain healthy skin by reducing inflammation and supporting skin barrier function. They may also help improve symptoms of certain skin conditions like eczema and psoriasis.

Including omega-3-rich foods in your diet, such as fatty fish, flaxseeds, chia seeds, walnuts, and hemp seeds, or taking omega-3 supplements if needed, can help ensure you get an adequate intake of these essential fatty acids and reap their many health benefits. However, it's important to consult with a healthcare professional before starting any supplementation regimen, especially if you have any underlying health conditions or are taking medications.

Essential Compounds - Antioxidant

What are Antioxidants?

Antioxidants are compounds that help protect the body against damage caused by free radicals. Free radicals are unstable molecules that can cause oxidative stress, a process linked to various chronic diseases and aging. Antioxidants neutralize free radicals by donating electrons, thereby preventing them from causing damage to cells, proteins, and DNA.

There are several types of antioxidants, including vitamins (such as vitamin C, vitamin E, and vitamin A), minerals (such as selenium and zinc), phytochemicals (found in plant-based foods), and enzymes (such as catalase and superoxide dismutase) produced by the body.

1. **Vitamin C (Ascorbic Acid):**
    - **Benefits:** Vitamin C is a powerful water-soluble antioxidant that helps protect cells from oxidative damage, supports immune function, promotes collagen synthesis for healthy skin, aids in wound healing, enhances iron absorption, and may reduce the risk of chronic diseases such as heart disease and certain cancers.
2. **Vitamin E (Tocopherols and Tocotrienols):**
    - **Benefits:** Vitamin E is a fat-soluble antioxidant that protects cell membranes from oxidative damage, acts as a free radical scavenger in lipid-rich areas of the body, supports immune function, promotes skin health, and may reduce the risk of age-related cognitive decline and cardiovascular disease.
3. **Beta-Carotene:**
    - **Benefits:** Beta-carotene is a provitamin A carotenoid antioxidant found in orange and yellow fruits and vegetables. It functions as a precursor to vitamin A, supports immune function, promotes healthy vision, helps maintain skin health, and may reduce the risk of certain cancers and cardiovascular disease.
4. **Selenium:**
    - **Benefits:** Selenium is a trace mineral that acts as a cofactor for antioxidant enzymes such as glutathione peroxidase. It helps protect cells from oxidative damage, supports thyroid function, boosts immune response, promotes reproductive health, and may reduce the risk of certain cancers and cardiovascular disease.
5. **Flavonoids:**
    - **Benefits:** Flavonoids are a group of polyphenolic compounds found in various plant-based foods, including fruits, vegetables, tea, and red wine. They possess antioxidant, anti-inflammatory, and anti-cancer properties, support cardiovascular

health, promote cognitive function, and may reduce the risk of chronic diseases such as diabetes and neurodegenerative disorders.

6. **Lycopene:**
    - **Benefits:** Lycopene is a carotenoid antioxidant found in red-colored fruits and vegetables, such as tomatoes, watermelon, and pink grapefruit. It exhibits potent antioxidant properties, helps protect against oxidative damage to cells and tissues, supports heart health, and may reduce the risk of certain cancers, particularly prostate cancer.
7. **Polyphenols:**
    - **Benefits:** Polyphenols are a diverse group of antioxidants found abundantly in plant-based foods, including fruits, vegetables, tea, coffee, cocoa, and red wine. They possess antioxidant, anti-inflammatory, anti-microbial, and anti-cancer properties, support cardiovascular health, promote cognitive function, and may contribute to longevity and overall well-being.
8. **Coenzyme Q10 (CoQ10):**
    - **Benefits:** CoQ10 is a fat-soluble antioxidant and a crucial component of the electron transport chain involved in cellular energy production. It helps protect cells from oxidative damage, supports heart health, enhances exercise performance, promotes skin health, and may reduce the risk of neurodegenerative diseases and migraine headaches.

Incorporating a variety of antioxidant-rich foods into your diet can help maintain optimal health, protect against oxidative stress, and reduce the risk of chronic diseases associated with free radical damage.

Back to Table of Contents

Free Radicals

What are Free radicals?

Free radicals are highly reactive molecules that contain one or more unpaired electrons in their outer shell. These unpaired electrons make free radicals highly unstable and reactive, as they seek to pair with electrons from other molecules in order to achieve stability. In the process of seeking to stabilize themselves, free radicals can cause damage to surrounding molecules by stealing electrons from them. This process, known as oxidative stress, can lead to cellular damage and contribute to the development of various diseases and aging processes.

Free radicals are generated as natural byproducts of cellular metabolism, particularly during processes such as respiration and energy production. Additionally, external factors such as exposure to environmental pollutants, radiation, cigarette smoke, and certain medications can also increase the production of free radicals in the body.

While some level of free radical production is normal and necessary for cellular function, excessive levels of free radicals can overwhelm the body's antioxidant defenses and lead to oxidative damage. Antioxidants are molecules that can neutralize free radicals by donating electrons without becoming destabilized themselves. Antioxidants can be obtained from dietary sources, such as fruits, vegetables, nuts, seeds, and certain spices, as well as produced by the body itself.

When free radicals are not properly neutralized by antioxidants, they can cause damage to cellular structures such as proteins, lipids, and DNA. This damage can disrupt cellular function and contribute to the development of various health conditions, including cardiovascular disease, cancer, neurodegenerative disorders, and aging-related conditions.

In summary, free radicals are highly reactive molecules that can cause damage to cells and tissues through oxidative stress. While some free radical production is normal and necessary for cellular function, excessive levels of free radicals can lead to oxidative damage and contribute to the development of various diseases and aging processes. Consuming a diet rich in antioxidants and minimizing exposure to factors that increase free radical production can help protect against oxidative damage and support overall health and well-being.

Oxidative Stress

What is oxidative Stress?

Oxidative stress is a physiological imbalance between the production of reactive oxygen species (ROS) or free radicals and the body's ability to neutralize them with antioxidants. Reactive oxygen species include molecules such as superoxide radicals, hydroxyl radicals, and hydrogen peroxide, which are generated as natural byproducts of cellular metabolism, particularly during processes such as respiration and energy production.

Under normal conditions, the body's antioxidant defenses, including enzymes such as superoxide dismutase (SOD), catalase, and glutathione peroxidase, as well as non-enzymatic antioxidants such as vitamin C, vitamin E, and glutathione, help neutralize reactive oxygen species and protect cells from oxidative damage. However, when the production of reactive oxygen species exceeds the body's antioxidant capacity, oxidative stress occurs.

Oxidative stress can lead to damage to cellular structures such as proteins, lipids, and DNA. This damage can disrupt cellular function and contribute to the development of various health conditions, including cardiovascular disease, cancer, neurodegenerative disorders, inflammatory conditions, diabetes, and aging-related conditions.

Several factors can contribute to oxidative stress, including:

1. **Environmental factors:** Exposure to environmental pollutants, radiation, cigarette smoke, and certain chemicals can increase the production of reactive oxygen species and contribute to oxidative stress.
2. **Lifestyle factors:** Poor diet, lack of exercise, excessive alcohol consumption, smoking, and chronic stress can all increase oxidative stress levels in the body.
3. **Disease conditions:** Certain diseases and health conditions, such as diabetes, obesity, autoimmune disorders, and neurodegenerative diseases, can also increase oxidative stress due to inflammation and impaired antioxidant defenses.
4. **Aging:** The aging process is associated with an increase in oxidative stress and a decline in antioxidant defenses, which may contribute to age-related diseases and the aging process itself.
5. **Dietary factors:** Consumption of a diet high in processed foods, refined sugars, unhealthy fats, and low in antioxidants can increase oxidative stress levels in the body.

In summary, oxidative stress is a physiological imbalance between the production of reactive oxygen species and the body's antioxidant defenses. It can lead to damage to cellular structures and contribute to the development of various diseases and aging processes. Minimizing exposure to factors that increase oxidative stress and consuming a diet rich in antioxidants can help protect against oxidative damage and support overall health and well-being.

Cardiovascular Disease (CVD)

What is cardiovascular disease?

Cardiovascular disease (CVD) refers to a group of conditions that affect the heart and blood vessels, often leading to complications such as heart attack, stroke, or peripheral artery disease. It is one of the leading causes of death globally, accounting for millions of deaths each year.

There are several types of cardiovascular diseases, including:

1. **Coronary artery disease (CAD):** CAD occurs when the blood vessels that supply oxygen-rich blood to the heart muscle become narrowed or blocked due to the buildup of plaque (a combination of cholesterol, fat, and other substances). This can restrict blood flow to the heart and lead to chest pain (angina), heart attack (myocardial infarction), or other complications.
2. **Stroke:** A stroke occurs when the blood supply to part of the brain is interrupted or reduced, depriving brain tissue of oxygen and nutrients. This can result in brain damage, disability, or death. There are two main types of stroke: ischemic stroke, which occurs when a blood clot blocks a blood vessel in the brain, and hemorrhagic stroke, which occurs when a blood vessel in the brain ruptures and causes bleeding.
3. **Peripheral artery disease (PAD):** PAD occurs when the blood vessels outside of the heart, usually in the legs, become narrowed or blocked due to atherosclerosis (the buildup of plaque). This can result in reduced blood flow to the limbs, leading to symptoms such as leg pain, numbness, or weakness, and increasing the risk of complications such as infection or tissue damage.
4. **Heart failure:** Heart failure occurs when the heart is unable to pump enough blood to meet the body's needs. This can result from conditions such as CAD, high blood pressure, or damage to the heart muscle (e.g., from a heart attack). Symptoms of heart failure may include shortness of breath, fatigue, swelling in the legs or abdomen, and difficulty exercising.
5. **Arrhythmias:** Arrhythmias are abnormal heart rhythms that can occur when the electrical impulses that regulate the heartbeat are disrupted. This can cause the heart to beat too fast (tachycardia), too slow (bradycardia), or irregularly. While some arrhythmias may be harmless, others can be life-threatening and require medical treatment.

Risk factors for cardiovascular disease include:

- High blood pressure (hypertension)
- High cholesterol levels
- Smoking
- Diabetes
- Obesity
- Physical inactivity
- Unhealthy diet

- Family history of CVD
- Age (risk increases with age)
- Gender (men are at higher risk than premenopausal women, though the risk equalizes after menopause)
- Socioeconomic factors (such as low income or education level)

Prevention and management of cardiovascular disease involve lifestyle modifications (such as regular exercise, healthy diet, smoking cessation, and weight management), medication (such as blood pressure or cholesterol-lowering medications), and, in some cases, medical procedures or surgery (such as angioplasty, stenting, or bypass surgery). Early detection and treatment of risk factors and underlying conditions are crucial for reducing the risk of cardiovascular disease and its complications. Regular check-ups with a healthcare provider can help assess and manage individual cardiovascular risk.

Here are some plant-based foods that are rich in key nutrients known to help manage certain cardiovascular disease such as:

High Blood Pressure

Managing high blood pressure through diet is a crucial aspect of overall health. Incorporating plant-based foods rich in essential nutrients can be beneficial for maintaining healthy blood pressure levels. Here are some plant-based foods that are rich in key nutrients known to help manage high blood pressure:

Leafy greens:

- Spinach, kale, Swiss chard, collard greens, and other leafy greens are excellent sources of potassium, magnesium, and dietary nitrates, which can help relax blood vessels and lower blood pressure.

Bananas:

- Bananas are rich in potassium, an essential mineral that helps regulate blood pressure by balancing sodium levels and promoting healthy blood vessel function.

Berries:

- Blueberries, strawberries, raspberries, and other berries are packed with antioxidants, including flavonoids and anthocyanins, which have been associated with lower blood pressure levels.

Beets:

- Beets are high in dietary nitrates, which the body converts into nitric oxide, a compound that helps relax blood vessels and improve blood flow, thereby lowering blood pressure.

Avocados:

- Avocados are rich in potassium, magnesium, and heart-healthy monounsaturated fats, which can help lower blood pressure and improve overall cardiovascular health.

Legumes:

- Beans, lentils, chickpeas, and other legumes are excellent sources of potassium, magnesium, fiber, and protein, all of which contribute to lower blood pressure levels and improved heart health.

Sweet potatoes:

- Sweet potatoes are rich in potassium and magnesium, as well as fiber and antioxidants, making them a nutritious choice for managing blood pressure and promoting overall health.

Oats:

- Oats are high in soluble fiber, which can help lower cholesterol levels and reduce blood pressure. They also contain magnesium and potassium, which further contribute to heart health.

Nuts and seeds:

- Almonds, walnuts, flaxseeds, chia seeds, and pumpkin seeds are rich in heart-healthy fats, magnesium, potassium, and fiber, all of which support lower blood pressure levels.

Garlic:

- Garlic contains compounds that may help relax blood vessels, improve blood flow, and lower blood pressure. Incorporating fresh or cooked garlic into meals can be beneficial for cardiovascular health.

Incorporating a variety of these plant-based foods into your diet, along with reducing sodium intake, maintaining a healthy weight, regular physical activity, and managing stress, can help support healthy blood pressure levels and overall cardiovascular health. It's also important to consult with a healthcare professional or registered dietitian for personalized dietary recommendations and guidance.

High Cholesterol

Managing high cholesterol levels through diet is an important aspect of cardiovascular health. Incorporating plant-based foods rich in essential nutrients can help lower LDL ("bad") cholesterol levels and improve overall lipid profiles. Here are some plant-based foods that are particularly beneficial for managing high cholesterol:

Oats and oatmeal:

- Oats are rich in soluble fiber, specifically beta-glucan, which helps reduce LDL cholesterol levels by inhibiting its absorption in the intestines. Consuming oats or oatmeal regularly can help lower cholesterol levels and improve heart health.

Legumes:

- Beans, lentils, chickpeas, and other legumes are excellent sources of soluble fiber, protein, and plant sterols, all of which help lower LDL cholesterol levels and improve overall lipid profiles.

Nuts and seeds:

- Almonds, walnuts, flaxseeds, chia seeds, and pumpkin seeds are rich in heart-healthy fats, fiber, and plant sterols, which help lower LDL cholesterol levels and reduce the risk of heart disease.

Avocados:

- Avocados are high in monounsaturated fats, which have been shown to help raise HDL ("good") cholesterol levels and lower LDL cholesterol levels. They are also rich in fiber and antioxidants, making them a heart-healthy addition to the diet.

Fatty fish:

- Fatty fish such as salmon, mackerel, sardines, and trout are rich in omega-3 fatty acids, which help lower triglyceride levels and reduce inflammation. Consuming fatty fish regularly can help improve lipid profiles and reduce the risk of heart disease.

Berries:

- Blueberries, strawberries, raspberries, and other berries are rich in antioxidants, including anthocyanins and flavonoids, which have been shown to help lower LDL cholesterol levels and reduce the risk of heart disease.

Whole grains:

- Whole grains such as brown rice, quinoa, barley, and whole wheat are rich in soluble fiber, which helps lower LDL cholesterol levels and improve heart health. Consuming whole grains regularly can help reduce the risk of heart disease.

Leafy greens:

- Spinach, kale, Swiss chard, and other leafy greens are rich in fiber, antioxidants, and plant compounds that help lower cholesterol levels and reduce the risk of heart disease.

Soy products:

- Soybeans, tofu, tempeh, and other soy products are rich in plant proteins, fiber, and phytoestrogens called isoflavones, which help lower LDL cholesterol levels and improve heart health.

Garlic:

- Garlic contains compounds that have been shown to help lower LDL cholesterol levels and reduce the risk of heart disease. Incorporating fresh or cooked garlic into meals can be beneficial for managing cholesterol levels.

Incorporating a variety of these plant-based foods into your diet, along with reducing saturated and trans fats, limiting dietary cholesterol, maintaining a healthy weight, regular physical activity, and managing stress, can help improve lipid profiles and reduce the risk of heart disease.

It's also important to consult with a healthcare professional or registered dietitian for personalized dietary recommendations and guidance.

Diabetes

Managing diabetes through diet is crucial for controlling blood sugar levels and preventing complications. Plant-based foods can be particularly beneficial for individuals with diabetes as they are typically low in saturated fats, rich in fiber, and provide essential nutrients. Here are some plant-based foods with essential nutrients that can help manage diabetes:

Leafy greens:

- Spinach, kale, Swiss chard, collard greens, and other leafy greens are low in calories and carbohydrates while being rich in fiber, vitamins, and minerals. They are excellent choices for managing blood sugar levels and supporting overall health.

Non-starchy vegetables:

- Vegetables such as broccoli, cauliflower, bell peppers, carrots, zucchini, and tomatoes are low in carbohydrates and calories but high in fiber, vitamins, and antioxidants. They can be included in meals to add flavor, texture, and nutrients without significantly affecting blood sugar levels.

Whole grains:

- Whole grains such as quinoa, brown rice, barley, oats, and whole wheat are rich in fiber, which helps slow down the absorption of glucose into the bloodstream and stabilize blood sugar levels. They also provide essential vitamins, minerals, and antioxidants.

Legumes:

- Beans, lentils, chickpeas, and other legumes are high in fiber, protein, and complex carbohydrates, making them excellent choices for managing blood sugar levels. They have a low glycemic index, which means they cause a gradual rise in blood sugar levels after consumption.

Berries:

- Berries such as strawberries, blueberries, raspberries, and blackberries are low in calories and carbohydrates but high in fiber, vitamins, and antioxidants. They can satisfy sweet cravings without causing significant spikes in blood sugar levels.

Nuts and seeds:

- Almonds, walnuts, flaxseeds, chia seeds, and pumpkin seeds are rich in healthy fats, protein, fiber, and essential nutrients. They can help stabilize blood sugar levels, reduce inflammation, and improve heart health when consumed in moderation.

Avocados:

- Avocados are rich in monounsaturated fats, fiber, and essential nutrients such as potassium and magnesium. They can help improve insulin sensitivity, reduce cholesterol levels, and promote heart health.

Sweet potatoes:

- Sweet potatoes are a nutritious source of carbohydrates, fiber, vitamins (such as vitamin A and vitamin C), and minerals. They have a lower glycemic index compared to white potatoes, meaning they cause a slower increase in blood sugar levels.

Cinnamon:

- Cinnamon is a spice that has been shown to help improve insulin sensitivity and reduce blood sugar levels. Adding cinnamon to foods and beverages can provide flavor and potential health benefits for individuals with diabetes.

Garlic and onions:

- Garlic and onions contain compounds that may help improve insulin sensitivity and reduce blood sugar levels. Incorporating them into meals can add flavor and potential health benefits for managing diabetes.

Incorporating a variety of these plant-based foods into your diet, along with portion control, regular physical activity, and blood sugar monitoring, can help manage diabetes and promote overall health and well-being. It's also important to consult with a healthcare professional or registered dietitian for personalized dietary recommendations and guidance.

Obesity

Managing obesity through diet involves choosing nutrient-dense foods that are low in calories but high in essential nutrients. Plant-based foods can be particularly beneficial for managing obesity as they are typically high in fiber, vitamins, minerals, and antioxidants while being lower in calories and saturated fats compared to animal products. Here are some plant-based foods with essential nutrients that can help manage obesity:

Leafy greens:

- Spinach, kale, Swiss chard, collard greens, and other leafy greens are low in calories and carbohydrates but high in fiber, vitamins, and minerals. They can help promote satiety and fullness while providing essential nutrients.

Non-starchy vegetables:

- Vegetables such as broccoli, cauliflower, bell peppers, carrots, zucchini, and tomatoes are low in calories and carbohydrates but high in fiber, vitamins, and antioxidants. They can be included in meals to add volume, flavor, and nutrients without significantly increasing calorie intake.

Whole grains:

- Whole grains such as quinoa, brown rice, barley, oats, and whole wheat are rich in fiber, which helps promote satiety and regulate appetite. They provide essential nutrients and can help stabilize blood sugar levels, reducing the risk of overeating.

Legumes:

- Beans, lentils, chickpeas, and other legumes are rich in fiber, protein, and complex carbohydrates, making them excellent choices for managing obesity. They help promote satiety, regulate blood sugar levels, and support weight management.

Berries:

- Berries such as strawberries, blueberries, raspberries, and blackberries are low in calories and carbohydrates but high in fiber, vitamins, and antioxidants. They can satisfy sweet cravings and provide essential nutrients without significantly increasing calorie intake.

Nuts and seeds:

- Almonds, walnuts, flaxseeds, chia seeds, and pumpkin seeds are rich in healthy fats, protein, fiber, and essential nutrients. They can help promote satiety, reduce cravings, and support weight management when consumed in moderation.

Avocados:

- Avocados are rich in monounsaturated fats, fiber, and essential nutrients such as potassium and magnesium. They can help promote satiety, reduce hunger, and support weight loss when included in a balanced diet.

Sweet potatoes:

- Sweet potatoes are a nutritious source of carbohydrates, fiber, vitamins (such as vitamin A and vitamin C), and minerals. They have a lower glycemic index compared to white potatoes and can help regulate blood sugar levels and promote satiety.

Non-dairy milk alternatives:

- Plant-based milk alternatives such as almond milk, soy milk, and oat milk are lower in calories and saturated fats compared to cow's milk. They can be used as substitutes in recipes or consumed as beverages to reduce calorie intake.

Herbs and spices:

- Herbs and spices such as cinnamon, ginger, turmeric, cayenne pepper, and black pepper can add flavor to meals without adding extra calories. They may also have metabolism-boosting or appetite-suppressing properties, supporting weight management efforts.

Incorporating a variety of these plant-based foods into your diet, along with portion control, regular physical activity, adequate sleep, and stress management, can help manage obesity and promote overall health and well-being. It's also important to consult with a healthcare professional or registered dietitian for personalized dietary recommendations and guidance.

Back to Table of Contents

Unhealthy Diet

Managing an unhealthy diet involves making healthier food choices rich in essential nutrients while limiting processed foods, refined sugars, unhealthy fats, and excessive salt intake. Plant-based foods can play a key role in improving dietary habits as they are typically high in fiber, vitamins, minerals, and antioxidants while being lower in calories and saturated fats compared to many animal products and processed foods. Here are some plant-based foods with essential nutrients that can help manage an unhealthy diet:

Leafy greens:

- Spinach, kale, Swiss chard, collard greens, and other leafy greens are rich in vitamins (such as vitamin A, vitamin C, and vitamin K), minerals (such as iron and calcium), and antioxidants. They can help improve overall nutrition and support a healthy diet.

Non-starchy vegetables:

- Vegetables such as broccoli, cauliflower, bell peppers, carrots, zucchini, and tomatoes are low in calories but high in fiber, vitamins, and antioxidants. They can add flavor, texture, and nutrients to meals while promoting satiety and fullness.

Whole grains:

- Whole grains such as quinoa, brown rice, barley, oats, and whole wheat are rich in fiber, vitamins, minerals, and complex carbohydrates. They provide sustained energy, promote satiety, and support digestive health.

Legumes:

- Beans, lentils, chickpeas, and other legumes are excellent sources of protein, fiber, vitamins, and minerals. They can help regulate blood sugar levels, reduce cholesterol levels, and support weight management.

Berries:

- Berries such as strawberries, blueberries, raspberries, and blackberries are low in calories but high in fiber, vitamins, and antioxidants. They can satisfy sweet cravings and provide essential nutrients without contributing to excessive calorie intake.

Nuts and seeds:

- Almonds, walnuts, flaxseeds, chia seeds, and pumpkin seeds are rich in healthy fats, protein, fiber, vitamins, and minerals. They can help reduce inflammation, support heart health, and promote satiety when consumed in moderation.

Avocados:

- Avocados are rich in monounsaturated fats, fiber, vitamins, and minerals. They can help improve cholesterol levels, reduce inflammation, and support overall health when included in a balanced diet.

Sweet potatoes:

- Sweet potatoes are nutritious root vegetables that are rich in fiber, vitamins (such as vitamin A and vitamin C), and minerals. They have a lower glycemic index compared to white potatoes and can help regulate blood sugar levels and promote satiety.

Herbs and spices:

- Herbs and spices such as garlic, ginger, turmeric, cinnamon, and black pepper can add flavor to meals without adding extra calories. They may also have anti-inflammatory, antioxidant, and metabolism-boosting properties.

Plant-based protein sources:

- Tofu, tempeh, seitan, edamame, and plant-based protein powders (such as pea protein or soy protein) are nutritious alternatives to animal protein sources. They are rich in protein, vitamins, minerals, and antioxidants and can be incorporated into a variety of dishes to improve overall nutrition.

Incorporating a variety of these plant-based foods into your diet, along with reducing processed foods, refined sugars, and unhealthy fats, can help manage an unhealthy diet and promote overall health and well-being. It's also important to practice mindful eating, portion control, and regular physical activity for optimal health outcomes. Consulting with a healthcare professional or registered dietitian can provide personalized dietary recommendations and guidance based on individual needs and preferences.

Nutrients Daily R*ecommendations*

Here's a comprehensive list of essential nutrients for optimal health along with their recommended daily intake:

Macronutrients:

- **Carbohydrates:** Provide energy for the body.
  - Recommended intake: **45-65% of total daily calories.**
- **Proteins:** Essential for building and repairing tissues.
  - Recommended intake: **0.8 grams per kilogram of body weight.**
- **Fats:** Important for cell structure, hormone production, and insulation.
  - Recommended intake: **20-35% of total daily calories.**

Vitamins:

- **Vitamin A:** Supports vision, immune function, and skin health.
  - Recommended intake: **700-900 micrograms for adults.**
- **Vitamin C:** Acts as an antioxidant, supports immune function, and aids in collagen synthesis.
  - Recommended intake: **75-90 milligrams for adults.**
- **Vitamin D:** Facilitates calcium absorption, important for bone health and immune function.
  - Recommended intake: **600-800 IU for adults.**
- **Vitamin E:** Acts as an antioxidant, supports immune function, and protects cell membranes.
  - Recommended intake: **15 milligrams for adults.**
- **Vitamin K:** Essential for blood clotting and bone metabolism.
  - Recommended intake: **90-120 micrograms for adults.**
- **Vitamin B-complex (B1, B2, B3, B5, B6, B7, B9, B12):** Essential for energy metabolism, nervous system function, and red blood cell production.
  - Recommended intake varies for each B-vitamin, typically ranging from a few micrograms to several milligrams.

Minerals:

- **Calcium:** Vital for bone and teeth health, muscle function, and nerve transmission.
  - Recommended intake: **1000-1200 milligrams for adults.**
- **Iron:** Essential for hemoglobin production and oxygen transport in the blood.
  - Recommended intake: **8-18 milligrams for adults.**
- **Magnesium:** Involved in over 300 biochemical reactions in the body, including energy metabolism and muscle function.
  - Recommended intake: **310-420 milligrams for adult males, 320-400 milligrams for adult females.**
- **Potassium:** Important for fluid balance, nerve transmission, and muscle contractions.

  - Recommended intake: **3400-4700 milligrams for adults.**
- **Sodium:** Essential for fluid balance, nerve function, and muscle contractions.
  - Recommended intake: **Less than 2300 milligrams per** day (lower for certain individuals such as those with hypertension).
- **Zinc:** Supports immune function, wound healing, and DNA synthesis.
  - Recommended intake: **8-11 milligrams for adult males, 8-9 milligrams for adult females.**

Other Essential Nutrients:

- **Water:** Essential for hydration, temperature regulation, and nutrient transport.
  - Recommended intake: **Approximately 3.7 liters (for adult males) to 2.7 liters (for adult females)** from all beverages and foods combined.

These recommended daily intakes are general guidelines and may vary depending on factors such as age, gender, activity level, and individual health status. It's essential to maintain a balanced diet that includes a variety of nutrient-rich foods to meet your body's needs for optimal health and well-being. If you have specific dietary concerns or health conditions, consult with a healthcare professional or registered dietitian for personalized recommendations.

Nutrient-Rich Food that Grows in less than 100 Days

Here are five nutrient-rich foods along with a brief overview of their growth process and approximate time to maturity:

1. **Arugula:**
    - Growth Period: Arugula is a fast-growing leafy green that can be ready for harvest in approximately 30 days.
    - Process: Arugula seeds can be directly sown into well-drained soil. Plant the seeds about 1/4 inch deep and 2 inches apart in rows or containers. Keep the soil consistently moist and provide partial shade in hot climates. Harvest arugula leaves when they reach the desired size, typically by cutting them near the base of the plant.
2. **Beets:**
    - Growth Period: Beets typically take around 50 to 60 days to mature, depending on the variety.
    - Process: Beets can be grown from seeds directly sown into well-prepared soil. Plant the seeds about 1/2 inch deep and 2 to 4 inches apart in rows spaced about 12 to 18 inches apart. Keep the soil consistently moist and provide full sun to partial shade. Harvest beets when they reach the desired size, usually when the roots are tender and about 1 to 3 inches in diameter.
3. **Carrots:**
    - Growth Period: Carrots usually take approximately 60 to 80 days to mature, depending on the variety.
    - Process: Carrot seeds should be sown directly into loose, well-drained soil. Plant the seeds about 1/4 inch deep and 2 inches apart in rows spaced about 12 to 18 inches apart. Keep the soil consistently moist, especially during germination. Thin seedlings to allow proper root development. Harvest carrots when they reach the desired size, typically when they are bright in color and about 1/2 to 1 inch in diameter.
4. **Cucumbers:**
    - Growth Period: Cucumbers generally take around 50 to 70 days to mature, depending on the variety.
    - Process: Cucumber seeds can be directly sown into warm, well-drained soil after the last frost date. Plant the seeds about 1 inch deep and 12 to 24 inches apart in rows spaced about 36 to 48 inches apart. Provide support for climbing varieties if needed. Keep the soil consistently moist and provide full sun. Harvest cucumbers when they are firm, crisp, and reach the desired size.
5. **Spinach:**
    - Growth Period: Spinach typically takes around 40 to 50 days to mature.

- Process: Spinach can be grown from seeds directly sown into well-drained soil. Plant the seeds about 1/2 inch deep and 2 inches apart in rows spaced about 12 inches apart. Keep the soil consistently moist and ensure the plants receive adequate sunlight. Harvest spinach leaves when they reach the desired size, usually when they are young and tender.

These foods are relatively quick to grow and offer a wealth of essential nutrients, making them excellent choices for home gardens or small-scale farming.

Back to Table of Contents

Conclusion

As we reach the culmination of our journey through "The Book of Life – Natural Healing," we reflect upon the profound insights and transformative wisdom that have illuminated our path towards optimal health and vitality. Through the exploration of natural ways to a healthy lifestyle, rooted in the abundance of plant-based foods, we have uncovered the keys to nourishing body, mind, and soul.

In these pages, we have delved into the myriad benefits of embracing a diet rich in fruits, vegetables, whole grains, nuts, seeds, and legumes – nature's pharmacy of essential nutrients. From the vibrant colors of antioxidant-rich berries to the nourishing power of leafy greens, each plant-derived food offers a symphony of flavors, textures, and nutrients that support our journey towards radiant health.

By incorporating essential nutrients such as vitamins, minerals, phytonutrients, and omega-3 fatty acids into our daily diet, we have embraced a holistic approach to wellness that nurtures every aspect of our being. We have learned that true health is not merely the absence of disease, but a state of vibrant vitality and well-being that emanates from within.

As we bid farewell to these pages, let us carry forth the wisdom of God gleaned from "The Book of Life – Natural healing" into our daily lives. Let us honor the earth and its bountiful offerings, savoring the flavors of wholesome, plant-based foods with gratitude and reverence. Let us cultivate mindfulness in our eating habits, sowing the seeds of health and vitality with each nourishing bite.

May "The Book of Life – Natural healing" serve as a beacon of inspiration and empowerment on your journey towards optimal health and wellness. May its empowering information guide you towards a life of balance, harmony, and abundance – a life nourished by the wisdom of nature and the transformative power of plant-based nutrition.

In closing, I extend my deepest gratitude first to God and to you, dear reader, for joining me on this journey of discovery and growth. May your path be illuminated by the radiant light of health, vitality, and joy.

With warmest wishes,
Niddia Alexander

Psalm 23

"The Lord is my shepherd; I shall not want.
He maketh me to lie down in green pastures:
He leadeth me beside the still waters. He restoreth my soul:
He leadeth me in the paths of righteousness for his name's sake.
Yea, though I walk through the valley of the shadow of death,
I will fear no evil: for thou art with me; thy rod and thy staff they comfort me.

Thou preparest a table before me in the presence of mine enemies: thou anointest my head with oil; my cup runneth over.

Surely goodness and mercy shall follow me all the days of my life: and I will dwell in the house of the Lord forever."

AMEN

Back to Table of Contents

www.ingramcontent.com/pod-product-compliance
Lightning Source LLC
LaVergne TN
LVHW082023200926
848481LV00010B/2908
* 9 7 9 8 9 9 9 7 3 0 6 6 4 *